This important new volume in the series Cambridge Reviews in Human Reproduction provides a wide-ranging and authoritative account of the uterus and its physiological role in fertility, normal pregnancy and delivery. Acknowledged authorities from around the world provide a detailed and timely account of uterine physiology. The volume encompasses a wealth of material including cell and developmental biology, structure, function, anatomy and endocrinology, and then goes on to cover clinically important issues such as the cervix during pregnancy, measurement of uterine contractions and initiation of labour. It will prove of particular value to those involved in the management of women with pre-term labour, as well as those concerned with the development of new procedures for the prevention or amelioration of this condition.

The Uterus

Cambridge Reviews in Human Reproduction

SERIES EDITORS

*Professor J.G. Grudzinskas, Dr J.L. Yovich, Professor J.L. Simpson,
Professor T. Chard*

This major new series on human reproduction will provide a comprehensive and integrated review of the reproductive process. The first six volumes concentrate on the essential reproductive events leading up to birth. The series will provide a synthesis of the scientific, clinical and physiological elements of reproductive process. Each volume will focus on a well-defined aspect of reproduction and provide a multidisciplinary though self-contained review.

Each volume will be prepared by an international and authoritative team of writers involving many of the world's leading experts. The series will be edited to the highest standard to insure an integrated and uniformly high level of presentation. An important feature of the series will be the inclusion of high-quality line illustrations.

The series will provide an essential source of information for all trainees in obstetrics, gynaecology, andrology and reproductive medicine and will also be of interest to reproductive biologists and geneticists, physiologists and endocrinologists.

Titles in the series:

THE UTERUS

The Uterus

Edited by

T. CHARD *and* J. G. GRUDZINSKAS

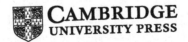

CAMBRIDGE
UNIVERSITY PRESS

Published by the Press Syndicate of the University of Cambridge
The Pitt Building, Trumpington Street, Cambridge CB2 1RP
40 West 20th Street, New York, NY 10011-4211, USA
10 Stamford Road, Oakleigh, Melbourne 3166, Australia

© Cambridge University Press 1994

First published 1994

A catalogue record for this book is available from the British Library

Library of Congress cataloguing in publication data

The Uterus–book 4/edited by T. Chard and J.G. Grudzinskas.
    p.   cm.–(Cambridge reviews in human reproduction)
            Includes index.
ISBN 0-521-41403-2 (hardback).–ISBN 0-521-42453-4 (pbk.)
1. Uterus–Physiology. 2. Pregnancy.   I. Chard, T.
II. Grudzinskas, J. G. (Jurgis gediminas) III. Series.
[DNLM: 1. Uterus–physiology.   WP 400 U89 1995]
            QP262.U86   1995
            612.6'2–dc20
              DNLM/DLC
    for Library of Congress   94-370   CIP

ISBN 0 521 41403 2 hardback
ISBN 0 521 42453 4 paperback

Transferred to digital printing 2003

We are particularly sad to record the death of Elizabeth Ramsey just before this volume went to press. She was probably the most outstanding of our contributors in the range of her knowledge and her reputation for fundamental contributions to this particular topic. She will be sadly missed and we dedicate this volume to her.

Contents

Contributors

J. D. APLIN
Research Floor, St Mary's Hospital, Manchester M13 0JH, UK

S. ARULKUMARAN
Department of Obstetrics & Gynaecology, National University of Singapore, National University Hospital, Lower Kent Ridge Road, Singapore 05111

S. BATRA
Department of Obstetrics & Gynaecology, University Hospital, S-221 85 Lund, Sweden

G. D. BRYANT-GREENWOOD
Department of Anatomy & Reproductive Biology, 1960 East West Road, University of Hawaii at Honolulu, Hawaii 96822, USA

A. A. CALDER
Department of Obstetrics & Gynaecology, Centre for Reproductive Biology, 37 Chalmers Street, Edinburgh EG3 9EW, UK

T. CHARD
Department of Reproductive Physiology, St Bartholomew's Hospital Medical College, West Smithfield, London EC1A 7BE, UK

R. E. GARFIELD
Department of Obstetrics & Gynaecology, University of Texas Medical Branch, 301 University Boulevard, Galveston, Texas 77555-1062, USA

T. KAWARABAYASHI
Department of Obstetrics & Gynaecology, School of Medicine, Fukuoka University, Fukuoka 814-01, Japan

L. D. KLENTZERIS
Department of Obstetrics & Gynaecology, Queens Medical Centre, University of Nottingham, UK

T. C. LI

Department of Obstetrics & Gynaecology, Jessop Hospital for Women, Leavygreave Road, Sheffield S3 7RE, UK

G. C. LIGGINS

Department of Obstetrics & Gynaecology, National Women's Hospital, Auckland, New Zealand

J. J. MORRISON

Department of Obstetrics & Gynaecology, Rosie Maternity Hospital, Robinson Way, Cambridge CB2 2SW, UK

E. M. RAMSEY

3420 Que Street NW, Washington, DC 20007, USA

C. ROMANINI

Clinica Ostetrica e Ginecologica, Universita Di Roma Tor Vergata, Policlinico Nuovo S. Eugenio, Ple Umanesimo 10, 00144 Roma, Italy

J.-C. SCHELLENBERG

Department of Obstetrics & Gynaecology, National Women's Hospital, Auckland, New Zealand

N.-O. SJÖBERG

Department of Obstetrics & Gynaecology, Malmo General Hospital, University of Lund, S-214 01 Malmo, Sweden

S. K. SMITH

Department of Obstetrics & Gynaecology, Rosie Maternity Hospital, Robinson Way, Cambridge CB2 2SW, UK

M. STJERNQUIST

Department of Obstetrics & Gynaecology, Malmo General Hospital, University of Lund, S-214 01 Malmo, Sweden

M. A. WARREN

Department of Biomedical Science, University of Sheffield, UK

C. YALLAMPALLI

Department of Obstetrics & Gynaecology, University of Texas Medical Branch, 301 University Boulevard, Galveston, Texas 77555-1062, USA

Editors' preface

The aim of this book is to provide a complete and up-to-date account of the anatomy, physiology and biochemistry of the uterus, with particular emphasis on the human, and on the relationship to clinical abnormalities of uterine function. The book begins with a historical perspective by Elizabeth Ramsey, a most fascinating account of some of the strange concepts of this organ which existed prior to the modern era. The second and third chapters are also contributed by Dr Ramsey: on the anatomy of the human uterus, and of its embryonic and fetal development. The latter is particularly relevant to some of the rare abnormalities found in children and adults. The structure and function of the uterine muscle are detailed by Garfield and Yallampalli, with particular emphasis on their own important contributions to our knowledge of gap junctions. Attention then turns to the endometrium, with a review of structure and ultrastructure by Warren and colleagues, and of biochemistry by John Aplin. Succeeding chapters deal with various functional aspects of the human myometrium. There is a full review of the electrophysiology by Kawarabayashi who has made many basic contributions to this topic. Biochemical aspects of control are then examined, with chapters on general hormonal control by Batra, on relaxin and oxytocin by Gillian Bryant-Greenwood and Tim Chard, and on the locally active agents such as neurotransmitters (Stjernquist and Sjöberg), and prostaglandins (Morrison and Smith). A thoughtful review by Schellenberg and Liggins summarizes the present rather unsatisfactory status of our knowledge about the onset of labour in the human, despite the obvious clinical importance of this topic. They particularly highlight the role of the cervix as, in a separate chapter, does Andrew Calder. The cervix may play as important a role in the process of delivery as the more obvious body of the uterus. Finally, chapters by Romanini and Arulkumaran summarize current procedures for the clinical and research measurement of uterine activity.

1

Concepts of the uterus: a historical perspective

E. M. RAMSEY

The first Stone Age Man who raised his face to the sky and cried, 'Where did I come from?' voiced a question which has perplexed wise men throughout the ages. In investigating it, theology and science have been closely intertwined, often inseparably, and much of anatomy has often been shrouded in superstition. That the chick comes from the egg, and the baby lamb from the body of the ewe, was readily apparent, but *How*? and *Why*? were the mysteries.

We may leave consideration of the 'Why' to theology and, for present purposes, even anatomy's 'How' may be narrowed to the role of the uterus. This is, itself, a large and engrossing subject, at all times integrally related to the prevailing attitude toward medicine as a whole.

Early concepts

Without delving into the misty realms of prehistory, when the gods were regarded as the sole source of health or sickness, and with the body itself and its organs playing no role in causation or cure, we may turn to the so-called Golden Age of *Greece* as a logical starting point for our account.

What was known, what was believed, about the uterus in the 4th century BC? At the outset, it is to be noted that the Hippocratic Corpus, embodying the thought of the great 'Father of Medicine' and his contemporaries, emphatically rejected belief that supernatural forces are involved in either causation or cure of disease. Rather the 'humours' existing in the human body and its environment maintain harmony (health) or, when in any way disturbed, create imbalance (sickness). Health can only be restored by correcting the imbalance. This, in turn, requires study of the patient's body and treatment of it. This radical shift by the Hippocratians may be hailed as the first early, tentative step toward modern medicine.

In the nascent study of anatomy and physiology, to which the Hippocratic

1

Table 1. *Chronology*

Century	Practitioner	Birth and death (active)	Place of birth; training; activity
BC			
Fourth	Hippocrates	460–377	Greece
	Aristotle	384–322	Greece
	Herophilus of Chalcedon	(300)	Greece; Alexandria; Rome
AD			
First	Rufus of Ephesus	(98–117)	Greece; Alexandria; Rome
Second	Soranus of Ephesus	(110)	Greece; Alexandria; Rome
	Galen	130–?200	Pergamon; Asia Minor; Alexandria; Rome
Ninth to 12th	School of Salerno		
14th	Mondino dei Luzzi	1275–?	Italy
15th	Leonardo da Vinci	1452–1519	Italy
	Berengario da Carpi	?1480–1550	Italy
16th	Vesalius	1514–1564	Brussels; Louvain and Paris; Padua
	Colombo da Cremona	1516–1559	Italy
	Eustachio	1520–1574	Italy
	Fallopio da Modena	1523–1562	Italy
18th	John and William Hunter	(1774)	England

concept gave impetus, the uterus was, of course, an object of attention. It was described as consisting of a number of cavities exhibiting angulation and horns, its lining studded with 'tentacles' or 'suckers'. One may wonder how anyone who had once held a uterus in his hand and made a simple sagittal section through it could so wrongly have conceived of its pattern – least of all Hippocrates himself who was skilled and learned as were many of his contemporaries. The crux of the matter is, of course, that early physicians did not hold the human uterus in their hands, many never even saw one. For many centuries, both law and religion forbade dissection of human bodies, and all concepts of reproductive tract anatomy were based on findings in animals, largely those with duplex or bicornuate uteri. As a result, extrapolation to the human produced this and many other erroneous and bizarre theories.

Aristotle, who followed shortly after Hippocrates (Table 1) and subscribed to most of the Hippocratic doctrine of humours, recognized this obstacle, frankly stating that he knew nothing of the reproductive tract of man and that his concept of the uterus as bicornuate and furnished with cotyledons similar to the Hippocratic tentacles was arrived at by analogy with the animals he had studied.

His studies were extensive and were combined with experimentation leading to numerous penetrating observations. Most of his drawings have been lost but a surviving sketch of a dogfish embryo attached to the maternal brood pouch shows how close he came to recognition of conditions prevailing in mammals. In the related field of chick embryo development, Aristotle laid the basis for embryological investigations by many centuries of future students and developed a classic terminology, some of which persists to this day – often causing confusion!

By the beginning of the Christian era, the Greek supremacy as a centre of learning had begun to wane and the torch of intellectual eminence passed to *Alexandria* in Egypt. Here, briefly, dissection of the bodies of executed criminals was permitted, and a trio of physicians made strides in the understanding of reproductive tract anatomy. The tradition of the bicornuate uterus was continued but uterine tubes were recognized, though Herophilus taught that they enter the urinary bladder. Rufus corrected this and modified earlier opinions of the shape of the uterus, describing it as similar to a 'cupping vessel'. He also differentiated a fundus with two cornua from the cervix, and both from the vagina.

The third of the outstanding Egyptians of the early Christian era was Soranus whose *Gynecology* was one of the great works of the early Christian centuries. It is chiefly a clinical textbook but does incorporate some of his anatomical studies. Although the book is not illustrated, a drawing in a text of the 9th century AD, which presents the earliest known representation of the anatomy of the uterus, embodies Soranus' concept of the organ (Fig. 1). Soranus held many progressive opinions but he also entertained some curious misconceptions, including identification of the cotyledons of Hippocrates and Aristotle as a species of nipple which provides opportunity for intrauterine suckling to accustom the fetus to a function in which it would need to be proficient at birth. Soranus identified the ovary but called it a female testis, as did his successors down to the 17th century. He was notable for his dispassionate objectivity. He fought against superstition and assailed many inherited opinions but always without rancour.

By the second century AD *Rome* had succeeded Alexandria as the lode-stone for men of learning, including physicians, but the cast of thought during the great years of the Empire was quite different from that prevailing in Greece and Egypt. This was particularly reflected in the biological sciences. Although the practice of medicine made great strides and gynaecology was an important facet of it, investigation of morphology and physiology took a back seat to the invention of surgical instruments and the elaboration of operative techniques. Pre-occupation with practicalities was a characteristic of the mode of Roman thought and it is not surprising that organization of a hospital system was one of Rome's great contributions to medicine in general.

Towering over the Roman period, the work and the fame of Galen set a

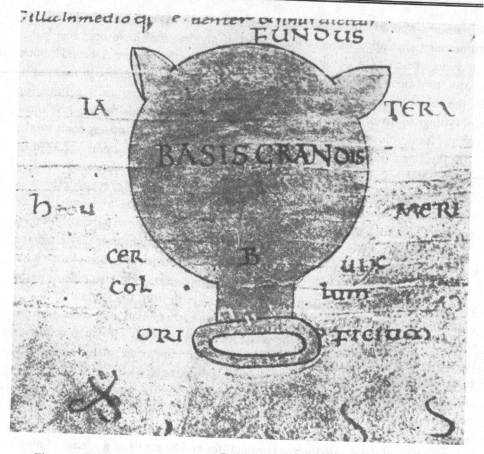

Fig. 1. Earliest known representation of the anatomy of the uterus. It embodies Soranus' conception of the organ and appears in a Muscio text of the ninth century. From Weindler (1908). Courtesy of the National Library of Medicine, Bethesda, MD.

standard against which European medicine measured itself for a thousand years following his death. His introduction of the concept of an anatomical and physiological basis of sickness rather than the operation of 'humours' was a great step forward. However, the extent to which his opinions came to be regarded for many centuries as definitive and exempt from improvement or debate had a stultifying effect upon research and creative thought.

Galen greatly extended knowledge of human structure and function although still hampered by the restrictions upon dissection of human bodies. He spent some time in Alexandria where he had access to the human observations made there in the brief interval when dissection was permitted and he extrapolated from his observation of animals and his experimentation upon them. Above all, he emphasized over and again that only with detailed knowledge of how the body works can disease be understood and treated.

As a practitioner, Galen was not particularly interested in gynaecology. For the uterus only, two points can be noted: he continued the belief that it is a multi-chambered organ (rather surprisingly as monkeys were one of the animals he studied) and to Aristotle's concept of endometrial cotyledons he contributed the idea that vessels opening into the crypts of the cotyledons transport menstrual blood.

Middle Ages

In the millennium following Galen's death, the intellectual brilliance which characterized Greece and Alexandria and classic Rome was supplanted by dusty scholasticism and blind dependence upon the dicta of ancient authorities. All avenues of thought were hampered by this attitude. Neither philosophic nor scientific problems were investigated on their merits but were solved by the satisfying pronouncements: 'according to Aristotle' or 'as Galen said'.

Typically, medical attention was heavily focused upon the doctrine of the multichambered uterus. To modern thought, it seems incredible that it was firmly believed that argument alone could settle such a matter. Perhaps some enlightened physicians did wish that they could take a quick look at an actual specimen, but recognizing the impossibility of gaining permission for such an ungodly and illegal procedure, they lined themselves up on one side or the other in the debate, espousing numerous chambers or only two or four, etc. The most popular choice invoked the magic number seven and stipulated that male embryos develop in the three right-hand cells, females in the left three, and hermaphrodites in the middle (Fig. 2). Another popular anatomic belief that generated endless discussion was that the female reproductive tract is the mirror image of the male; the vagina, a penis turned inside out; the uterus, analogous to the scrotum; and so forth.

At just one place, the old spark was kept alive during the Dark Ages. Salerno in Sicily became the nucleus of a small amount of continued scientific investigation. Not much, however, was done in the field of human reproduction, and no advances in understanding of the uterus are recorded.

Renaissance

After the long, dark years of medieval stagnation, what Nuland calls 'the Reawakening' and others 'the Revival of Learning' did not come as a sudden revelation marked by a single dramatic event. The 1453 fall of Constantinople

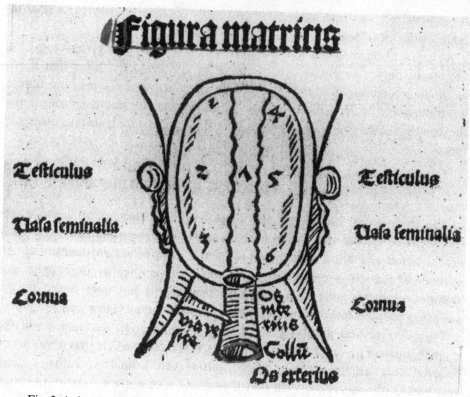

Fig. 2. A drawing illustrating the doctrine of the seven-chambered uterus. From Hundt (1501). Courtesy of the National Library of Medicine, Bethesda, MD.

is often cited as an initiating factor through the influx into Europe of Byzantine and Arabic learning, but there had been numerous evidences of awakening long before that. The founding of universities, the first one at Salerno in the 9th century followed by many throughout Europe and especially in Italy during the enlightened regime of the Venetian Republic, reflected growing interest in rediscovered Greek learning and in the cultivation of objective study and investigation, plus unhampered discussion of new ideas.

The burgeoning spirit of the Renaissance was reflected brilliantly in the graphic arts and, in the hands of skilled and famous artists, book illustrations became scientific reports in themselves, as Figs. 3 to 8 illustrate. The artists devoted great care and effort to achieving accuracy in their depictions, often doing extensive dissection themselves or sometimes, as in the case of such men as Leonardo da Vinci and Vesalius, both scientific and artistic genius resided in the same great man.

Medicine participated actively in the general intellectual ferment, greatly assisted by relaxation of the ban on human dissection. The much-debated doctrine of the multi-chambered uterus was slowly undermined as physicians at last held the uterus in their hands. Galen's influence persisted in somewhat altered and increasingly attenuated form. Fervent disciples, known as Galenists, still solved all problems and answered all questions with the decision 'according to Galen'. Others recognized abundant errors in Galen's observations and pronouncements yet honoured the soundness of his concept of the anatomic and physiological basis of disease and deplored the debasing and misinterpretation of his work and philosophy.

Among the great names that appear in the record of the early centuries of the Renaissance, many are associated with advances in knowledge of the uterus. Mondino dei Luzzi, who was one of the first to conduct a public dissection, in 1315 at the University of Bologna, published a book which included a representation of the female genital tract much as we know it today, though tubes and ovaries are not shown (Fig. 3). He believed the uterus to be divided into compartments, but introduced the new idea that the organ is fixed in the pelvis and does not migrate about the abdominal cavity, as previously believed. He followed an opinion then current that vessels from the uterus carried menstrual blood to the mammary glands to be converted into milk in pregnancy.

Leonardo da Vinci's writings and his famous sketches reflect the ideas current in his day as well as his own. Ovaries, tubes and ligaments were now recognized, although the breast-to-uterus vessels were still identified (Fig. 4). In this drawing, the uterus is depicted as lobular but not as sub-divided. From the beautiful drawing in Fig. 5, it can be confidently deduced that Leonardo considered the cavity of the pregnant uterus to be single.

One of Leonardo's contemporaries, Berengario da Carpi, was the first to assert unequivocally that the uterus has only a single chamber. He stated it in a delightfully quotable phrase, 'Es purum mendacium dicere ...'. It is a pure lie to say that the uterus has seven cavities. In the illustration shown in Fig. 6, the subject points to her single chambered uterus on the table beside her. Her foot is firmly planted on a pile of books in which, presumably, the multiple chamber theory is described. Another contemporary, Nicholas Massa, was equally firm in his opinion, stating 'decepti sunt etiam ...' deceived are they who believe that the uterus contains several cells. But as evidence that old ideas die hard, Dryander, a few years later, published a charmingly naive drawing (Fig. 7) in which a dimple at the fundus of the uterus is said to denote the presence of a septum dividing the uterine cavity.

Within this same richly productive century, one of the high points of Renaissance anatomy was reached in the work of Vesalius. Born in Brussels, educated at Louvain and Paris, Vesalius eventually settled in Padua. His career

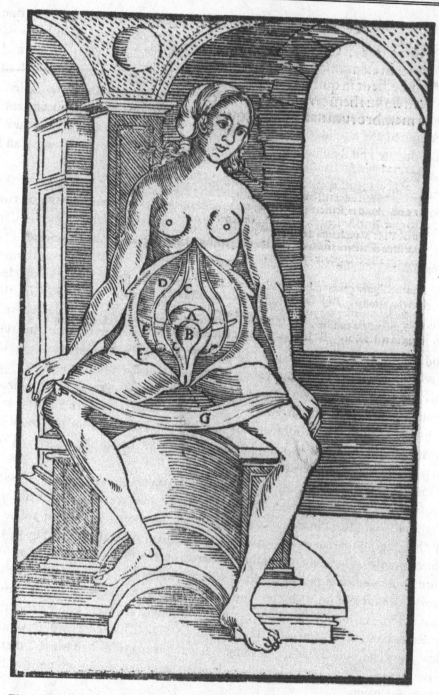

Fig. 3. Female genital tract according to Mondino as illustrated in a 1541 German translation of his work. Note indentation at fundus of uterus, indicating compartmentalization. From Mondino dei Luzzi, per J. Dryandrum (1541). Courtesy of the National Library of Medicine, Bethesda, MD.

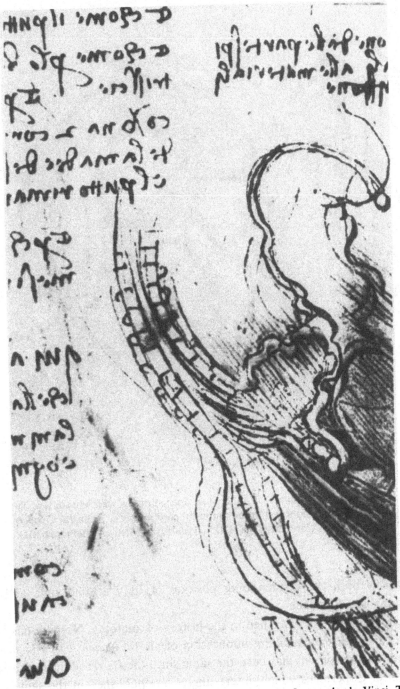

Fig. 4. Organs of the female genital tract as drawn by Leonardo da Vinci. The uterus is lobular though not sub-divided. The 'milk vein' is clearly shown. From the *Quaderni d'Anatomia* (1513). Courtesy of the National Library of Medicine, Bethesda. MD.

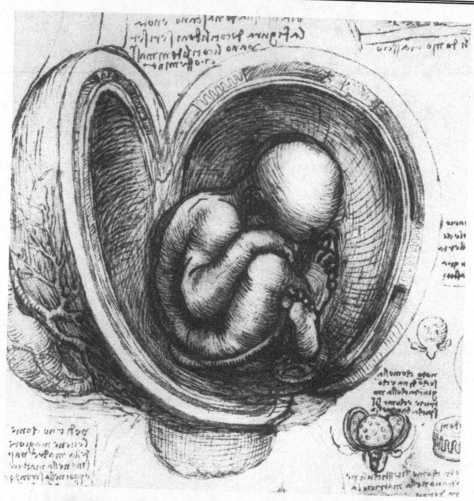

Fig. 5. Drawing by Leonardo da Vinci of an opened uterus with fetus *in situ*. The rim of the placenta and a coil of the umbilical cord are seen. From the *Quaderni d'Anatomia* (1513). Courtesy of the National Library of Medicine, Bethesda, MD.

demonstrates both the commanding position of Italy at that time and the internationalism of science.

Vesalius' work was a watershed in the history of anatomy. Nothing has been the same since the epochmaking publication of his *De humani corporis fabrica* any more than astronomy has been the same since the *De revolutionibus orbium coelestium* of Copernicus which, interestingly, was published in the same year, 1543. The *Fabrica* was based on personally conducted anatomical studies including a famous dissection in 1540 at Bologna where Mondino had also conducted a demonstration two centuries before. We know that Vesalius dissected

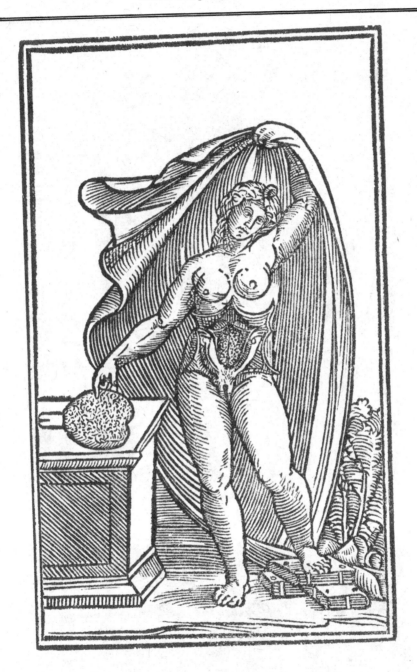

Fig. 6. Female genital tract as illustrated by Berengario da Capri. Note clear representation of the single cavity in the uterus. From Berengario (1521). Courtesy of the National Library of Medicine, Bethesda, MD.

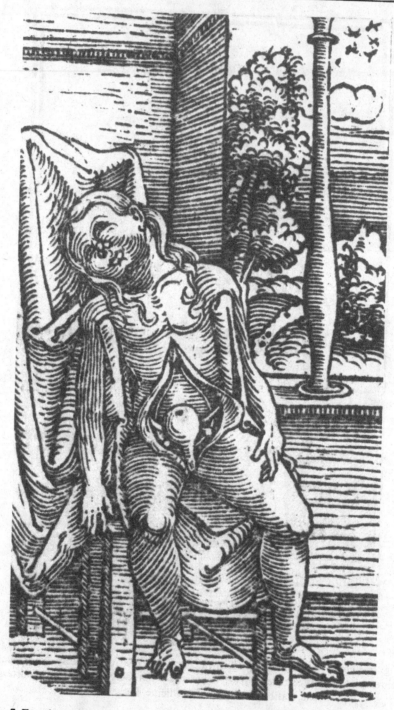

Fig. 7. Female genital tract shown by Dryander. The 'dimple' at the fundus of the uterus denotes the presence of a septum dividing the cavity. From Dryander (1547). Courtesy of the National Library of Medicine, Bethesda, MD.

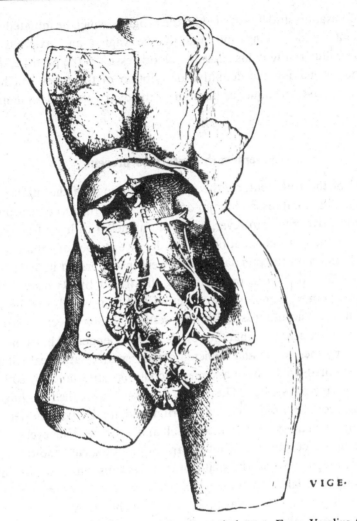

Fig. 8. Vesalius' illustration of the female genital tract. From Vesalius (1543). Courtesy of the National Library of Medicine, Bethesda, MD.

the female cadaver, for the frontispiece of the *Fabrica* shows him presiding over such a dissection.

Within the seven volumes of the *Fabrica*, each section devoted to description of a specific anatomical topic (bones, muscles, blood vessels, nerves, reproductive organs) (Fig. 8), etc., Vesalius presented the entire human body in superb illustrations of meticulous accuracy, accompanied by an illuminating text in particularly beautiful Latin. His gift as a teacher is manifested on every page though he constantly urged readers to do their own dissecting and provided practical instructions for doing so. It is recorded that students flocked to Vesalius' lectures from every country in Europe, including also Britain, Poland and Russia.

Three of Vesalius' students carried on the progress which he initiated: Colombo da Cremona by describing and naming the vagina and external genitalia; Eustachio by illustrating in his Atlas the blood vessels of the pelvis; and Fallopio da Modena by making the definitive description of the tubes which bear his name. He also gave 'the aqueous humour of the ovary' its modern name 'corpus luteum'.

Seventeenth century to present

By the end of the 16th century, the gross morphology of the uterus had been established in all essentials, and major attention was turned to other components of the reproductive tract. However, one 'great name' or rather a fraternal pair of great names remains to be mentioned. The decisive studies of John and William Hunter in London on the pregnant uterus were incorporated in Williams's 1774 treatise, *The Gravid Uterus*, magnificently illustrated by Rymsdyk. In it, the long-standing debate as to whether maternal and fetal vessels are anastamosed end to end in the placenta was definitively settled by their injection experiments. These showed unequivocally that the vessels are independent. Almost incidentally there are briefly mentioned and depicted certain small anatomical components, previously unnoted, which have assumed increasing importance in 20th century analysis of uterine physiology. These (Fig. 9) which they called 'curling arteries' pursue a spiral course through the endometrium and are the dynamic determinants of physiological activity in the menstrual and reproductive cycles. To their malfunctioning are currently attributed various pathological conditions affecting the course of pregnancy and the well-being of the fetus and newborn infant.

Modern and especially contemporary studies of the uterus concern themselves more particularly with the cellular biology and biochemistry, ultra-structure and endocrine control of the components of the uterine wall. These state-of-the-art matters are set forth in various of the chapters of this book, but do not belong in a historical review.

Perspectives

It will have been noted in the course of this brief account of the growing knowledge of the human uterus that, in each era, the prevailing mode of thought in other fields of knowledge profoundly influenced medical and scientific opinion. Such matters as availability of subjects for study, tools and facilities for experimental use and similar physical conditions were often limiting factors, but how results were interpreted was conditioned most of all by the leading philosophical attitudes of the time. Recognition of this factor must restrain us from passing judgment

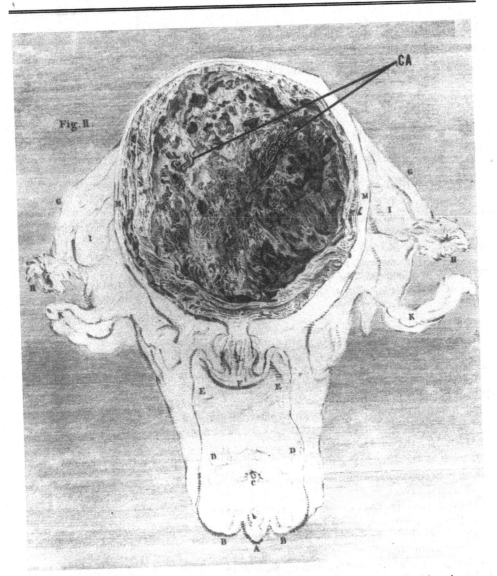

Fig. 9. William Hunter's demonstration of curling arteries of the endometrium in an injected specimen. CA, curling arteries. Drawing by Rymsdyk. From Hunter (1774). Courtesy of the National Library of Medicine, Bethesda, MD.

upon theories and deductions which seem naive or biased to 20th century observers. That the uterus has seven chambers is no more naive a theory than that a given number of angels can dance upon the head of a pin. Both concepts prevailed at a certain time and represented conclusions reached by intelligent and earnest students. One wonders what our 21st and 22nd century successors will make of the conclusions reached by workers of our own 'Computer Age'.

We may hope that they will at least detect in us the same sincerity and dedication as motivated the Hippocratic and Galenic pioneers of our heritage; the same buoyant enthusiasm, genius and skill as Leonardo and Vesalius possessed.

References

Standard texts on the history of medicine. These works supply background and basic information about individuals

Castiglioni, A. (1958). *A History of Medicine*, tr. and ed. by E. B. Krumbhaar, 2nd edn, Knopf, New York.

Garrison, F. H. (1961). *An Introduction to the History of Medicine*, 4th edn, Saunders, Philadelphia.

Mettler, C. C. & Mettler, F. A. (1947). *History of Medicine: A Correlative Text Arranged According to Subjects*, Blakiston, Toronto.

Nuland, S. B. (1988). *Doctors: The Biography of Medicine*, Knopf, New York.

Singer, C. & Underwood, E. A. (1962). *A Short History of Medicine*, 2nd edn, Clarendon Press, Oxford.

Histories of the reproductive tract

Barbour, A. H. F. (1887–1888). Early contributions of anatomy to obstetrics, Trans. *Edinburgh Obstetrics Society*, **13**, 127–54.

Peillon, G. (1981). *Étude Historique sur les Organes Génitaux de la Femme*, O. Berthier, Paris.

Ricci, J. V. (1943). *The Genealogy of Gynecology*, Blakiston, Philadelphia.

Works dealing in greater depth with specific individuals, discoveries, and theories

Albini, B. S. (1791). *Explicatio Tabularum Bartholomaei Eustachii*, Joannes and Hermannus Verbeek, Leyden.

Berengario, J. (1521). *Capri Commentaria cum Amplissimis Additionibus super Anatomia Mundini*, Impressum per Hieronymum de Benedictis, Bonaniae.

Corner, G. W. (1963). Exploring the placental maze. The development of our knowledge of the relationship between the blood stream of mother and infant *in utero. American Journal of Obstetrics and Gynecology*, **86**, 408–18.

da Vinci, L. (1513). *Quaderni d'Anatomia. III. Organi della Generazione-Embrione*, Dodici Fogli della Royal Library di Windsor, Casa Editrice Jacob Dyburad, Christiana.

Dryander, J. (1547). *Arzenei Spiegel gemeyner Inhalt derselbigen, wes beded einem Leib unnd Wundtartzt, in der Theoric, Practic und Chirurgei zusteht*, Christian Ehenolph, Franckfurt am Meyn.

Hundt, M. (1501). *Antropologium de Hominis Dignitate*, Baccalarium Wolfgangum Monacenem, Liptzick.

Hunter, W. (1774). *The Gravid Uterus*, Baskerville, Birmingham.

Hunter, W. (1794). *An Anatomical Description of the Human Gravid Uterus, and Its Contents*, J. Johnson, London.

Kudlein, F. (1965). The seven cells of the uterus: The doctrine and its roots. *Bulletin of the History of Medicine*, **39**, 415–23.

Massa, N. (1559). *Anatomiae liber introductoris*, Venet.

Mondino dei Luzzi (1541). *Anatomia Mundini*, per Joannem Dryandrum. In officina Christiani Egenolph, Marburg.

Ramsey, E. M. (1982). *Uterine and Placental Blood Flow*, ed. by Atef H. Moawd, MD and Marshall D. Lindheimer, MD, Mason Publishing USA, Inc.

Ramsey, E. M. (1989). *Biology of the Uterus*, 2nd edn, ed. by Ralph M. Wunn, MD and William P. Jollie, PhD, Plenum Publishing Corp.

Soranus (1956). *Gynecology*, tr. by O. Temkin, Johns Hopkins Press, Baltimore.

Vesalius, A. (1543). *De Humani Corporis Fabrica*, Basilae (facsimile, Brussels, 1964).

Weindler, F. (1908). *Geschichte der Gynäkologisch–anatomischen Abbildung*, Zahn and Jaensch. Dresden.

2

Anatomy of the human uterus

E. M. RAMSEY

It is the purpose of this chapter to present in concise résumé the fundamentals of gross and microscopic uterine anatomy by way of background for the highly detailed and *avant garde* matters presented in the chapters to follow. It is not proposed to tap the large body of information required by obstetricians and gynaecologists, surgeons, classical anatomists and others with specific technical interests. Pertinent reference works supplying these needs, as well as those of medical students, are briefly listed in this chapter's bibliography (pp. 39–40).

The newer ultramicroscopic studies are a world apart from the body of information upon which Henry Gray based his great classic in 1858, and even from the many revisions which, in the hands of a succession of distinguished editors, have brought the original up to date. But knowledge of the simple basics is still the essential starting point. It would be impossible, for example, to follow a discussion of the biochemical components of the endometrium of pregnancy without prior knowledge of what the endometrium of pregnancy is, or to appreciate an analysis of the hormonal control of myometrial function without an initial introduction to the location, amount, character and other basic aspects of the myometrium. With this specific purpose in mind, an attempt will be made to supply basic information in usable form.

In describing the human uterus, one parameter, in addition to the usual anatomy and physiology, must be taken into consideration: that is time.

For most of the organs of the body the intra-uterine gestation period suffices to bring them to the mature and functional state. The kidneys, the lungs, the skeletal musculature, etc., are ready to function at birth. Indeed, modern pre-natal studies have shown that fetal organs are already functioning *in utero*. After birth, the organs grow *pari passu* with the individual's own increase in size, but extensive qualitative changes do not occur except in the organs of the reproductive tract at puberty.

In the case of the uterus, the situation is particularly complicated for, with the maturing of the female endocrine system, puberty ushers in not a single definitive change but a repetitive series of cyclic changes which recur throughout reproductive life. As a result, various components of uterine structure are greatly affected by the stage of the cycle at any given time.

In the following description, it will be convenient to follow the two divisions of uterine function set out in Chapter 3 at the point where the oviparity/viviparity conversion is discussed: first, the role of the uterus in replacing the protection afforded oviparous animals by the egg shell and, second, its role as the channel for supply of maternal nutrients to the embryo in the absence of yolk. In addition, two special roles of the uterus in pregnancy must be noted: one, the formation by the uterine lumen of a nidus for the embedding of a fertilized egg; and the other the action of the musculature in assisting the evacuation of the fetus at parturition.

Protection, nidation, evacuation

For generations, by unwritten tradition, every textbook describing the uterus commences with the statement that it is a 'pear-shaped' organ. Its rounded end is directed upward and comprises the fundus and body of the uterus, the elongated lower end forms the cervix.

The major female organs of generation, together with their mutual relationships and orientation to other pelvic organs, are shown in Fig. 1.

Ligaments

The uterus fits rather loosely into the bony pelvis where it is maintained in place by several ligaments. The importance of the ligaments is augmented in pregnancy when the organ increases in size many times and escapes the pelvic confinement.

Five sets of bilateral ligaments perform these functions. The broad ligaments and the round ligaments both connect the uterus to the sidewalls of the pelvis by reflexions of the peritoneum which covers the uterus and pelvic organs. The broad ligaments are flattened sheets which divide the pelvic cavity into anterior and posterior compartments. The round ligaments extend into the inguinal canal making additional attachments there. The cardinal ligaments, which are particularly important, are composed of condensations of subserosal fascia and extend from the uterus to the pelvic wall. They provide support for the middle and upper third of the vagina and cervix and, together with the uterosacral ligaments, prevent prolapse of the uterus. The folds of the cardinal ligaments enclose the ureters and the blood vessels supplying the uterus, especially the

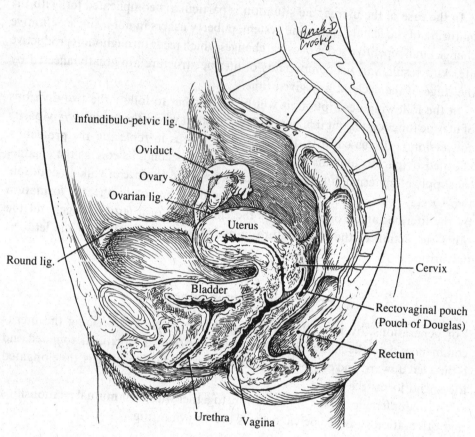

Fig. 1. Sagittal section of the pelvis of a mature woman showing the chief female reproductive organs, their mutual relations and their orientation to other pelvic organs. (After Ranice W. Crosby.)

major branches of the hypogastric artery. The uterosacral ligaments, which are also condensations of subserosal fascia, extend from the sacrum around the rectum to the cervix. The uterovesical ligaments, composed of connective tissue, attach the bladder to the lower uterine segment.

Two more structures assisting in the stabilization of the organs of the female pelvis are the infundibulo-pelvic ligaments and the ovarian ligaments. The former are folds of peritoneum which are attached to the ovarian fimbriae of the Fallopian tubes and are directed upward over the iliac vessels. They contain the ovarian vessels. The ovarian ligaments lie within the broad ligaments and attach the ovaries to the lateral angles of the uterus. They are cordlike structures containing some muscle fibres.

Fallopian tubes

It will be recalled that, in early development, the right and left Müllerian ducts grow toward each other, and that in the 10th week their lower two-thirds fuse. From this fused portion the uterus, cervix and part of the vagina are formed. The upper thirds of the Müllerian ducts do not fuse but remain independent, forming the Fallopian tubes (oviducts).

The manner in which the tubes join the uterine fundus is clear from Figs. 1 and 2. The tubes vary in length from some 8 to 14 cm. Each consists of four parts. The interstitial portion is embedded in the uterine wall and runs diagonally upward from the uterine cavity. The isthmus, the narrowest portion of the tube, adjoins the uterine wall and in turn passes into the ampulla, which is the widest portion. The final segment is the infundibulum, usually referred to as the fimbriated end. It is funnel shaped and forms the opening to the abdominal cavity.

The wall of the tube consists of a muscular outer coat and an inner mucous membrane. The constituent cells of the muscularis are arranged as an outer longitudinal layer and an inner circular one. The muscle of the tube undergoes rhythmic contractions which vary in magnitude and in rate throughout the ovarian cycle. They are most frequent and intense when ova are traversing the tube *en route* from the ovary to the uterus. Contractions are weakest and slowest during pregnancy. The mucosa is continuous with that lining the uterus. Cilia characterize the lining epithelium and are most abundant at the fimbriated end. During the ovarian cycle changes roughly similar to those occurring in the uterus appear (see p. 25) but are less marked. There is a moderate amount of decidual reaction during late pregnancy. Elastic tissue, blood vessels and lymphatics are abundant throughout the walls of the Fallopian tubes and there is extensive sympathetic innervation. The role of the latter is not fully understood (Woodruff & Pauerstein, 1969).

Uterus

The uterus has two distinct parts: the body or corpus and the cervix. Its wall has three layers: an outer covering, the serosa; a middle muscular layer, the myometrium; and an inner mucous membrane, the endometrium. The organ varies in size from 2.5–3.5 cm in length in the prepubertal child to 6–8 cm in the nulliparous adult to 9–10 cm in multiparous women. Uterine weights in nulliparae are normally between 50 and 70 g and, in multiparae, 80 g or over. At term, the uterus achieves 500 to 1000 times greater capacity than in the nulliparous state, reflecting a weight increase up to 1100 g. The change in relative size of uterine body and uterine cervix is shown in Fig. 2. Note the two sharp constrictions,

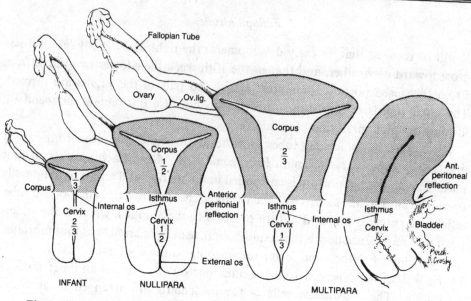

Fig. 2. Drawings illustrating comparative sizes of pre-pubertal, mature non-parous and parous uteri. The relative proportions of uterine corpus and cervix are seen to change with age and parity. Frontal and sagittal sections are presented. (After Ranice W. Crosby.)

first where the uterine corpus meets the cervix, the internal os; and secondly where the cervix meets the vagina, the external os. Observe also the manner in which the cervix protrudes into the vagina creating two vaginal folds, the anterior and posterior vaginal fornices. The posterior fornix is longer than the anterior.

The serosal layer of the uterine wall is a continuation of the peritoneal epithelium that entirely covers the uterus except at its lateral margins where it is diverted to clothe the broad ligaments and at an area just above the bladder where it walls off the rectouterine pouch or cul-de-sac (the pouch of Douglas).

The uterine functions of protection, nidation and evacuation are chiefly lodged in the myometrium and endometrium. The protective and expulsive functions of the myometrium are accomplished first by the sheer bulk of the smooth muscle composing it and then by the pattern of arrangement of the muscles. The myometrium is the thickest of the layers composing the uterine wall. The concentration of muscle is greatest in the fundus with lesser amounts in the lateral walls than in the anterior and posterior areas. The concentration at the myometrial–endometrial surface is greater than that where myometrium and serosa meet. The amount of muscle decreases caudally in the uterine wall until there is only about 10% of muscle in the cervix, the remainder being fibrous connective tissue.

The detailed arrangement of the muscular tissue throughout the uterus is highly effective, especially for evacuation of contents. In the fundus, there is an outer covering of muscle which is extended into the ligaments plus an internal muscular layer from which fibres enclose the orifices of the tubes and the internal cervical os, acting as sphincters in those regions. In both layers, there is an elaborate network of muscle cells. The individual muscle bundles are surrounded by connective tissue sheaths containing a small amount of elastic tissue. Blood vessels, lymphatics and nerves course in the sheaths. Between these layers, both of which are relatively narrow, lies the main portion of the musculature. This, again, is a dense network of interlacing fibres penetrated by blood vessels. The constituents are so arranged that they both promote evacuation and, by the orientation of individual cells toward one another, constrict adjacent blood vessels and assist haemostasis at delivery.

In the enlargement of the uterus in pregnancy, the myometrium is the main component. During the first trimester, myometrial growth is accomplished by an increase in the number of muscle cells (hyperplasia) accompanied to a lesser degree by increase in the size of the cells (hypertrophy). The latter process takes over in the remainder of the first half of pregnancy. Then at mid-gestation this process too slows to a halt at the time that Reynolds (1947) characterized as 'conversion'. Thereafter, as he showed in the rabbit and subsequently confirmed in primates, uterine enlargement is accomplished by stretching alone; this, in turn, is occasioned by the increase in fetal size and in the volume of amniotic fluid.

Myometrial activity, in the form of sporadic, low amplitude contractions, commences early in pregnancy. These contractions are usually painless and non-rhythmical. By mid-pregnancy they can be detected on bimanual palpation. They slowly increase in frequency, rhythmicity and strength as pregnancy progresses and by the final two weeks may simulate labour. First observed by Braxton Hicks in 1873, they are still known by his name.

The endometrium is far from idle during these episodes of myometrial adjustment. Its evolution through the phases of the non-pregnant cycle is controlled by the action of the ovarian hormones which are themselves under the control of the pituitary. Fig. 3 shows these relationships in graphic form.

The endometrium commences as a simple mucous membrane derived from the coelomic epithelium lining the Müllerian ducts. In the peri-natal and pre-pubertal periods the glandular elements and their supporting stroma proliferate and gradually mature. At menarche, when pituitary and ovarian stimulation has become coordinated and effective, menstruation is initiated and recurring cycles commence. Each cycle has three parts. The first is the follicular or proliferative phase which is characterized by oestrogen induced thickening of the stroma and increased number and complexity of glands. The second part, the luteal or

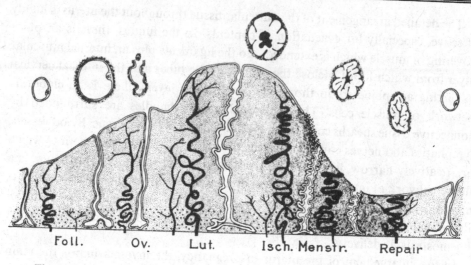

Fig. 3. Schematic representation of the relation between the changes in the ovary and in the endometrium during the menstrual cycle. From G. W. Bartelmez (1957). *American Journal of Obstetrics and Gynecology*, **74**, 931.

secretory phase, is controlled by production of progestational hormones by the corpus luteum (Fig. 4). During this phase, the glands become 'corkscrew' in course and their epithelium 'saw-toothed' or jagged. The lining cells of the glands contain secretory granules and the lumina are distended by a PAS positive secretion. The connective tissue cells of the stroma become swollen and a little interstitial fluid accumulates. Glycogen is deposited in the gland cells and in the interstitial fluid. This picture is that of a very early stage of the decidual reaction which is characteristic of the endometrial stroma in pregnancy. Note, therefore, that similar change may appear premenstrually in a non-pregnant subject, an important point to be considered in examination of operative specimens. In the third part of the cycle, with regression of the corpus luteum in the absence of pregnancy, there is involution of the endometrial tissue and onset of menstrual bleeding.

In the human, ovulation usually occurs on or about day 17 of the cycle, and implantation of the fertilized ovum takes place 6–7 days later. These events halt the regression of the corpus luteum which thereafter undergoes further development as do the endometrial changes initiated in the secretory phase of the menstrual cycle. Three distinct layers become apparent in the endometrium of pregnancy: a zona compacta close to the uterine lumen and surrounding the mouths of the glands; a zone spongiosa surrounding the deeper secretory portions of the glands and a zona basalis adjacent to the myometrium. There are relatively few glands in the basalis though in many cases a sparse scattering of them may even be seen

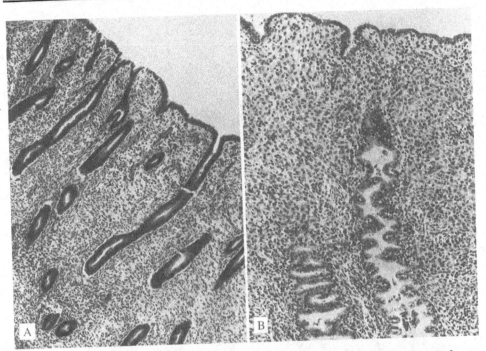

Fig. 4. Photomicrographs of the human non-pregnant endometrium. A. Day 6 of the menstrual cycle. Proliferative phase showing simple tubular glands. H and E. ×32. B. Day 26. Secretory phase. Glands run a 'cork-screw' course; lining epithelium is 'saw toothed'. H and E. ×58. From I. A. R. More (1987). *Haines and Taylor Obstetrical and Gynaecological Pathology*.

in the muscularis. The secretory activity of the glands is progressively enhanced and at the same time the swelling of the stroma, i.e. the decidual reaction, is increased until eventually the situation depicted in Fig. 5 is achieved. The stromal swelling presses upon the glands so that, by mid-pregnancy, they are compressed to the point of atrophy and functional activity ceases. At term, a few residual fragments of glands may remain which, having no access to the uterine lumen to permit drainage, become cystic. The compacta and spongiosa are the two layers that are shed at parturition. The so-called line of separation, a rather loose and jagged line, lies between the spongiosa and basalis.

The foregoing changes, largely determined by hormonal factors emanating from the pituitary and ovary, are supplemented by action of the trophoblast. This tissue, of fetal origin, is a component of the wall of the embedding and developing ovum. Long considered to be simply an invasive tissue effecting the implantation and attachment of the fertilized egg, the manifold activities of the trophoblast are becoming recognized on the basis of extensive studies in a number

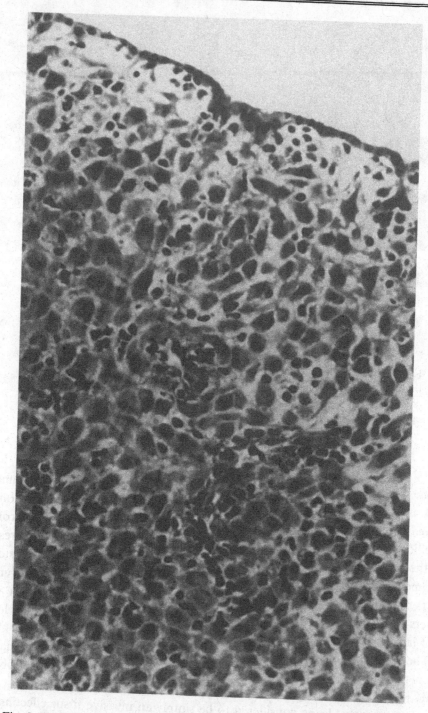

Fig. 5. Photomicrograph of a portion of a human secretory endometrium, Day 27, showing decidualized stroma cells. Note partially obliterated spiral artery which is compressed by swelling of stroma and accumulation of interstitial fluid. H and E. ×300. Source as in Fig. 4.

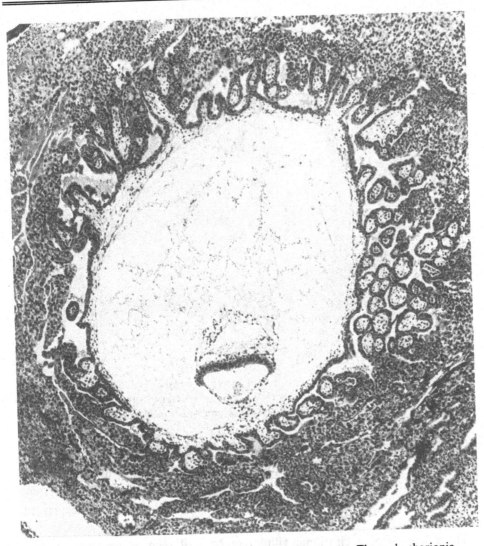

Fig. 6. Photomicrograph of a 16 day human embryo *in situ*. The early chorionic villi are starting to penetrate the surrounding endometrium in which the blastocyst is embedded. Carnegie No. 7802. H and E. ×33.5.

of animals, especially the related primates. The dominant role of the trophoblast in pregnancy and the mechanism of its activity form the basis of many of the reports in subsequent chapters of this book.

Immediately after implantation, the embedding ovum sends projections into the surrounding endometrium, the chorionic villi (Fig. 6). The villi become elaborate, interlacing fronds with intercommunicating spaces or lacunae between them constituting 'the intervillous space'. In it, maternal blood circulates supplied by the endometrial spiral arteries (see p. 29). By the end of the first trimester of

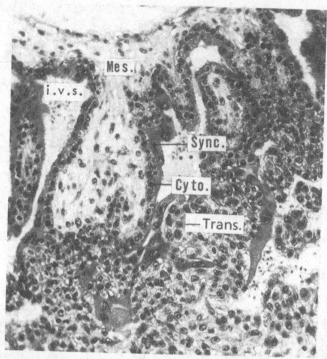

Fig. 7. Photomicrograph of a portion of the 16 day blastocyst shown in Fig. 5. × 250. (After Carnegie Institution of Washington.) Cyto: cytotrophoblast; i.v.s.: intervillous space; Mes: mesoderm; Sync: syncytium; Trans: transitional trophoblast.

pregnancy, when the placenta is fully formed, the villi number in hundreds and are concentrated at the base of the placenta where attachment to the uterus is effected. The villi, together with the intervillous space, constitute the placenta proper.

The make-up of a chorionic villus can be well seen at an early stage of development in Fig. 7. It should be remembered that all of the tissues are of fetal origin. First, there is the mesodermal core which is continuous with the mesodermal lining of the gestation sac. In this core there are fetal vessels of all calibres which are continuations of the vessels within the fetal body itself. These vessels reach the chorionic villi via the umbilical cord. Secondly, there is the trophoblast which is of three types, the cytotrophoblast, the transitional trophoblast and the syncytiotrophoblast. The cytotrophoblast consists of complete cells with characteristic intracellular membranes and mature nuclei. The cells are orientated in neat rows or sheets. These cells are the invaders which promote attachment of the egg, and are also the parents of the syncytiotrophoblast (usually referred to simply as the syncytium). The components of the syncytial layer lack cell borders. The nuclei are clumped and vary in size and shape and staining properties. It is this layer of trophoblast that is of special interest, for it has many activities, including secretory ability. The relationship between cyto- and syncytiotrophoblast has been convincingly established by identification of transitional forms and by ultramicroscopic studies (Kurman, Main & Chen, 1984).

As the trophoblast penetrates ever more widely into the endometrium, it digests or engulfs the maternal structures it encounters: stroma, glands, capillaries and veins and finally the tips of spiral arteries, establishing free communication with the source of maternal nutrition. In this way the replacement of the yolk of oviparous animals is achieved. This will be more fully considered in the following section. Meanwhile, it should be noted that the maternal blood in the intervillous space and the fetal blood in the fetal vessels within the mesodermal core are not in direct communication. Transfer of maternal nutrients and fetal products of metabolism occurs across the tissues of the chorionic villus and the endothelium of the fetal capillaries. The placental circulation in man and the higher primates is thus of the haemochorial type.

Nutrition

To replace the nutrition afforded to oviparous animals by egg yolk, viviparous animals depend upon nutrients derived from the mother's blood stream. The placenta is the vehicle which effects the transfer. Overall consideration of this organ of dual origin, maternal and fetal, is not germane to the present discussion and will be dealt with elsewhere. However, the manner in which the placental circulation is connected to the maternal circulation is within the scope of this chapter; it is the blood vessels of the uterine wall which make the connection.

As in the case of the other components of the uterus, the uterine vasculature has been extensively investigated in the present century, and the studies have been particularly facilitated by the similarity between the rhesus monkey and other primates, including man.

The uterine blood supply is largely derived from the aorta, via the uterine and the iliac arteries. Minor or variable contributions are made by the inferior mesenteric, middle sacral, inferior epigastric, external pudendal and ovarian arteries. The contribution of the ovarian arteries may sometimes be considerable; up to one-third of the total has been reported in the monkey though less in man. Fig. 8 shows the pattern of vascular distribution within the uterine wall. Branches of the uterine artery enter the wall at a sharp angle and proceed through the outer myometrium to the middle third without significant branching. In the middle third, they form an arcuate wreath to which branches of both right and left halves contribute. From the wreath small branches (not depicted in the

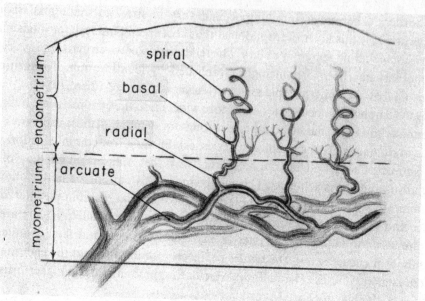

Fig. 8. Schematic representation of uterine arteries. After H. Okkels and E. T. Engle (1938). *Acta Pathologica Microbiologica Scandinavica*, **15**, 150.

drawing) are distributed throughout the myometrium. The radial arteries are large stems which come off the wreath at right angles and travel toward the uterine lumen. As they pass the myometrial–endometrial junction they become known as endometrial spiral arteries. The name change was conferred in earlier times to reflect a supposed difference in the composition of their walls from those of the radial stems of which they are the continuation. This is no longer considered to be the case, but the term is retained as descriptive of both the course and the configuration of the endometrial segments of the vessels. Since several other arteries in the reproductive and other organs which pursue a convoluted course are also loosely referred to as 'spiral arteries', it is well to specify 'endometrial spiral' when referring to these particular vessels.

Just after entering the endometrium, the spiral arteries give off small branches, the basal arteries, which ramify in the deepest layer of the endometrium. The composition of the walls of these two types of vessel is strikingly different. The spiral arteries, carrying forward the basic structure of the parent radial and arcuate arteries, contain extensive elastic and fibrous tissues and some muscle. They are surrounded by a sheath of dense connective tissue constituting the so-called Columns of Streeter. The basal arteries, on the other hand, are essentially muscular with little   elastic and fibrous tissue and they have no fibrous sheath (Fig. 9).

The venous drainage of the uterus is particularly noteworthy in the endometrium where an extensive network of vessels of all calibres is distributed throughout.

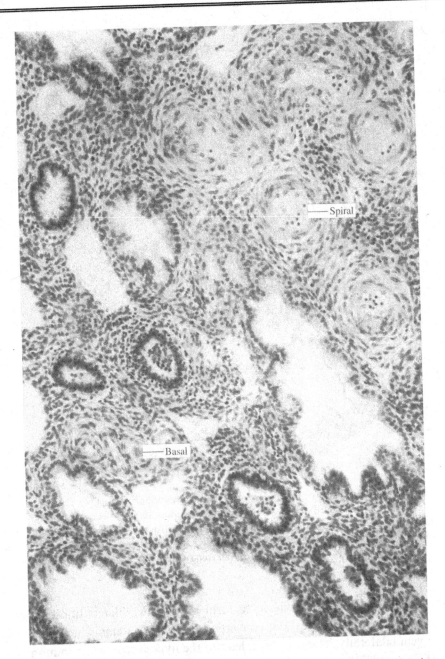

Fig. 9. Photomicrograph of an area in a human secretory endometrium showing the difference between an endometrial spiral artery, right, and an endometrial basal artery, left. Carnegie No. 8602. H and E. ×68.

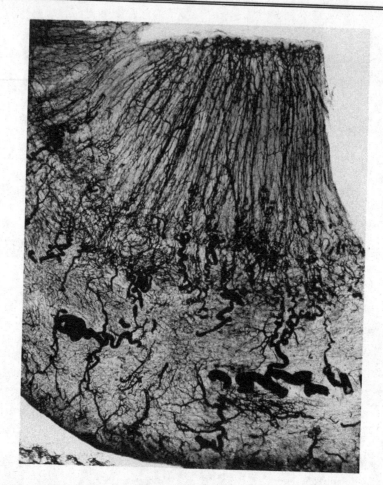

Fig. 10. A cross-section of the uterine wall of a rhesus monkey on Day 12 of the menstrual cycle. A spiral artery displays minimal coiling in the lower third of the endometrium. Its straight distal end reaches almost to the surface epithelium. India ink injection. Monkey B338. × 15. From G. W. Bartelmez (1957*b*). *Carnegie Contributions to Embryology* **36**, 153.

Many of the smaller veins coalesce to form prominent, dilated sinuses. From these, vessels of increasing calibre converge upon major stems which enter the uterine vein bilaterally. These, in turn, lead to the hypogastric and common iliac veins (Daron, 1937).

It is at this point that the 'time element' enters the picture. As with all the tissues of the uterine wall, following the menstrual slough there is a period of repair. Regeneration of the torn blood vessels is accomplished while the ovarian follicle is growing and elaborating oestrogen. As the endometrial diameter slowly increases the spiral arteries grow toward the uterine lumen. The familiar expression

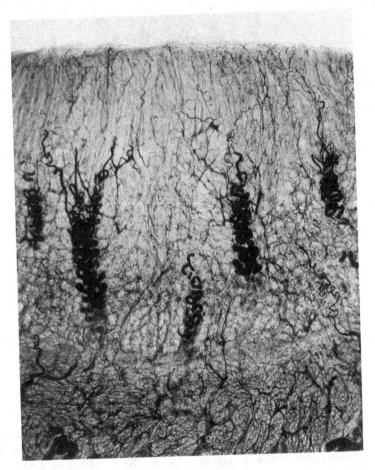

Fig. 11. A cross-section of the endometrium and inner layer of the myometrium of a monkey on Day 17. Abundant coils of several arteries are seen in the middle third of the endometrium. Their straight distal ends reach 3/4 of the way to the surface. India ink injection. Monkey B309. × 15. Same source as Fig. 10.

'grow toward' is something of a misnomer. What really happens is that the arterial stumps give rise to capillary sprouts which proliferate toward the surface of the endometrium. Muscle and elastic tissues are gradually formed around them converting them into arterioles and arteries, though a capillary bed persists in the immediately subepithelial layer of the endometrium.

As they grow, the arteries become increasingly convoluted, in part because the arterial growth is greater than the endometrial thickening so that the arteries become compressed in the manner of a bedspring (Figs. 10 and 11).

The deepest portions of the spiral arteries, together with the adjacent segments of radial arteries, reveal an activity which has an important influence upon the

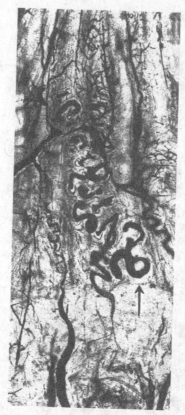

Fig. 12. A cross-section of the myometrial–endometrial junction (↑) in a monkey on the 11th day of the menstrual cycle showing constriction of a spiral artery and its parent radial artery. India ink injection. Monkey B323. × 60. Same source as Fig. 11.

course of the menstrual and reproductive cycles. First noted by Daron (1936) in injected specimens and confirmed by Markee (1940) in *in vivo* studies of intraoccular endometrial transplants (both in monkeys) the phenomenon consists of intense vasoconstriction of the vessels at or close to the myometrial–endometrial junction (Fig. 12). The constrictions do not occur synchronously throughout the endometrium but intermittently and independently. Localized ischaemia resulting from temporary shutdown of blood supply is now regarded as the basis of the necrosis, bleeding and slough of menstruation. The constrictions continue to occur throughout pregnancy, and are an important factor in regulating volume and pressure of maternal blood supply to the placenta (see p. 37).

The basal arteries are unresponsive to hormonal stimuli and take no part in the changes noted in the spiral arteries. They are not damaged in the menstrual slough and remain unchanged throughout the whole cycle, maintaining their sole

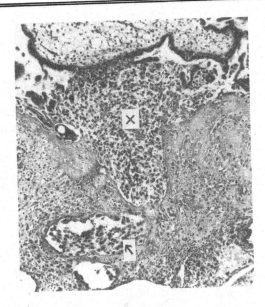

Fig. 13. Cytotrophoblast streaming from the wall of a chorionic villus plugs the lumen of a spiral artery at its point of entry to the intervillous space of the placenta (×). There is only partial occlusion of the deeper portions of the artery (↑). Human specimen. 12th week of pregnancy. University of Virginia U32-2. ×83.

function of nourishing the basal (outermost) layer of the endometrium and preserving it as a seed bed for reconstruction of the destroyed superficial layers after menstruation or pregnancy.

A full appreciation of the potential of the spiral arteries requires some consideration of their role in pregnancy. If implantation of a fertilized ovum occurs, the developments in the arterial structure and pattern which were commenced in the second, pre-menstrual, half of the non-pregnant cycle continue. As the result of the growth of the spiral arteries toward the uterine lumen and simultaneous infiltration of the endometrium by trophoblast cells from the wall of the implanted blastocyst, a meeting of the two occurs within the first week to ten days of the pregnancy. The trophoblast penetrates the terminal capillary tips of the spiral arteries, or in some cases engulfs them. As a result, maternal blood seeps into the lacunar (intervillus) spaces in the trophoblastic shell of the growing conceptus. As time passes, trophoblastic invasion becomes increasingly aggressive and cells enter the lumina of the arteries, often creating obstruction (Fig. 13). From these trophoblastic plugs invasion of the vessel walls occurs and, in addition, there is invasion from without by trophoblast cells dispersed throughout the stroma (Fig. 14). The trophoblast replaces the muscle and elastic tissue of the arterial walls rendering them flaccid and non-contractile. The presence of

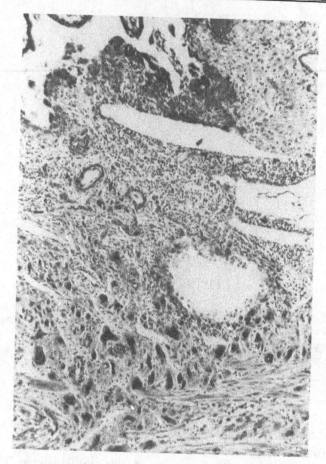

Fig. 14. Photomicrograph of a pregnant human endometrium showing trophoblast cells invading the uterine stroma at the placental base and extending into the muscularis: $11\frac{1}{2}$ weeks. Same source as Fig. 13. U8. ×120.

trophoblast prevents them from being so weak as to be prone to rupture, but extensive dilation occurs under the impact of maternal blood pressure.

By the 12th week of pregnancy, the dilatation has involved most of the endometrial portion of the spiral arteries which connect with the placenta and a variable amount of the parent radial arteries. Actual 'lakes' of arterial blood are formed at the base of the placenta (Fig. 15). Subsequently, the trophoblast disappears from the deeper portions of the vessel walls and is replaced by fibrous tissue (Fig. 16). There is some evidence (Brosens, Robertson & Dixon, 1967) of a second wave of trophoblastic invasion into arterial walls occurring around mid-pregnancy. This invasion is restricted to the deeper stretches of the arteries. Here again the trophoblast disappears and fibrosis is the end result.

ARTERIES

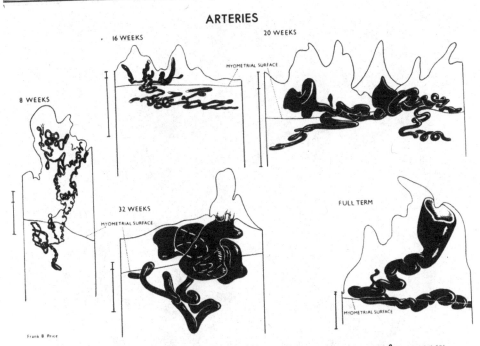

Fig. 15. Drawings of human uteroplacental arteries at various stages of pregnancy, based on three-dimensional models constructed from serial sections. Dotted line indicates myometrial–endometrial junction; smooth line the base of the placenta. From E. M. Ramsey and J. W. S. Harris (1966). *Carnegie Contributions to Embryology*, **38**, 59.

Two physiological consequences of the trophoblastic action are: first, diminution of the pressure of maternal blood reaching the intervillous space of the placenta; secondly, establishment in the lakes of a pool in which can be accommodated the vastly increased volume of maternal blood which the placenta requires, versus the small amount which flows through the non-pregnant vascular network. The importance of the constrictions in the basal portions of the spiral arteries and adjacent segments of the radial arteries is readily apparent. Adequate pressure and volume regulation, which the terminal portions of the arteries can no longer perform, is achieved by the deeper, still functioning basal stems. This action is essential for normal pregnancy and for control of hemorrhage at parturition. Lack of such regulation characterizes some pathological clinical entities (Robertson, Brosens & Dixon, 1975).

The mechanism of the circulation of blood through the intervillous space of the placenta has long been a matter of concern and speculation. Various complicated theories elaborated in the past by Grosser, Stieve, Spanner and others (see Ramsey, 1956) have been supplanted in this century as modern techniques

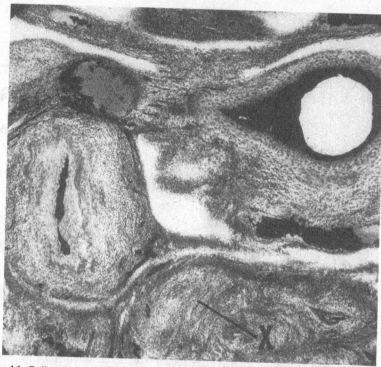

Fig. 16. Coils of two spiral arteries underlying the placenta in a pregnant rhesus monkey showing replacement of vessel wall by trophoblast on the right and by fibrosis on the left. Below, the vessels show physiological constriction. 102nd day of pregnancy. Carnegie no. C-679, B125. H and E. ×25.

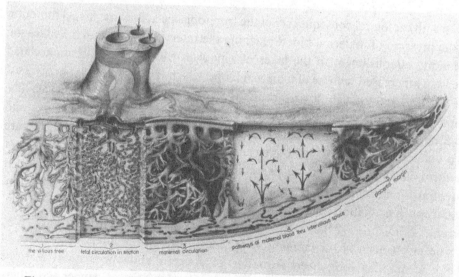

Fig. 17. Composite drawings of the primate placenta showing its structure and circulation. (Drawing by Ranice W. Crosby. From *Carnegie Yearbook*, 1961–1962.)

have made possible physiological methods of study. In particular, the use of non-human primate models has permitted *in vivo* studies. Thus, it can now be stated that the head of maternal systemic blood pressure which propels blood into the intervillous space in characteristic fountain-like spurts is the motivating force and that it is adequate to carry blood through the space and into the maternal veins draining it without diversion or 'short-cutting' (Fig. 17). The venous drainage is accomplished through venous orifices located at intervals all along the base of the placenta, not at the margin alone, as Spanner supposed to be the case (see Ramsey, 1956).

References

General references

Danforth's Obstetrics and Gynecology (1990). Ed. by J. R. Scott, P. J. DiSaia, C. B. Hammond and W. N. Spellacy, 6th edn, J. B. Lipincott, Philaelphia, PA, USA.

Gray's Anatomy (1989). Ed. by P. L. Williams, R. Warwick, M. Dyson and L. H. Bannister, 37th edn, Churchill Livingstone, Edinburgh, UK.

Haines and Taylor Obstetrical and Gynaecological Pathology (1987). Ed. by H. Fox, 3rd edn, Churchill Livingstone, Edinburgh, UK.

Hamilton, W. J. & Mossman, H. W. (1972). *Hamilton, Boyd and Mossman's Human Embryology*, 4th edn, Heffer, Cambridge, UK.

O'Rahilly, R. (1983). *Basic Human Anatomy*, WB Saunders, Philadelphia, PA, USA.

O'Rahilly, R. & Muller, F. (1992). *Human Embryology and Teratology*, Wiley-Liss, New York, USA.

Williams Obstetrics (1989). Ed. by F. G. Cunningham, P. C. MacDonald and N. F. Grant, 19th edn, Appleton & Lange, Norwalk, Connecticut, USA.

Wynn, R. M. & Jollie, W. P. (1989). *Biology of the Uterus*, 2nd edn, Plenum, New York, USA.

Specific references

Bartelmez, G. W. (1957*a*). The phases of the menstrual cycle and their interpretation in terms of the pregnancy cycle. *Americal Journal of Obstetrics and Gynecology*, **74**, 931–55.

Bartelmez, G. W. (1957*b*). The form and the functions of the uterine blood vessels in the rhesus monkey. *Carnegie Contributions to Embryology*, **36**, 153–82.

Brosens, I., Robertson, W. B. & Dixon, H. G. (1967). The physiological response of the vessels of the placental bed to normal pregnancy. *Journal of Pathology and Bacteriology*, **93**, 569.

Daron, G. H. (1936). The arterial pattern of the tunica mucosa of the uterus in *Macacus rhesus. American Journal of Anatomy*, **58**, 349–420.

Daron, G. H. (1937). The veins of the endometrium (*Macacus rhesus*) as a source of the menstrual blood. *Anatomical Records*, **67**, suppl. 13.

Goerttler (1930). Die Architektur der Muskelwand des menschlichen Uterus und ihre funktionelle Bedeutung. *Morphologische Jahrbuch*, **65**, 45. Also *Americal Journal of Obstetrics and Gynecology*, **44**, 952.

E. M. Ramsey

Kurman, R. J., Main, C. S. & Chen, H.-C. (1984). Intermediate trophoblast: a distinctive form of trophoblast with specific morphological, biochemical and functional features. *Placenta*, **5**, 349–69.

Markee, J. E. (1940). Menstruation in intraocular endometrial transplants in the rhesus monkey. *Carnegia Contributions to Embryology*, **28**, 219–308.

More, I. A. R. (1987). The normal human endometrium. In *Haines and Taylor Obstetrical and Gynaecological Pathology*, ed. H. Fox, vol. I, Churchill Livingstone, Edinburgh, UK.

Okkels, H. & Engle, E. T. (1938). Studies on the finer structure of the uterine blood vessels of the *Macacus* monkey. *Acta Pathologica Microbiologica Scandinavica*, **15**, 150–68.

Ramsey, E. M. (1956). Circulation in the maternal placents of the rhesus monkey and man. *American Journal of Anatomy*, **98**, 159–90.

Ramsey, E. M. & Harris, J. W. S. (1966). Comparison of utero placental vasculature and circulation in the rhesus monkey and man. *Carnegie Contributions to Embryology*, **38**, 59–70.

Reynolds, S. R. M. (1947). Uterine accommodation of the products of conception: Physiologic considerations. *American Journal of Obstetrics and Gynecology*, **53**, 901–13.

Robertson, W. B., Brosens, I. & Dixon, G. (1975). Uteroplacental vascular pathology. *European Journal of Obstetrics, Gynecology and Reproductive Biology*, **5**, 47–65.

Robertson, W. B. (1987). Pathology of the pregnant uterus. In *Haines and Taylor Obstetrical and Gynaecological Pathology*, ed. H. Fox, vol. II, Chapter 44, Churchill Livingstone, Edinburgh, UK.

Woodruff, J. D. & Pauerstein, C. J. (1969). *The Fallopian Tube*, Williams and Wilkins, Baltimore, Maryland, USA.

3

Development of the human uterus and relevance to the adult condition

E. M. RAMSEY

Introduction

When, in the course of animal evolution, oviparity was supplanted by viviparity, it became necessary to replace the protection afforded to the embryo by the shell and membranes of the egg and the nourishment provided by the egg yolk. For most viviparous animals, the wall of the mother's brood pouch or uterus supplies protection while nourishment comes from the maternal blood via the placenta.

The dominant role of the uterus in these arrangements is at once apparent. The thickness of the uterine wall, combined with the intra-abdominal location of the organ within the bony pelvis, in most species, is insulation against external trauma and the vasculature of the wall provides the channels through which maternal blood is carried to and from the placenta.

The transition from oviparity to viviparity, however, was not an immediate, clear-cut nor even a total one. Vestigial remnants of primitive structures characteristic of ancestral animals are found in the course of development of individuals of advanced forms, and many of them are functionally important at particular embryological stages.

These circumstances led to the formulation by Haeckel in the 19th century of the so-called Law of Recapitulation or Biogenesis which stated that 'ontogeny (development of the individual) recapitulates phylogeny (development of the race)'. Modern embryological study, revealing the ontogenetic sequence in a wide variety of species, has not found evidence that each embryo actually passes through all the stages its ancestors traversed or, in the familiar catch phrase, 'climbs up the family tree'. Thus, modification of the strict Biogenetic Law is now necessary. Modification but not abandonment, for the vestigial remnants of primitive structures indicate that some recapitulation is indeed operative. De Beer in his treatise, *Embryos and Ancestors*, restates the law in the following currently acceptable form: 'The embryo of the descendant passes through modified stages of the ancestral ontogeny.' This is still an incomplete explanation of the developmental course taken by any particular individual, but it does have value as a general principle and its details can be modified as newly acquired evidence requires.

The necessity for familiarity with the embryological development of the uterus emerges from these considerations and attention will now be directed to this.

Embryology of the uterus

The uterus develops as an integral part of the genito-urinary system and can best be understood in that context. The widely accepted opinion that this topic is among the most difficult of medical fields to comprehend loses its validity if four underlying considerations are recognized at the outset.

1. There is a close relation between the developing urinary and reproductive systems. Some early excretory organs are later used by both systems or diverted to reproductive tract functions alone.
2. Reproductive tract structures appear in sexually undifferentiated form. Subsequently, they are modified to conform to the individual's genetic sex although residual remnants of structures appropriate to the opposite sex may persist.
3. Development of structures occurs in consecutive but often overlapping waves, commencing high in the abdominal cavity and progressing downward toward the pelvis.
4. External genitalia are derived in part from the hindgut or cloaca.

These basic propositions are summarized in the chart in Fig. 1, which shows the chronologic relations between developmental events in the four systems involved in urogenital tract formation. The transfer or disappearance of certain structures as development progresses is indicated by arrows carrying through successive weeks. The vertical subdivision of the third column, labelled 'Ducts', demonstrates the early coexistence of structures of both future male and future female types and their later separation into organs of sex specificity. The chart also usefully shows the time element, so that if one has particular interest in conditions prevailing at a special time, a horizontal line drawn across the chart at that time provides a quick, initial overview of structures to be found at that age.

Urogenital structures

Pronephros

The first anlage is a urinary tract organ, the pronephros or primitive kidney, which appears bilaterally early in the third or fourth week post-conception. It is

Age	Glands	Urinary Tract	♂ Ducts ♀		External Genitalia
3–4 weeks	Primordial germ cells	Pronephros (non-functional) Tubules and ducts	Pronephric		
4–9 weeks		Mesonephros or Wolffian body (temporary fuction) Tubules and ducts	Mesonephric or		Cloaca
5th week	Urogenital ridge				
6th week	Indifferent gonad: germinal and core epithelium	Mesonephros or kidney (permanent) Tubules and ducts	Paramesonephric or Müllerian		Cloaca subdivides genital tubercle
7th week	Male type cords				Anal and urethral membranes rupture
8th week	Testis and Ovary				
9th week			Müllerian ducts fuse at tubercle		Urethral and labioscrotal
10th week			Müllerian ducts degenerate	Wolffian ducts degenerate	folds, phalus and
11th week			Seminal Vesicles, epididymis, vas deferens		glans
12th week	Ovary descent complete			Walls form	Sex distinguishable
5 months	Testes at inguinal ring			Sinus epithelium grows in vaginal cleft	
8 months Term	Testis descent complete			Rapid uterine growth	

Fig. 1. Chart showing interrelations and time sequence of events in development of genitourinary system. From Ramsey, E. M. (1986). In Danforth, D. N. & Scott, J. R., eds (1986). *Obstetrics and Gynecology*, 5th edn, p. 107.

an example of the third of the basic propositions noted above, in that it is first seen high in the abdominal cavity and in subsequent development progresses toward the pelvis. The first step is a bilateral bulging of mesoderm into the primitive abdominal cavity, forming the genital ridges (Fig. 2). Into these ridges

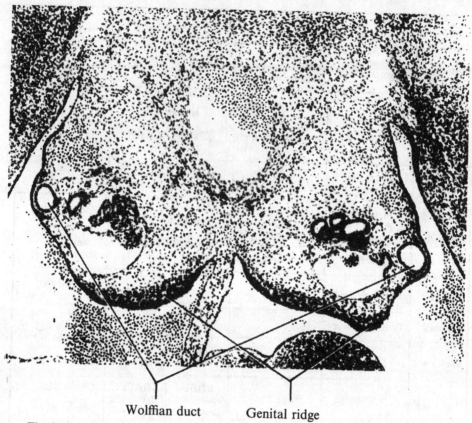

Wolffian duct   Genital ridge

Fig. 2. Part of transverse section through 7-week embryo, showing thickening of coelomic epithelim and condensation of underlying mesenchyme forming genital ridge. Carnegie No. 6524, Section 48M3M4. ×148. From Gillman, J. (1948). *Contributions to Embryology*, **32**, 114.

coelomic epithelium invaginates forming numerous tubules whose medial ends meet and fuse to form the pronephric ducts. As the pronephros progresses toward the pelvis, tubules in the higher locations degenerate simultaneously with the appearance of new ones lower down. The pronephric ducts, on the other hand, do not degenerate but persist and continue to grow toward the cloaca, eventually entering it. The pronephros is probably non-functional in the human.

Mesonephros

The second kidney, the mesonephros, arises in the fourth week in the subdiaphragmatic location and replaces the pronephros. It is composed of tubules which progressively degenerate as new ones are formed lower down and the lining of the tubules is again derived from coelomic epithelium which has invaginated the mesodermal core. The mesonephros does not form a duct of its own; instead, it appropriates the pronephric duct which thereafter is known as the mesonephric or Wolffian duct. The mesonephric duct persists in the adult male as the vas deferens but degenerates in the female around the 10th week (Fig. 1). The mesonephros probably has at least a rudimentary function, but, like the pronephros, it degenerates and is replaced by the definitive kidney, the metanephros.

Metanephros

The metanephric tubules, arising in the same manner as the pronephric and mesonephric tubules, appear in the sixth or seventh week but form rather lower in the abdominal cavity than those of the first two kidneys. The metanephric ducts are not simple takeovers of the Wolffian duct; instead, they are independent developments from outpouchings of the lower end of the Wolffian duct, the so-called ureteric buds. These grow upwards (not downward like other formations), eventually invaginating the metanephros and connecting with the tubules. The metanephric ducts eventually form the definitive ureters and they are therefore strictly urinary tract features.

Uterus

The structures that have been described so far are only indirectly ancestral to the uterus itself. They are included because their vestigial remnants may give rise to congenital anomalies.

Müllerian duct

Closer attention will now be paid to the direct ancestors of the uterus. In the sixth week, at about the time when the permanent kidney is appearing, a new duct is formed bilaterally, unrelated to the kidney, by proliferation of coelomic epithelium lateral to the upper end of the mesonephric (Wolffian) duct. This is, at first, a blind cord which grows downward toward the pelvis. Subsequently it becomes canalized and is known as the paramesonephric or Müllerian duct. By virtue of its origin as a derivative of coelomic epithelium, the lining of the Müllerian duct is the same as that of the urinary tract structures which have a similar origin. Both the Wolffian and this new Müllerian duct originate during the 'neuter' stage of embryonic development, i.e. before sexual differentiation is grossly observable, and therefore they are common to both males and females. As already stated, in

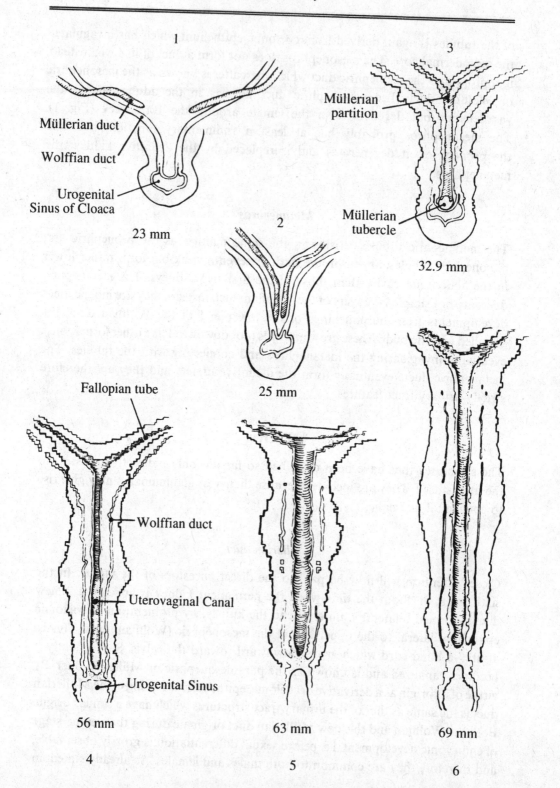

1

Müllerian duct

Wolffian duct

Urogenital
Sinus of Cloaca

23 mm

2

25 mm

3

Müllerian
partition

Müllerian
tubercle

32.9 mm

Fallopian tube

Wolffian duct

Uterovaginal Canal

Urogenital Sinus

56 mm

4

63 mm

5

69 mm

6

the male the Wolffian duct persists in post-natal life as the vas deferens, but in the female it degenerates around the tenth week. The future of the Müllerian duct is the reverse. In the male, it degenerates in the tenth week but persists in the female giving rise to the uterus (Fig. 1).

The right and left Müllerian ducts grow toward each other, crossing over the Wolffian duct anteriorly until they meet in the midline in the ninth week (Fig. 3). The point of crossing is known as the uterotubal junction because the portions of the Müllerian ducts above it form the uterine (Fallopian) tubes while the portions below it form the uterus. The Fallopian tube portions remain independent, each opening into the peritoneal cavity via a fimbriated end. The lower portions gradually fuse and progress toward the cloaca, at first as a solid cord ending at the Müllerian tubercle which lies against the upper wall of the cloaca. Eventually, the medial walls of the fused Müllerian ducts are absorbed to form a single cavity comprising the uterine cavity and the vaginal canal. In the fifth month the Müllerian tubercle likewise becomes canalized establishing continuity of the uterine cavity with the cavity of the cloaca.

Urogenital sinus and its derivatives

Meanwhile, changes are taking place in the cloaca and adjacent regions. The cloaca, as seen in Fig. 4, is in fact the blind end of the hindgut into which reproductive, excretory and intestinal tracts all open in early stages. The cloaca and its derivatives are lined with gut endoderm, in contrast to the other structures discussed here which are lined with epithelium of coelomic origin.

In the sixth week a septum forms dividing the cloaca in two, establishing independent urogenital and intestinal compartments or sinuses. These are at first closed receptacles separated from the exterior by the urogenital and rectal membranes. Rupture of these membranes provides orifices of exit from the sinuses. Almost simultaneously there appear in the future perineal region, i.e. on the exterior surface of the body, a midline protuberance and paired lateral swellings (Fig. 5). The first is the genital tubercle, the forerunner of the phallus. The lateral swellings constitute precursors, in the female, of the genital folds and, in the male, of the labioscrotal folds. In the female, the groove between the folds forms the inner portion of the vestibule of post-natal life. The rupture of the urogenital membrane occurs in the depth of the vestibule and the resulting orifice converts

Fig. 3. Drawings to show fusion of paramesonephric (Müllerian) ducts to form uterus and vagina in human embryos. From Koff, A. K. (1933). *Contributions to Embryology*, **24**, 59–90.

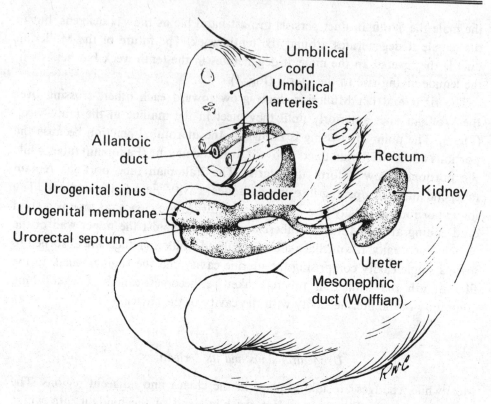

Fig. 4. Drawing to show relations of cloaca and its derivatives. From Ramsey,
E. M. (1986). In Danforth, D. N. & Scott, J. R., eds (1986). *Obstetrics and Gynecology*,
5th edn., 114. Drawn by Ranice W. Crosby.

the whole former urogenital sinus into an open trough. Perineal ectoderm grows
into the trough; junction with the urogenital sinus endoderm (cloacal) occurs on
the inner aspect of the genital folds.

The Müllerian epithelium throughout the genital tract becomes columnar, thus
constituting a characteristic mucosa in the Fallopian tubes, the endometrium, the
cervix and the upper portion of the vagina. The cloacal endoderm of the lower
portion of the vagina becomes stratified squamous. The junction between the
two types of epithelium may result in a number of pathologic processes in the adult.

Anomalies

The smooth developmental sequence outlined in the foregoing section pre-
supposes the timely disappearance of certain structures which are rudimentary
in human and related primates but persistent and functional in lower animals.
The disappearance is not always complete and rudimentary structures may persist,

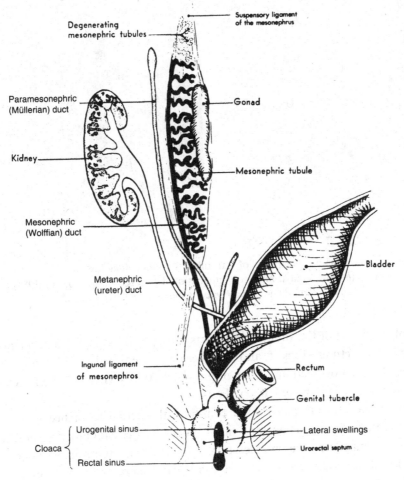

Fig. 5. Schematic diagram showing plan of urogenital system at an early stage while still sexually undifferentiated. From Corliss, C. E. ed. (1976). *Patten's Human Embryology*, 358.

in larger or smaller fractions, giving rise to the 'vestigial remnants' which were discussed at the beginning of this chapter. These remnants form the basis of many malformations observed in adults and are the major source of anomalies of the uterus. Although these remnants usually lack functional activity, they still have clinical importance, as well as evolutionary significance, for any of them may lead to cyst formation, inflammation or even malignancy.

Vestigial remnants arise by one or other of two basic processes. First, the simple failure of rudimentary structures to disappear entirely, or, secondly, the failure of structures to fuse in orderly fashion.

In the first category, failure to disappear, both pronephros and mesonephros

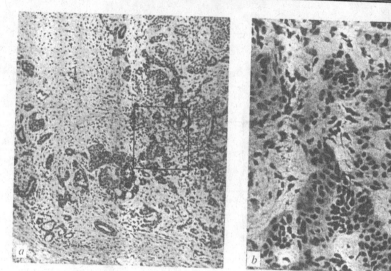

Fig. 6. Microscopic appearance of paratubal Wolffian duct remnants. (*a*) Low power view, (*b*) same area at higher magnification. From Kurman, R. J., ed. (1987). *Blaustein's Pathology of the Female Genital Tract,* 3rd edn, 431.

are involved. Some of the tubules and ducts may persist as isolated segments of the original structures (Figs. 5 and 6). These small epithelium-lined fragments have long been recognized and their origin identified by virtue of their location along the course of the rudimentary ducts.

Although persisting fragments are common, the actual incidence is hard to assess since they are usually asymptomatic. When, as occasionally happens, their epithelium displays its inherent secretory properties and the fragments become cystic, clinical attention is aroused. The cysts may become very large, dilated by accumulated secretion, and subject to infection. Neoplastic degeneration is not common but can occur.

A fairly constant location of the vestigial remnants in the adult female is the epoophron which lies adjacent to the ovary. It is composed of remnants of the upper portion of the mesonephric (Wolffian) duct and its tubules. Less constantly, the central segment of the Wolffian duct gives rise to the paroophron which is found in the broad ligament, while derivatives of the terminal portion occur adjacent to or incorporated in the cervix or vagina. In the latter location they are known as Gartner's ducts and may be clinically active.

Sometimes clusters of rudimentary ducts are encapsulated by fibrous connective tissue creating the semblance of a tumour. These may be entirely unnoticed by a patient or may cause symptoms necessitating surgical removal of the mass.

Although the paramesonephric (Müllerian) ducts are permanent structures which do not form vestigial remnants they do give rise to anomalous structures

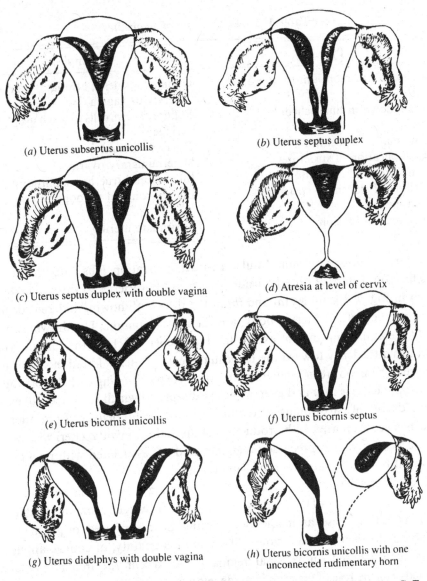

(a) Uterus subseptus unicollis

(b) Uterus septus duplex

(c) Uterus septus duplex with double vagina

(d) Atresia at level of cervix

(e) Uterus bicornis unicollis

(f) Uterus bicornis septus

(g) Uterus didelphys with double vagina

(h) Uterus bicornis unicollis with one unconnected rudimentary horn

Fig. 7. Schematic drawings of various types of abnormal uteri. From Corliss, C. E. ed. *Patten's Human Embryology*, McGraw Hill Book Co.

through elaboration of small branches or outpouchings. These appear as cysts which may contain clear serous fluid or inspissated matter. These characteristically appear in the tissues surrounding the Fallopian tubes and as such are lumped together as paratubal cysts (Fig. 6). The most common such structure is the hydatid of Morgagni which may be found attached to one of the fimbriae of the Fallopian tube.

Table 1. *Types of origin of anomalies*

Type	Example
1. Failure of primordium to appear	Gonadal agenesis; atresia of uterine cervix or vagina
2. Breakdown in time schedule	Failure of germ cells to reach urogenital ridge
3. Anomalies of position	Ovary in labium majus
4. Reduplication of structures	Supernumerary ovaries
5. Chromosomal aberration	Intersex and true hermaphroditism
6. Failure of transitory structure to disappear	Epoophron and paroophron
7. Anomalies of fusion	Bicornuate uterus

By far the most common Müllerian duct aberration falls into the second classification, failure of orderly fusion. The possible varieties of this anomaly are shown in Fig. 7. Examples (*a*) and (*b*) in the drawing, showing different degrees of partitioning of the uterine body, are the most common. The drawings in (*e*) and (*f*) resemble (*a*) and (*b*) except for the deeper notch in the fundus which illustrates a tendency toward the bicornuate form of uterus found in subprimate Eutheria. These too are not uncommon. Complete partitioning with double vagina as in example (*g*) is rare and even rarer is example (*c*) which resembles (*g*) except for the degree of partitioning of the fundus. In type (*g*) delivery from alternate horns has been reported with production of up to three infants. Uteri with atresia of the cervix or vagina preclude pregnancy and are associated with retention of menstrual blood (hematometra or hematocolpos).

To complete the account of anomalies occurring in the genitourinary tract, mention must be made of those whose origin is not in vestigial remnants (Table 1).

Merely listing these anomalies and noting their supposed origin begs the question as to their ultimate cause. The same uncertainty, of course, applies to the anomalies based on vestigial remnants. As recent research has enlarged knowledge of the role of genetics in all developmental processes, many malformations formerly attributed to miscellaneous factors are now being gathered into the genetic category. With further progress the specific genetic factors responsible for normal development will be identified together with the aberrations which underlie abnormalities, both benign and malignant.

References

Some of the cited works which deal with embryological development in general also have chapters or sections which emphasize phylogeny or anomalies. The given passages are noted in parentheses following the bibliographic data.

Amoroso, E. C. (1968). The evolution of viviparity. *Proceedings of the Royal Society of Medicine,* **61**, 1188–200.

Amoroso, E. C. (1981). Viviparity. In *Cellular and Molecular Aspects of Implantation.* ed. S.R. Glasser and D. W. Bullock, pp. 3–25, Plenum, New York.

Arey, L.B. (1965). *Developmental Anatomy.* 7th edn. WB Saunders Co., Philadelphia.

Corliss, C. E. (1976). *Patten's Human Embryology.* New York: McGraw-Hill Book Co. (366–269 Anomalies).

Cunningham, F. G., MacDonald, P. C. & Gant, N. F. (1989). *Williams Obstetrics.* 18th edn. Appleton & Lange, Norwalk, Connecticut. (729–736 Anomalies).

Danforth, D. N. & Scott, J. R., eds. (1986). *Obstetrics and Gynecology.* 5th edn. J.B. Lippincott Co., Philadelphia. (116–118 Anomalies).

DeBeer Sir G. (1958). *Embryos and Ancestors.* 3rd edn. The Clarendon Press, Oxford.

Grine, F. E., Fleagle, L. B. & Martin, L. B., eds. (1987). *Primate Phylogeny.* US edn. Academic Press Inc., San Diego CA.

Gruenwald, P. (1941). Relation of the growing Müllerian duct to the Wolffian duct and its importance for the genesis of malformations. *Anatomical Research,* **81**, 1–19.

Hamilton, W. J. & Mossman, H. W. (1972). *Hamilton, Boyd and Mossman's Human Embryology.* 4th edn. W. Heffer & Sons Ltd, Cambridge (Chapter XVII, Phylogeny).

Hill, J.P. (1932). Developmental history of the Primates. *Philosophical Transactions of the Royal Society,* **B221**, 45–178.

Kurman, R. J. (ed) (1987). *Blaustein's Pathology of the Female Genital Tract.* 3rd edn. Springer Verlag, New York.

Mossman, H. W. (1989). Comparative anatomy. In *Biology of the Uterus.* ed. R. M. Wynn and W. P. Jollie, pp. 19–34, Plenum Medical Book Company, New York (19–34 Phylogeny).

Mossman, H. W. (1987). *Vertebrate Fetal Membranes.* New Brunswick, NJ: Rutgers University Press, New Brunswick, NJ (122–123 Phylogeny).

O'Rahilly, R. & Müller, F. (1992). *Human Embryology & Teratology.* Wiley-Liss, Incl, New York (217–219 Anomalies).

Ramsey, E. M. (1986). Embryology and developmental defects of the female reproductive tract. In *Obstetrics and Gynecology,* ed. D.N. Danforth & J.R. Scott, 5th edn, pp. 106–19.

Reynolds, S. R. M. (1949). *Physiology of the Uterus.* 2nd edn. Paul B. Hoeber, Inc., New York.

Scott, J. R., DiSaia, P. J., Hammond, C. B. & Spellacy, W. N., eds. (1990). *Danforth's Obstetrics and Gynecology.* 6th edn. J. B. Lippincott Company, Philadelphia.

Wynn, R. M., Jollie, W. P., eds. (1989). *Biology of the Uterus.* 2nd edn. Plenum Medical Book Company, New York (19–34 Phylogeny).

4

Structure and function of uterine muscle

R. E. GARFIELD AND C. YALLAMPALLI

Introduction

Knowledge of the anatomy of the myometrium and the relationship of muscle cells to other components of the uterus is essential for understanding uterine function. The structure and function of the uterine muscle has been examined by our laboratory and many others (Garfield, 1984; Garfield, Blennerhassett & Miller, 1988; Broderick & Broderick, 1990).

The constituents of the uterine wall are remarkably similar to elements found in other organs containing a preponderance of smooth muscle such as the gastrointestinal tract, airways, and blood vessels. However, unlike other smooth muscle organs the myometrium is normally functional for only a brief period following a lengthy gestation. In this review we will consider the structure of the myometrium and the factors which regulate uterine contractility during pregnancy. This is necessary for comprehension of the mechanisms which maintain the uterus in a quiescent state throughout pregnancy and then convert the muscle to an active and reactive state during labour.

The uterus becomes increasingly contractile and reactive to excitatory agents at the end of gestation and eventually reaches a state in which it expels the fetus and other products of conception. This contractile state (labour) is achieved when contractions of different regions of the uterine wall become stronger, more frequent, and synchronous. Coordination of these contractions is believed to be required for the normal progression of parturition, and the absence of this activity throughout pregnancy is essential for adequate nourishment of the developing fetus (Csapo, 1981).

In approximately 5 to 10% of pregnant women the uterus begins to contract early. Some cases of pre-term labour can be related to pathological conditions while others have no apparent underlying causes. Spontaneous pre-term labour is the number one problem confronting the obstetrician. The inability to control pre-term labour may be attributed in part to the lack of understanding of uterine contractility. It is also difficult to diagnose labour. During both the term and pre-term situations the physician is sometimes faced with the decision to either inhibit or induce/augment labour. Unfortunately there is no objective manner in which to evaluate the labour state. Frequent contractions and/or state of the cervix are used as indicators of labour. However, neither is an adequate objective parameter since contraction frequency gives no information about synchrony or force of contractility and cervical dilation or effacement sometimes occurs independent of uterine contractions.

Contractions of the uterus depend upon the underlying electrical activity. The frequency, duration, and magnitude of uterine contractions are dependent on the frequency of action potential discharge, the duration of the train of action potentials within each muscle cell, and the total number of cells simultaneously and synchronously active (Marshall, 1962). Therefore, the propagation of potentials from pacemaker regions or from areas influenced by stimulatory agents to adjacent and distant cells is of fundamental importance to the events controlling excitability and contractility. The observation that gap junctions appear between myometrial cells during the onset and progression of labour was a major breakthrough in our understanding of circumstances that control this process. In this review we will concentrate on this aspect and emphasize how control of this process contributes to the maintenance of pregnancy and the initiation of labour. We will also discuss our recent studies of nitric oxide inhibition of uterine contractility.

Structure of the myometrium

There are numerous reviews of the structure of the uterus and the myometrium (Garfield, 1984; Garfield & Somlyo, 1985; Broderick & Broderick, 1990). Of great importance to functional considerations, are the features of the muscle cells which regulate intracellular calcium and thus control contractility. Also significant is the presence of other cells in the uterus which may modulate the contractile function of myometrium. The composition of the muscle and makeup of the uterine wall which reflect these two aspects will be emphasized below.

Organization of the myometrium

The composition of the myometrium is heterogeneous. The myometrium consists predominantly of muscle cells but also contains fibroblasts, blood and lymphatic vessels, immune cells, and a large proportion of connective tissue.

The uterine wall is usually composed of at least three distinct layers. The innermost layer, the endometrium, lines the lumen of the organ and consists of

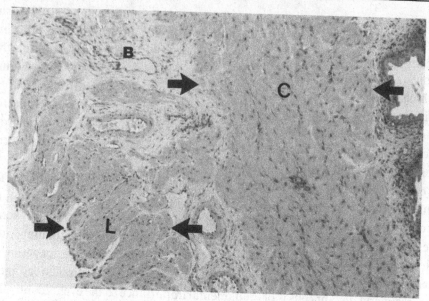

Fig. 1. Light micrograph of a cross-section through the uterine wall from a pregnant rat. Note the thickness of the smooth muscle layers indicated by arrows (longitudinal (L) and circular (C)) as well as the vascular plexus containing blood vessels (B) between the layers (× 75).

columnar epithelium and underlying stromal tissue. The myometrium makes up the other two layers: the outer longitudinal muscle layer and the inner circular layer. Fig. 1 shows a light micrograph of a cross-section of the rat uterus showing the two layers of the myometrium.

The outer longitudinal muscle layer of the myometrium consists of a network of bundles of smooth muscle cells that are generally oriented in the long axis of the uterus (Csapo, 1962; Garfield & Somlyo, 1985). The bundles interconnect and form a network over the surface of the uterus. Each bundle is composed of smooth muscle cells arranged in the long axis of the bundle. Muscle cells of the circular muscle layer are arranged concentrically around the longitudinal axis of the uterus. The muscle cells in the circular layer are arranged more diffusely and the bundle arrangement, if present, is not as apparent as that of the longitudinal layer. There are functional and structural studies indicating that the longitudinal layer is continuous with the circular layer (Finn & Porter, 1975; Osa & Katase, 1975). A low magnification electron micrograph of a cross-section through portions of several bundles of longitudinal muscle layer is shown in Fig. 2. The extracellular space between the muscle cells is occupied by collagen and other cells. During pregnancy the uterus increases tremendously in size to accommodate the growing fetus (Fig. 3). Growth of the myometrium during pregnancy is thought

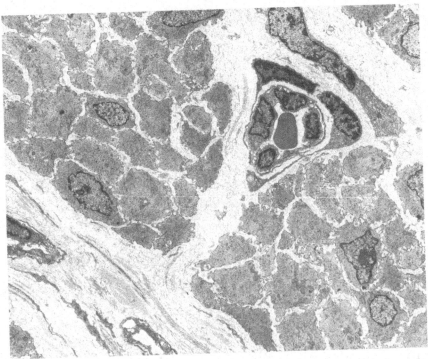

Fig. 2. Low magnification electron micrograph of the uterus from a rabbit showing longitudinal muscle cells cut in cross-section × 4800.

to be primarily accounted for by increases in number of cells (hyperplasia) which precedes implantation and then increases in size of muscle cells (hypertrophy) during the remainder of gestation (Carsten, 1968).

The muscle cell

Smooth muscle cells of the myometrium are generally thought to be long, spindle shaped cells, but may be irregularly shaped. The cells are largest during the later stages of gestation and their size and number are regulated by steroid hormones and distention (Carsten, 1968). The cells range in size from 5 to 10 μm in diameter in the centre of the cell and from 300 to 600 μm in length (Csapo, 1962; Finn & Porter, 1975). The average volume of a human myometrial smooth muscle cell has been estimated at 21 000 mm^3 (Kao, 1977) which would translate into a surface area estimate of about 23 000 mm^2 based upon a volume to surface area ratio of 0.9. The size of smooth muscle cells probably varies considerably between different species. The muscle cells of the human uterus are considerably larger than those of the mouse although quantitative studies have not been done.

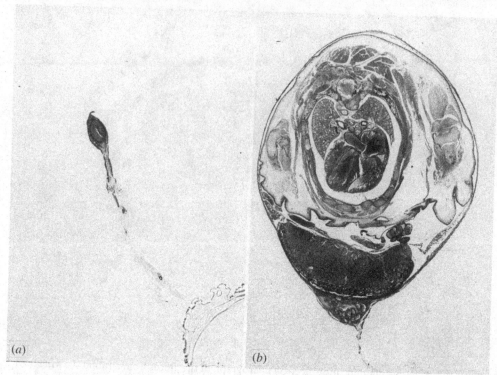

Fig. 3. Photographs of cross-sections through entire uterus from rat uteri at day 6 of pregnancy (*a*) and at term (*b*). Note the increase in diameter of the uterus at term (*b*) showing a section through the uterus containing the fetus and placenta. × 3.8.

Contracted cells are shorter, but larger in the middle, whereas relaxed and distended cells are long and narrow. Generally, the cells are round or oval in the relaxed state when viewed in the transverse orientation and appear serrated when contracted isotonically.

The plasma membrane of the smooth muscle cell is the barrier that divides the intracellular compartment of the muscle cells from their extracellular environment. This membrane is responsible for the excitable properties of the muscle cells. The plasma membrane, as in other cells, is a trilaminar structure of approximately 8 nm in thickness (Matlib *et al.*, 1979; Singer & Nicholson, 1972). The plasma membranes of uterine smooth muscle cells form various types of cell-to-cell contacts including gap junctions. The concept of cell-to-cell communication is discussed in more detail below.

Uterine smooth muscle cells have an extensive system of sarcoplasmic reticulum consisting of a network of tubules and sacs within the cytoplasm (Fig. 4). The volume of the sarcoplasmic reticulum is not known but in other smooth muscles

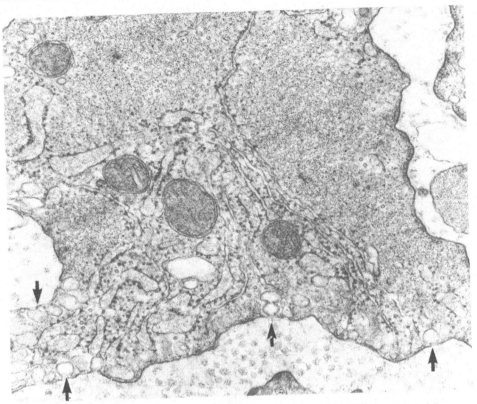

Fig. 4. Transverse section through a myometrial cell from pregnant guinea-pig uterus. Note the continuity between granular and agranular sarcoplasmic reticulum and the close association between vesicles (arrow), reticulum, plasma membrane and mitochondria. × 34 400.

ranges from 2 to 7.5% of the cell volume (Somlyo, 1980). The granular reticulum and agranular reticulum are continuous and the agranular reticulum makes close contact with surface vesicles, plasma membrane (Fig. 4, Garfield & Somlyo, 1985) and gap junctions (Garfield, Merrett & Grover, 1980).

The major known functions of the sarcoplasmic reticulum are those of a storage site of activator calcium (see below; smooth endoplasmic reticulum) and a site for protein synthesis (rough endoplasmic reticulum). The increased prominence of the rough endoplasmic reticulum observed in uterine smooth muscle following oestrogen treatment or pregnancy presumably reflects increased protein synthesis (Bergman, 1968; Ross & Klebanoff, 1967). Isolated enriched fractions of microsomes, plasma membranes, and sarcoplasmic reticulum membranes from uterine smooth muscle and other smooth muscle accumulate calcium (Grover *et al.*, 1980). The fact that uterine smooth muscles contract *in vitro* when placed in calcium-free solutions, and contract when skinned with

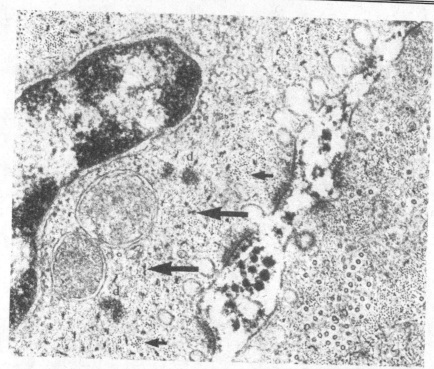

Fig. 5. Transverse section of a portion of a myometrial cell from non-pregnant human uterus showing contractile filaments. Actin (small arrows) and myosin (large arrows) filaments and dense bodies (D) present in the cytoplasm. × 61 000.

saponin in response to inositol triphosphates (IP3), supports the concept of an internal source of calcium for uterine contraction (Edman & Schild, 1962; Savineau, Mironneau & Mironneau, 1988; Izumi et al., 1990).

Contraction of smooth muscle cells is thought to occur, as in skeletal muscle, through the interaction of myosin and actin filaments (Somlyo, 1980). At least three distinct types of filaments have been identified in uterine smooth muscle (Garfield, 1984). These include the thick (15 nm diameter, myosin), thin (6–8 nm, actin) and intermediate (10 nm, desmin or vimentin filaments, Fig. 5). Microtubules are also prominent within the cytoplasm of smooth muscle cells (Fig. 5).

Myometrial cells also contain a variety of other important organelles such as nuclei, mitochondria, Golgi, etc., which are also present in most animal cells (Garfield & Somlyo, 1985; Broderick & Broderick, 1990). However, since these organelles generally have only indirect effects on control of contractility they will not be described here. For more detailed analysis of these elements, one should consult general reviews of the uterus or smooth muscle (Garfield & Somlyo, 1985; Broderick & Broderick, 1990; Gabella, 1981).

Control of Ca²⁺: basis for contraction

Normally, contractions of the pre-term uterus are local and asynchronous and fail to generate effective force. At term, contractions become increasingly more frequent, synchronous and intense, producing powerful propulsive contractions in order to propel the fetus through the birth canal (Csapo, 1981; Garfield, Blennerhassett & Miller, 1988). The conversion of myometrium from an inactive state during early pregnancy to an active state during labour is central to the understanding of uterine contractility. Equally important is the mechanism by which the myometrium recruits contractile units to produce a forceful contraction.

The ability of myometrial cells to contract depends upon the distribution of ions across their plasma membranes. The ionic distribution in uterine smooth muscle, as in other excitable tissues, is such that sodium and calcium ions are higher outside the cell than inside, whereas potassium ions are higher within the cells (Kao, 1989). These ionic gradients allow the muscle cells to respond when small changes in permeability result in significant movements of ions down their electrochemical gradients.

The ions are distributed so that the resting membrane potential (difference between inside and outside) is about -45 mV (range -40 to -60 mV), but varies depending upon the hormonal state. Excitation in the form of action potentials or spikes occurs when the membrane permeability is changed, and ions move down their respective electrochemical gradients through membrane channels.

The basis for a uterine contraction lies in the electrical and chemical changes that occur within the muscle cells. Phasic contractile activity is a direct consequence of the underlying electrical activity of the muscle cells (Marshall, 1962; Kao, 1989). The sequence of contraction and relaxation of the myometrium results from the cyclic depolarization and repolarization of the muscle cell in the form of action potentials. The driving force for myometrial contractility is thought to be provided by propagated action potentials (Fig. 6) that arise from pacemaker regions (Marshall, 1962; Kao, 1989). As in other excitable tissues, the action potential in uterine smooth muscle results from voltage- and time-dependent changes in membrane ionic permeabilities (the ionic theory of excitation). The depolarizing phase of the action potential is due to an inward current carried mainly by Ca^{2+} ions but also by Na^+ ions (Fig. 7). The outward current, causing repolarization, is carried by K^+ ions and consists of a fast (voltage-dependent) and a slow (Ca^{2+} activated) component (Kao, 1989). The frequency and intensity of contractions are directly proportional to the regularity and duration of action potentials in each muscle cell and total number of cells that are active (Marshall, 1962). The contractile event of uterine smooth muscle is initiated by a rise in the intracellular free ionized Ca^{2+} to approximately 10^{-5} M from a resting level of

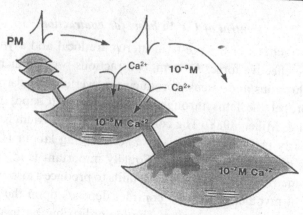

Fig. 6. Diagram of a group of myometrial cells interconnected by low-resistance pathways. Action potentials, as recorded by microelectrodes, are initiated in pacemaker cells (PM) and propagate to coupled cells. As the action potential passes, it increases Ca^{2+} ions intracellularly from about $10^{-7}M$ to $10^{-5}M$ to produce a contraction. Thus, presence of intracellular pathways indirectly controls the availability of Ca^{2+} to the muscle cells.

about 10^{-7} M (Figs. 6 and 7) (Kao, 1989). The source of this activator Ca^{2+} is extracellular (Ca^{2+} ions that flow into the cell down their electrochemical gradient through potential dependent Ca^{2+} channels in response to a change in membrane permeability when the membrane potential reaches about -35 mV) or intracellular (Ca^{2+} ions released from intracellular storage sites) or a combination of both (Lao, 1989; Kuriyama, 1961). Therefore, the mechanism that controls the propagation of action potentials between muscle cells from pacemaker regions indirectly regulates the availability of intracellular Ca^{2+} ions. Conversely, a reduction of intracellular free Ca^{2+} (either as a result of efflux into the extracellular space or re-uptake into intracellular storage sites) terminates contraction (Grover, 1986).

Pacemaker cells are thought to be responsible for initiation of spontaneous electrical activity in uterine smooth muscle. Pacemaker cells are autonomously active smooth muscle cells in which the resting membrane potential varies (~ -50 mV), as compared with non-pacemaker cells (Lodge & Sproat, 1981). Spontaneous oscillations (pacemaker potentials) in the membrane potential of pacemaker cells lead to action potentials when the threshold for firing is reached. The electrical activity which arises from the pacemaker areas then excites surrounding non-pacemaker regions.

It has been proposed that any muscle cell can act as a pacemaker cell (Marshall, 1962). It has been shown that non-pacemaker regions can become pacemakers by the application of oxytocin, acetylcholine, or prostaglandins but not by simply depolarizing the membrane with high K^+ solutions (Lodge & Sproat, 1981).

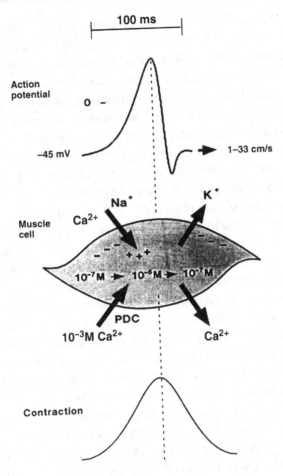

Fig. 7. Diagram to show the changes in membrane potential (top), influx and efflux of ions (middle) and mechanical event (contraction, bottom) during passage of an action potential over a single myometrial cell. (PDC = potential dependent channel.)

Stretching of the uterine wall also induces pacemaker activity (Lodge & Sproat, 1981; Marshall, 1962). Pacemaker potentials are independent of nerve activity, because nerve blocking agents fail to prevent them. However, neuronal or hormonal influences may modulate the activity of the pacemaker cells and induce or suppress activity and impose directionality.

In the myometrium, an action potential depolarization opens voltage-dependent Ca^{2+} channels allowing Ca^{2+} ions to enter the muscle cell and interact with the myofilaments (electromechanical couplings, Figs. 6 and 7). The Ca^{2+} ions from a single action potential can initiate a twitch contraction (Fig. 6) (Marshall, 1962). However, when action potentials are repetitively discharged (for example, in spike bursts) the contraction amplitude is increased because the intracellular level of free Ca^{2+} is increased and because the increments in tension triggered by individual spikes can summate. When action potentials are discharged at a rate higher than about 1 cycle per second, a fused tetanic type contraction is generated (Marshall, 1962; Kao, 1989). Thus, the frequency and duration of spike discharge can control the contraction height and duration, respectively. In this way, the frequency of pacemaker discharge determines the rate and intensity of uterine contractions. However, increases in contractile force in the muscle may be achieved by a more or less synchronous stimulation of large areas of the myometrium by increases in conduction of action potentials, as opposed to a faster rate of stimulation of individual cells. The ability of muscle cells to propagate action potentials is related to the resting membrane potential (about $-45\,mV$), the ability of ions to pass through the membranes, as well as the extent of intercellular coupling. Cells more easily elicit action potentials when they are more positive and nearer their threshold. Action potentials develop with more difficulty when cells are more negative (hyperpolarized). Therefore, the level of excitability of the muscle cells as well as the extent of electrical coupling between the cells significantly influences the ability of the muscle to contract. Intrinsic substances from either the endocrine, nervous, and immune systems or from the application of pharmacological agents which either change the membrane potential, initiate pacemaker activity, influence ionic exchange, or modulate electrical propagation, can have important consequences.

Despite a variety of experimental approaches, most investigators of myometrial contractility have ultimately concluded that propagation of electrical signals between muscle cells plays a major role in the excitation–contraction process (Bozler, 1938; Kuriyama, 1961; Marshall, 1962: Csapo, 1981). Most also have found that electrical coupling is greatest during parturition and that is either higher or lower, respectively, after oestrogen or progesterone treatment of non-pregnant animals (Bozler, 1941; Csapo, 1981; Marshall, 1962). However, it is only recently that the system for cell-to-cell conduction propagation has been described (see below).

Intercellular communication

Propagation

A specialized mechanism of conduction must be present between the cells to coordinate their activity because the myometrium is composed of billions of small muscle cells (Csapo, 1981). Bozler (1938) was one of the first to indicate that rhythmic contractions can only be understood by postulating some mechanism of conduction which coordinates the activity of these elements. The innervation of the uterus was not considered to be of importance in regulating myometrial activity (Reynolds, 1949), because procedures which interfere with nerve impulses fail to change the outcome. Furthermore, there is no recognized specialized conduction pathway comparable to the Purkinje fibre system of the heart present in the myometrium. Additionally, the effects of stimulants on contractility cannot account for synchronous patterns of contractility during labour. For these reasons, electrical activity must propagate from cell-to-cell to coordinate the individual myometrial muscle cells (Abe, 1968; Finn & Porter, 1975; Csapo, 1981). The manner by which this activity is conducted between the smooth muscle cells and the factors which regulate this process are essential to an understanding of the mechanisms which maintain pregnancy and initiate parturition.

Gap junctions as sites of propagation

Gap junctions are intercellular channels that link cells to their neighbours by allowing the passage of inorganic ions and small molecules. They have been found between cells in every tissue and organ examined and are essentially ubiquitous in the animal kingdom (Peracchia, 1980; Saez *et al.*, 1993). In the electron microscope, they appear in regions of close apposition between cells as zones of paired, parallel membranes of unusually smooth outline separated by a narrow space of constant width – the 'gap' (Figs. 8 and 9).

Gap junctions consist of channels which connect the interiors of two cells. The channels are composed of proteins, termed connexins, which span the plasma membranes to form a pore (Saez *et al.*, 1993). Each gap junction can be made up from a few hundred to thousands of channels, and each channel is constructed from six connexin proteins in one cell aligned symmetrically with six connexins in the adjacent connected cell. The gap junction proteins have been cloned and antibodies have been prepared to the connexins. In the myometrium a 43 kD protein, termed connexin 43, is thought to be the major component of the gap junction (Beyer *et al.*, 1989). Connexin 43 is a protein composed of 382 amino acids with at least two sites for phosphorylation (Fig. 10). Connexin 43 is also found in other tissues including between muscle cells of the heart where it is thought to be required for synchronizing cardiac contractility (Kanter, Safitz & Beyer, 1992). The channels formed by connexins serve as sites for electrical coupling because the resistance in the gap junction channel is lower than the membrane resistance and therefore changes in charge within a cell, as during an action potential, will preferentially flow between cells (Fig. 11).

In all species studied, the onset and progression of labour contractile activity during term or pre-term labour is invariably associated with the presence of large

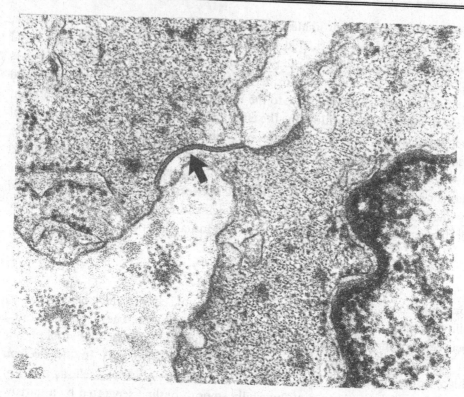

Fig. 8. Intermediate magnification micrograph of portions of two myometrial cells from rabbit during parturition showing a gap junction (arrow). × 71 000.

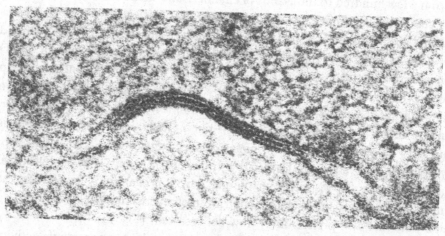

Fig. 9. High magnification micrograph of a gap junction. Note 7-lined appearance. × 250 000.

Connexin 43

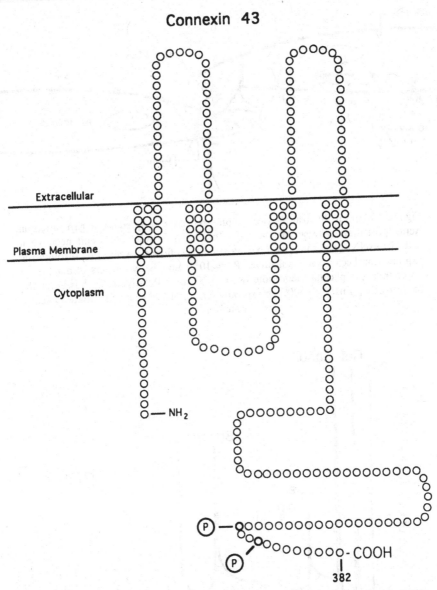

Fig. 10. Schematic representation of connexin 43. The protein is composed of 382 amino acids that crosses the plasma membrane four times with both the carboxyl and amino termini located in the cytoplasmic compartment. There are two serine residues on the carboxyl end that may be phosphorylated.

numbers of gap junctions between the myometrial cells (Fig. 12) (Garfield, Sims & Daniel, 1977; Garfield *et al.*, 1978). Moreover, improved electrical and metabolic communication (see below) between uterine smooth muscle cells is associated with the formation of junctions, supporting the hypothesis that the

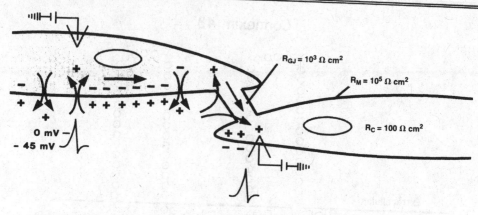

Fig. 11. Diagram illustrating two myometrial cells coupled by a gap junction. Action potentials traverse over the surface of a cell (left) by a local circuit mechanism with the exchange of ions (see text). Positive ions flow between cells through the gap junction because the resistance ($R_{GJ} = 10^3 \Omega$ cm^2) is two orders of magnitude lower than the plasma membrane ($R_M = 10^5 \Omega$ cm^2). Positive ions thus enter the coupled cell (right) ($R_C = 100\Omega$ cm^2) producing depolarization and initiate an action potential.

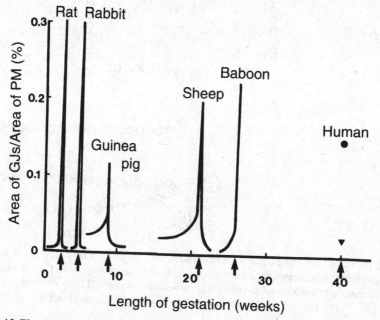

Fig. 12. The change in myometrial gap junctions (GJs) at term in several mammalian species. Area of gap junctions as a percentage of the plasma membrane (PM) is compared with the length of gestation for the rat, guinea pig, sheep, and baboon. Human data: ●: at term and in labour: ▼, at term but not in labour. Note that during labour (arrows) there is a dramatic increase in gap junctions and that following delivery, gap junctions decrease.

gap junctions permit the myometrium to behave as a functional syncytium during parturition. The presence of gap junctions and cell-to-cell communication represents the biophysical basis for synchronous and effective uterine contractile activity during labour.

Evidence from our studies and that of others suggests the presence of specific physiological mechanisms for regulating structural and functional coupling in the myometrium. Below we describe the possible mechanisms involved in the control of coupling in uterine smooth muscle: (1) the presence of the gap junctions and hence the extent of structural couplings; (2) the permeability of the gap junctions, and hence the extent of functional coupling in the myometrium and (3) the degradation of the gap junctions.

Gap junctions occupy a significant percentage of the area of the uterine smooth muscle cell plasma membrane (ca. 0.1–0.4%) only during term or pre-term labour as quantified by electron microscopy (Fig. 12), immunoblots (Fig. 13) and immunocytochemistry (Fig. 14). The junctions are increased when the muscle is functionally active during pregnancy (Garfield *et al.*, 1982; Garfield, Blennerhassett & Miller, 1986). Gap junctions are absent or present in low frequency and small size in non-pregnant, as well as pre-term and post-partum animals (Garfield *et al.*, 1977, 1978, 1979; Beyer *et al.*, 1989; Risek *et al.*, 1990; Hendrix *et al.*, 1992). In pregnant animals, the junctions begin to form about one day prior to the onset of labour. Gap junctions are always present in large numbers (ca. 1000 per cell) and increased size (ca. 250 nm) during normal delivery but disappear within 24 hours after parturition (see Fig. 12; Garfield *et al.*, 1988). This pattern of altered structural coupling in the myometrium is particularly prominent in rats and rabbits (Garfield *et al.*, 1978; Puri & Garfield, 1982; Deminanczuk, Towell & Garfield, 1984). Sheep and guinea pigs (Garfield *et al.*, 1979; Garfield, Puri & Csapo, 1982) differ slightly in that they have higher numbers of gap junctions prior to term (see Fig. 12). The gap junction profile in women during pregnancy and normal delivery is not known, but junctions are present in greater numbers in tissues from women undergoing Caesarean section and in labour compared with those not in labour as demonstrated by electron microscopy (Fig. 12) and using antibodies to connexin 43 for immunoblots or immunocytochemistry (Garfield & Hayashi, 1981; Tabb *et al.*, 1992). It is also significant that gap junctions are invariably present in myometrial tissues from animals undergoing premature labour either as a result of experimental manipulation or pathology (Garfield, Kannan & Daniel, 1980; Garfield *et al.*, 1978; Garfield *et al.*, 1982; MacKenzie & Garfield, 1985). Moreover, if the development of gap junctions is delayed then pregnancy is prolonged (Garfield *et al.*, 1978; Garfield *et al.*, 1982; Garfield, Gasc & Baulieu, 1987). Thus, myometrial gap junctions are dynamic and transitory structures whose presence is clearly associated with the conversion

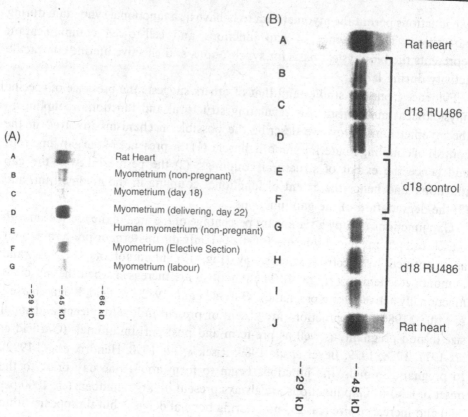

Fig. 13. (a) Immunoblots (50 mg protein each lane) of rat heart and of myometrial samples from rats (non-pregnant, day 18 of gestation and during term delivery) and humans (non-pregnant, elective Caesarean section and parturient. (b) Immunoblots (50 mg protein each lane) of rat heart (lanes A, J) and tissues from six different rats delivering prematurely at day 18 of gestation (lanes B, C, D and G, H, I) compared to tissues from two control rats at day 18 of gestation (lanes E and F). Note the distinct division of each blot into three regions and the increased density of blots from animals delivering prematurely.

of the uterus into an active organ just prior to parturition. Gap junctions appear to be necessary for effective labour because there is no known exception to this phenomenon.

Electrical coupling

Studies of the electrical role of the gap junctions between myometrial cells are not easily accomplished because of the small sizes of cells and their complex arrangement. Direct measurement of electrical spread of current is not possible because injected current rapidly dissipates in all directions. However, the following

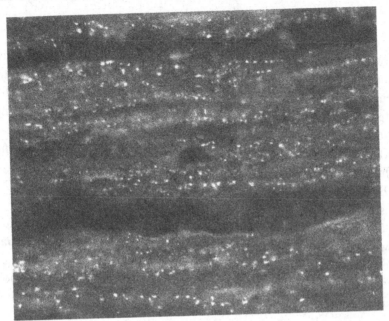

Fig. 14. Myometrial gap junctions in rat uterus during delivery as demonstrated with connexin 43 antibody staining and secondary antibody fluorescence. Each bright spot represents a gap junction as an aggregation of connexin proteins. × 925.

indirect studies indicate that myometrial cells are better coupled electrically during labour at term or pre-term when gap junctions are elevated:

(a) correlation of gap junctions, labour and electrical/contractile activity (Garfield *et al.*, 1988; Demianczuk, Towell & Garfield, 1984; Verhoeff *et al.*, 1985; Miller, Garfield & Daniel, 1989);

(b) increased space constant (Sims, Daniel & Garfield, 1982);

(c) decreased impedance (Sims *et al.*, 1982);

(d) increased propagation distance of spontaneous and evoked potentials (Miller *et al.*, 1989);

(e) increased conduction velocity (Miller *et al.*, 1989);

(f) increased synchrony of burst of action potentials (Miller *et al.*, 1989);

(g) decrease in input resistance (Blennerhassett & Garfield, 1991; Sakai, Blennerhassett & Garfield, 1992*a,b*; Sakai, Tabb & Garfield, 1992*c*);

(h) increased responsiveness to contractile agonists (Garfield & Beier, 1989; Chwalisz *et al.*, 1991).

Moreover, the above studies show that, when the junctions are decreased or closed, coupling is similarly reduced. These studies provide strong support for the proposal that gap junctions control electrical coupling between myometrial cells.

Metabolic coupling

We have also evaluated coupling by examining diffusion of radioactive and fluorescent dyes. Because the probes are considerably larger than electrolytes, measurement of diffusion between cells represents metabolic co-operation between cells. Our studies indicate that, when the gap junctions are elevated during term or pre-term labour, there are dramatic increases in:

(a) diffusion of deoxyglucose between myometrial cells (Cole, Garfield & Kirkaldy, 1985; Cole & Garfield, 1986);

(b) diffusion of Lucifer yellow and carboxyfluorescein (Blennerhassett & Garfield, 1991; Sakai et al., 1992a,b,c).

Also, studies of cultured myometrial cells show that, when gap junctions are present, fluorescent dyes can rapidly diffuse between cells (Sakai, Tabb & Garfield, 1992d); when the gap junctions are closed diffusion between cells is inhibited. We conclude that the myometrium is better coupled electrically and metabolically when the gap junctions are elevated, and that these contribute to the ability of the uterus to contract synchronously during labour.

Gap junctions as sites of hormonal control of labour

Hormones control the presence of gap junctions

Our studies and those of others (see Garfield et al., 1988) suggest that the changes in steroid hormones and prostaglandins that precede or accompany labour regulate the presence of the gap junctions. These studies describe how changes in hormone levels are translated into a structural change in the muscle.

The changes in the steroid hormones that occur before labour may activate the synthesis of the myometrial gap junctions through genomic mechanisms (Garfield et al., 1978, 1980). Evidence that progesterone suppresses the junctions is suggested from the following observations: (1) progesterone normally declines in rats and rabbits (Csapo, 1981) at term prior to the development of gap junctions and labour. If progesterone levels are maintained by injections of the hormone, animals do not develop junctions and they do not go into labour (Garfield et al., 1980, 1982; Garfield, 1987); (2) ovariectomy leads to premature progesterone withdrawal, appearance of junctions and labour. Progesterone treatment after ovariectomy prevents all three effects (Garfield et al., 1982); (3) progesterone will inhibit the oestrogen induced development of the junctions in non-pregnant animals (MacKenzie & Garfield, 1985); (4) antiprogesterone compounds induce pre-term development of the junctions and progesterone receptor agonists with high affinity will prevent this effect (Garfield et al., 1987); (5) progesterone will suppress gap junction development in vitro provided oestrogens are present

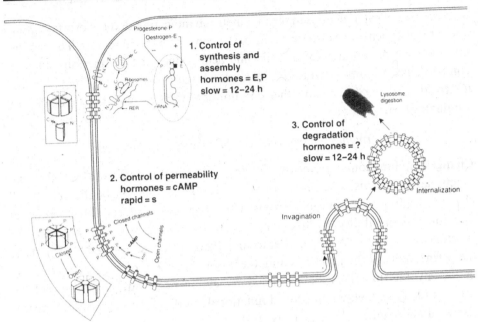

Fig. 15. Schematic illustration of two myometrial cells showing sites for the control of the synthesis, permeability, and degradation of the junctions. Oestrogen (E), progesterone (P), and possibly the prostaglandins regulate site 1. An increase in cAMP closes the junctions (site 2). Degradation of the junctions involves invagination, internalization, and digestion (site 3).

(Garfield *et al.*, 1980). The role of progesterone in inhibiting gap junction synthesis is shown in Fig. 15.

Oestrogens promote the synthesis of gap junctions in the myometrium and in other target tissues which possess steroid receptors (MacKenzie & Garfield, 1985). That oestrogens stimulate the formation of gap junctions is proven by the following observations: (1) oestrogens rise prior to labour (Csapo, 1981) and injections of oestrogens into pregnant animals stimulates the premature appearance of gap junctions and labour (MacKenzie & Garfield, 1985); (2) injections of oestrogens into immature, mature and ovariectomized rats induces gap junctions (MacKenzie & Garfield, 1985); (3) oestrogens promote gap junctions in tissues incubated *in vitro* (Garfield *et al.*, 1980); (4) anti-oestrogen compounds such as tamoxifen prevent the oestrogens from stimulating the increase in gap junctions (MacKenzie & Garfield, 1985); (5) mRNA extracted from oestrogen treated rats induces the formation of gap junctions in cells which normally lack gap junctions (Dahl, Azarnia & Serner, 1980). Oestrogens may stimulate the synthesis of gap junctions by interacting with its receptor and stimulating the gene for the gap junction protein (Fig. 15).

Prostaglandin synthesis inhibitors such as indomethacin and meclofenamate alter the area of gap junctions in the myometrium indicating that the prostaglandins and/or leukotrienes are also involved in the control of the junctions. The manner in which the metabolites of arachidonic acid influence the junctions must be complex since, in some conditions, prostaglandin inhibition reduces gap junctions (Garfield et al., 1980) and in other conditions (MacKenzie & Garfield, 1985) it stimulates their presence.

Hormones control the permeability of gap junctions

Changes in junctional permeability may occur with alterations in the gap junctional connexins, such as all-or-none closure or dilation of the cell-to-cell channel, leading to a state of decreased or enhanced coupling. Modulation of junctional permeability by hormones or neurotransmitters and a variety of substances has been described (Peracchia, 1980; Spray & Bennett, 1985). That the permeability of the junctions and, therefore, the extent of functional coupling in the myometrium may be regulated by endogenous mechanisms has been demonstrated (see below). Improved functional coupling should promote greater electrical and contractile synchrony in the uterine wall and enhance the rate of intra-uterine pressure development and more effective labour. Gap junction closure would be equivalent to the absence of gap junctions and reduce synchrony leading to ineffective labour and a prolongation of pregnancy.

We have used a 2-deoxyglucose (2DG) diffusion technique to study the influence of several agents on coupling in the myometrium of parturient rats (Cole et al., 1985; Cole & Garfield, 1986). Our studies suggests that the permeability of the junctions in the parturient myometrium is decreased by intracellular Ca^{2+}, pH and cAMP. Elevated cAMP produced by treatment with dibutyryl- or 8-bromo-cAMP reduced cell–cell diffusion in 2DG in the myometrium, and this can be mimicked by inhibiting phosphodiesterase activity with theophylline or by stimulating adenylate cyclase with forskolin. That cAMP may play a role in regulating functional coupling in the myometrium is significant in that relaxin, prostacyclin (PI_2) and B_2-adrenoceptor agonists appear to influence labour and parturition and exert inhibitory effects on the myometrium by elevating intracellular cAMP. Moreover, in experiments with porcine relaxin, carbacyclin (a stable PGI_2 analogue) and isoproterenol (a non-specific β-adrenoceptor agonist) the diffusivity of 2DG was found to be significantly lower in treated than in control tissues. We have also recently demonstrated myometrial uncoupling by cAMP by measuring electrical resistance (Sakai, Tabb & Garfield, 1992c, 1992d). These data indicate that there are specific receptor and secondary messenger-mediated physiological mechanisms for controlling cell–cell conduction in the myometrium independent of the systems controlling structural coupling (see Fig. 15).

A rise in cAMP in myometrial cells is well known to inhibit contractility (Kao, 1989). A cAMP-mediated uncoupling mechanism may be involved in maintaining pregnancy in instances of premature junction formation and/or in species such as the guinea pig, sheep and possibly human, in which low but significant numbers of gap junctions are present throughout pregnancy (see above). Perhaps the high levels of relaxin and prostacyclin observed in pre-term pregnant animals act to elevate intracellular cAMP and, alternatively, prevent synchronous activity in the myometrium. A decline in these hormones or their receptors, or antagonism of their action by oxytocin or stimulatory prostaglandins (e.g. PGF_2 or PGE_2), may facilitate a shift to patent gap junction channels and the development of syncytial behaviour.

There is evidence that phosphorylation of connexins controls gating of gap junction channels (see Saez *et al.*, 1993). cAMP-dependent protein kinases may regulate phosphorylation (Saez *et al.*, 1993). At present, there is no evidence for such a mechanism in myometrial cells but it is likely that the effects of cAMP in closing the junctions (see above) is mediated in such a manner. Western blots of Cx 43 in myometrial tissues (Fig. 13) show characteristic banding patterns typical of phosphorylated and unphosphorylated forms of the protein (Tabb *et al.*, 1992). The mechanisms regulating phosphorylation and conditions favouring phosphorylation need further study.

Transjunctional voltage can change the permeability of gap junctions. Connexins display characteristic sensitivities to transjunctional voltage that are symmetric about potentials of O mV, so that either hyperpolarization or depolarization of either coupled cell closes the junctions. There is voltage dependence for gating of connexin 43 in gap junctional channels of cardiac muscle cells (Wang *et al.*, 1992). The possibility that voltage changes in myometrial cells could control propagation offers another level of regulation of contractility. Perhaps myometrial gap junctions are all in the open state at a given membrane potential but then close at the highest point of depolarization to coordinate a burst of action potentials.

Control of the decline of gap junctions following parturition

Changes in the synthesis of gap junctions are important determinants in regulating the presence of the junctions in the myometrium. However, destruction or degradation of junctions may also play a role. Gap junctions decline rapidly following delivery. Immediately post-partum the signal for synthesis may be withdrawn (i.e. decrease in oestrogens and prostaglandins) and junction degradation may proceed by the formation of annular contacts followed by internalization and endocytosis (Garfield *et al.*, 1980; Fig. 15). It remains to be demonstrated what substances are involved in stimulating or inhibiting this process. Inhibition of the breakdown of gap junctions may have the same effect as stimulating their formation and a stimulation of degradation should have the opposite effects. This system needs to be further characterized; however, degradation is not easy to quantify with any method.

Gap junctions as sites for the coordination of action of agents which either stimulate or inhibit labour

Substances that stimulate or inhibit the myometrium can influence the muscle cells in ways that may or may not affect the gap junctions. However, stimulants and inhibitors do not normally work independently of the gap junctions and the propagation of action potentials. The influx and efflux of Ca^{2+} ions in the muscle cells during the passage of the action potentials, and the opening of voltage-dependent Ca^{2+} channels, are responsible for the increases and decreases in tension (electromechanical coupling, see above). This mechanism can be modified by endogenous or exogenous hormones, neurotransmitters, and other agonists and antagonists to either increase or decrease the excitability of the muscle. Additionally, pharmacomechanical coupling (i.e. the ability of endogenous substances to influence contractility) may account for the actions of some agents. However, pharmacomechanical coupling in the myometrium usually occurs only with electromechanical coupling and the propagation of action potentials because contraction of the myometrium is action potential dependent. Thus, the effects of excitatory and inhibitory agents are superimposed upon the driving force that is supplied by the presence and propagation of action potentials. Examples of the role of gap junctions in the action of stimulants and inhibitors are illustrated below.

Myometrial cells contain many systems that regulate the influx of Ca^{2+} and other ions (Kao, 1989). The systems involved in raising intracellular Ca^{2+} levels include (a) voltage or potential-dependent channels (see above); (b) passive influx; (c) receptor-operated channels, which may or may not be coupled to the generation of IP_3; and (d) release from sarcoplasmic reticulum (Fig. 16). The voltage-dependent channels are the primary source of activator Ca^{2+} ions. The propagation of action potentials from pacemaker regions is essential for activating these channels. Without intercellular coupling, either from the absence of gap junctions or their closure, action potentials would not propagate and the myometrium would not contract. Thus, the presence of gap junctions indirectly controls the availability of Ca^{2+}.

Contractile agonists can interact with the above systems to increase Ca^{2+} inside the muscle cells and effect contraction. The most common action might be through effects on receptor-operated channels or to release internal Ca^{2+}

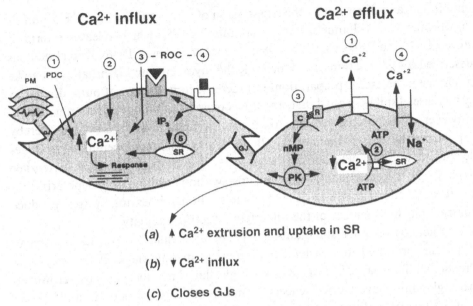

Ca²⁺ influx   Ca²⁺ efflux

(a) ▲ Ca²⁺ extrusion and uptake in SR

(b) ▼ Ca²⁺ influx

(c) Closes GJs

Fig. 16. Diagram to illustrate the relationship between gap junctions (GJs) and other systems. The influx and efflux pathways for Ca^{2+} ions are shown in two separate cells coupled together via gap junctions and to a pacemaker (PM). Although both pathways exist within every myometrial cell, they are illustrated separately to emphasize the importance of gap junctions. Shown are many different mechanisms for influencing the levels of internal Ca^{2+} ions to stimulate (e.g. potential-dependent channels [PDC], receptor-operated channels [ROC], IP_3 generation and release from sarcoplasmic reticulum [SR]) or to inhibit (e.g. receptor-R=C-mediated nucleotide-nMP [cAMP or cGMP] and protein kinase [PK] interaction, uptake into sarcoplasmic reticulum, extrusion from the cell by active and passive mechanisms and closure of gap junctions) myometrial contraction. The most important mechanism involved in phasic contraction is the opening of PDCs during the passage of an action potential. Gap junctions are involved in regulating both contraction and inhibition. The effects of agents that affect contractility may affect any of the pathways but generally their actions are superimposed upon the ability of action potentials to propagate between cells.

(pharmacomechanical coupling). However, the general effects of these agents are to increase the membrane potential or the ability of action potentials to propagate and thereby increase the excitability of the muscle cells. In this manner, action potentials propagate more easily between cells because the membrane potential is closer to its threshold. Contractile agonists do not, by themselves, drive the myometrium to contract. Their action is superimposed upon the driving force provided by propagated action potentials (Fig. 16).

An example of the effects of a contractile agonist is demonstrated by the action of oxytocin. Oxytocin binds to specific receptors to increase internal Ca^{2+} by (a) inhibiting Ca^{2+} extrusion by the suppression of Ca^{2+}-ATPase (the Ca^{2+} pump), (b) opening Ca^{2+} channels, and (c) stimulating IP_3, which releases internally stored Ca^{2+} ions (Fig. 16) (Kao, 1989; Riemer & Roberts, 1986). Kao (1989) has described a 4-fold action of oxytocin on the myometrium: (a) initiation of spike discharge in quiescent preparations, (b) increase in frequency of burst discharge, (c) increase of spikes in any burst, and (d) increase in amplitude of action potential. However, oxytocin's net action is to raise intracellular levels of Ca^{2+} and thereby depolarize the cells (Marshall, 1962) or it may facilitate opening of voltage-dependent ion channels during the process of excitation by action potentials (Kao, 1989). Increased action-potential propagation resulting from depolarization and its other effects are the basis of oxytocin's action. It does not, by itself, produce contractions independent of the underlying electrical activity.

The actions of other stimulants are probably similar to oxytocin. Marshall (1962) has proposed that carbachol depolarizes myometrial cells like oxytocin. Prostaglandins may also operate through the same mechanisms. However, prostaglandins have varied effects, some producing relaxation and others contraction. In addition, prostaglandins have immediate and delayed effects. Prostaglandins are involved in the formation of gap junctions. Therefore, the delayed contractile effects of prostaglandins could be mediated through the stimulation of gap junction synthesis (MacKenzie & Garfield, 1985), and their immediate contractile action may be similar to that of oxytocin.

Obviously gap junctions are also involved in relaxation of the myometrium. Ca^{2+} ions are the key to contraction-relaxation. The efflux of Ca^{2+} and lowering of intracellular Ca^{2+} to promote relaxation is regulated by several mechanisms. These include extrusion of Ca^{2+} by the Ca^{2+} pump, Na^+/Ca^{2+} exchange system, uptake of Ca^{2+} into the sarcoplasmic reticulum and steps involving cyclic nucleotides (Fig. 16). Many substances can indirectly affect these systems but like contractile agonists they do not function independently of gap junctions and the propagation of action potentials.

Lack of conducted action potentials and inactivity of the myometrium are promoted by decreases in (1) pacemaker activity, (2) excitability of the muscle cells and (3) cell-to-cell coupling. Any agent that suppresses the generation of action potentials, closes gap junctions or decreases their number inhibits the electrical events and thereby reduces contractility. These contractile antagonists may act to prevent activity not by causing relaxation of the myometrium but by inhibition of the propagation of action potentials. Generally, β-noradrenergic agonists act by increasing cAMP and stimulate Ca^{2+} efflux and K^+ conductance resulting in a hyperpolarization of the myometrium and thus take the resting membrane potential further from the threshold for excitation. Their net action is thus to inhibit the ability of action potential propagation throughout the tissue.

However, the most important action of β-agonists and similar substances which increase cAMP levels is probably to close myometrial gap junctions and thus prevent propagation rather than to change the membrane potential or the efflux of Ca^{2+}. These agents therefore promote inactivity of the myometrium rather than causing direct relaxation. Furthermore, β-agonists at low concentrations cause a cessation of spike activity without hyperpolarization (Kao, 1989). Thus, the primary mechanism of action of β-agonists may be to decrease junctional permeability. Since the action of agonists and antagonists, either inhibitory (hyperpolarizing the myometrium) or stimulatory (depolarizing the muscle), are dependent upon the status of gap junctions, the presence of the junctions and their functional state will dramatically influence the contractile patterns the agent produces.

Summary of gap junction studies

We have attempted to review the evidence that gap junctions play an essential role in the gradual evolution of uterine contractility during labour. Our studies suggest that the synthesis, permeability and degradation of myometrial junctions are physiologically regulated by hormones (Fig. 15). Thus, there are several targets for the control of the junctions and the possible management of term or pre-term labour.

Nitric oxide inhibition of myometrial contractility

Nitric oxide is an important and ubiquitous effector molecule that plays a significant role in the regulation of various physiological processes. It is involved in relaxation of various smooth muscles including vascular (Furchgott & Vanhoutte, 1989; Ignarro & Kadowitz, 1985; Moncado, Palmer & Higgs, 1991), intestinal (Sanders & Ward, 1992), tracheal (Li & Rand, 1991) and corpus cavernosus (Pickard, Powell & Zar, 1991). However, there are no studies that indicate oxide might regulate uterine contractility except that nitroglycerin and sodium nitroprusside have been shown to inhibit contractions (Diamond, 1983) and it is now recognized that these two compounds are nitric oxide donors.

We have examined the possibility that nitric oxide might be one of the factors that mediate uterine relaxation during pregnancy (Yallampalli *et al.*, 1993, 1994*a,b*; Izumi *et al.*, 1993). We tested the effects of L-arginine, the substrate for nitric oxide, on uterine contractility of strips of tissues from pregnant rats *in vitro*. L-Arginine caused a rapid and substantial relaxation of spontaneous activity of the uterine strips from rats at mid- to near-term gestation (Fig. 17). The relaxation effects were reversed by L-nitro-arginine methyl ester (L-NAME), an inhibitor of

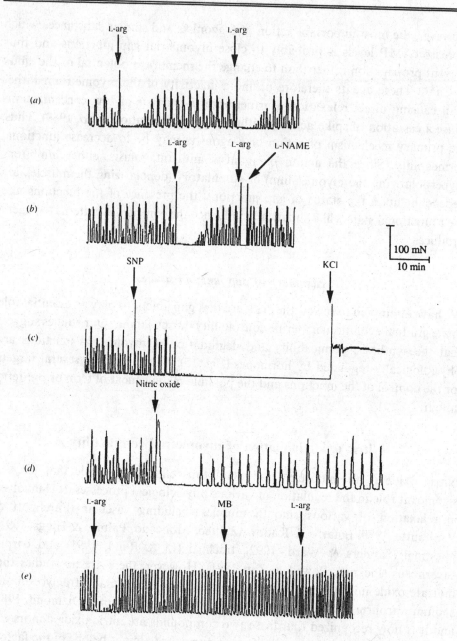

Fig. 17. The effects of L-arginine, L-NAME, sodium nitroprusside, nitric oxide, and methylene blue on spontaneously contracting uterine strips from rat uterus obtained on day 18 of pregnancy. Application of L-arginine to a muscle bath caused immediate relaxation (10–15 min duration) (*a*). The effect of L-arginine was antagonized by L-NAME when added during an L-arginine-induced relaxation (*b*). Effects of sodium nitroprusside (*c*) and nitric oxide (*d*). Inhibition of L-arginine effects with methylene blue (*e*). These are typical recordings and each upstroke from baseline represents a contraction.

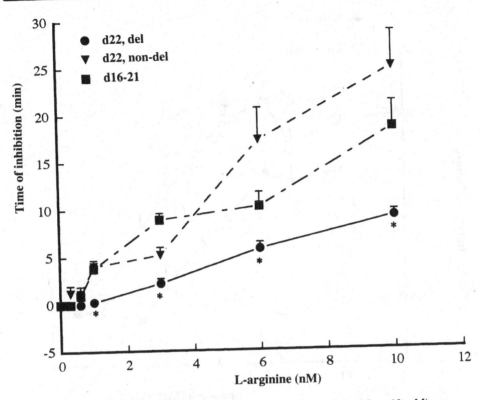

Fig. 18. Dose-dependent relaxation effects of L-arginine (0.1 mM to 10 mM) on spontaneously contracting uterine strips from rats at days 16–21 of gestation and on day 22 with and without delivery. The duration of inhibition of spontaneous uterine contractions is dose dependent. The effects of L-arginine from concentrations of 1 mM are significantly ($P < 0.01$) decreased during spontaneous delivery compared to days 16–21. Each data point represent mean ±S.E.M. The total number of strips studied at each time period was 8–16 from 4–6 animals per group.

nitric oxide synthase (Fig. 17). Sodium nitroprusside, a nitric oxide donor, completely abolished spontaneous contraction (Fig. 17). Nitric oxide gas, when added to the muscle bath, produced significant relaxation of spontaneous activity. Methylene blue, an inhibitor of guanylate cyclase, also prevented the inhibitory effects of L-arginine. These results strongly support the existence of an L-arginine–nitric oxide–cGMP system for regulating uterine relaxation.

However, the effects of L-arginine and nitric oxide on tissues from delivering animals were substantially decreased. Fig. 18 shows responses (dose of L-arginine–nitric oxide system versus duration of inhibition) to L-arginine of tissues during pregnancy and delivery. The inhibitory action of L-arginine was considerably lower during delivery; nitric oxide may contribute to the maintenance of uterine quiescence during pregnancy but not during delivery.

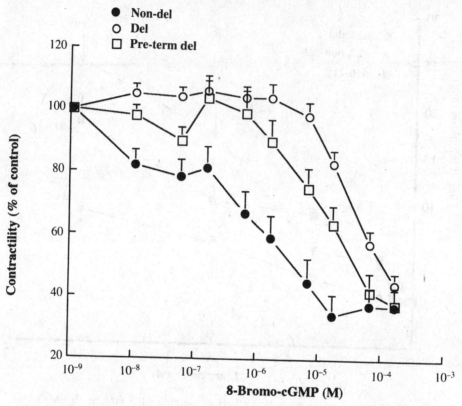

Fig. 19. Effect of 8-bromo-cGMP on uterine strips from rats at day 18 of pregnancy (closed circles), day 18 pregnancy during pre-term birth following antiprogesterone treatment (ZK299, Schering) (open squares), and during spontaneous birth at term (open circles). Note that, during both term and pre-term labour, the dose–response relationship to cGMP is shifted to a less sensitive state.

Because the effects of L-arginine and nitric oxide were decreased at term delivery compared to pre-term we reasoned that the generation of cGMP might be lower during delivery, that guanylate cyclase produces less cGMP during delivery or that cGMP is less effective during delivery. When we tested the ability of 8-bromo cGMP to inhibit uterine contractions, we found that during delivery, at term or pre-term the responses were greatly attenuated versus pre-term non-delivery (Fig. 19). This data clearly indicate that the ability of cGMP to produce relaxation is greatly reduced during term delivery. The fact that an antiprogesterone (ZK299, Schering) produced similar changes to those at term shows that the decrease in sensitivity of cGMP may be controlled by progesterone (Fig. 19). Other substances which inhibit uterine contractility may also act through cGMP and be expected to decline during labour.

If nitric oxide is necessary for maintenance of the uterus in the quiescent state

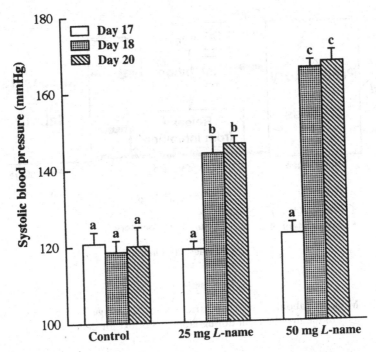

Fig. 20. Effect of L-nitro-arginine methylester (L-NAME) on systolic blood pressure of pregnant rats. Blood pressure was measured on day 17, before the osmotic minipumps were subcutaneously implanted, day 18 and day 22 of gestation. Animals received 25 or 50 mg L-NAME per day in saline or saline only (control). Each bar represents mean ±SEM for 8–10 rats per group. Bars with different letters at the top differ significantly ($P < 0.01$).

during pregnancy, then manipulations of the nitric oxide–cGMP system might alter gestational length. We treated pregnant rats at day 17 through to term with L-NAME and nitroglycerin. To our surprise, neither compound altered the timing of parturition: all animals delivered spontaneously at term. However, all L-NAME treated animals developed severe hypertension (Fig. 20) and classic features of pre-eclampsia (Yallampalli & Garfield, 1993) including growth retardation and proteinuria. These studies suggest that nitric oxide is involved in the generation of pre-eclampsia; treatment with nitric oxide donors might alleviate the symptoms.

The observation that nitric oxide synthase inhibitors and donors did not initiate early labour or prevented term labour suggests that nitric oxide may not be essential for the maintenance of pregnancy. However, nitric oxide may play a significant role in uterine quiescence, and nitric oxide donors might be effective in suppressing uterine contractility. Nitric oxide may inhibit uterine contractility prior to conversion of the myometrium to an active muscle to produce labour

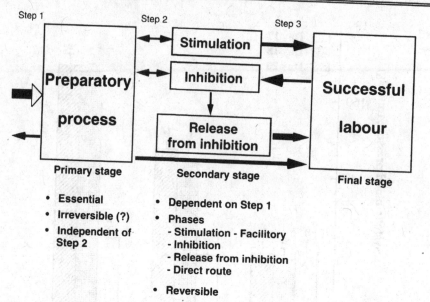

Fig. 21. Model of labour. Shown are various steps and stages in the conversion of the myometrium during labour. See text for details.

contractions (Fig. 21). Labour occurs when the muscle is activated by changes in steroid hormones and the addition of gap junctions for electrical coordination.

Nitric oxide donors may be ineffective in preventing labour because they act at a step prior to conversion to the active stage and because of a decrease in the cGMP relaxation system (Fig. 21). On the other hand, nitric oxide synthase inhibitors may increase spontaneous contractions but not initiate labour because they too act prior to the conversion step. Nitric oxide would not be expected to inhibit labour because there is a decrease in the responsiveness of the cGMP effector system.

Control of labour

Initiation of labour

The initiation or onset of labour occurs when an inactive and quiescent uterus is transformed to an active state which responds to stimulation. Theories of events which initiate labour include:

1. progesterone withdrawal (Csapo, 1961);
2. changes in oestrogen/progesterone ratios (Bedford *et al.*, 1972);
3. increase in oxytocin receptors (Soloff, Alexandrova & Fernstrom, 1979);
4. increase in prostaglandins (see Thorburn & Challis, 1979);
5. fetal stimulus (Liggins, 1967);

6. decrease in innervation (Thorbert, 1979);
7. increase in gap junctions (Garfield, Sims & Daniel, 1977; see above).
8. Withdrawal of inhibition by nitric oxide (Yallampalli *et al.*, 1993, 1994*a,b*)

The theories are not mutually exclusive. Most theories consider changes in the uterine content of steroid hormones as a common event. For example, oxytocin might initiate labour following an increase in receptors controlled by oestrogens and progesterone (Soloff *et al.*, 1979). Prostaglandins also lead to luteolysis and decreases in progesterone but some prostaglandins have direct stimulatory effects on the myometrium. Increased prostaglandin synthesis precedes labour and may be stimulated by oestrogens and inhibited by progesterone (Thorburn & Challis, 1979). The theory that gap junctions regulate the onset of labour includes control by progesterone and oestrogens. None of the theories, except that involving the gap junctions, accounts for conversion of the muscle to contract in the synchronous and forceful manner required for labour.

The initiation of labour might be the first step leading to labour or it might be construed as the final common event that activated the muscle. Several pathways may lead to labour (Liggins, 1979), and no pathway has been shown to be necessary and sufficient for labour in all species. However, the presence of gap junctions has been shown to be necessary for labour in all species. The final common pathway must be regarded as the step which initiates labour contractions. The theory that the presence of gap junctions initiates labour consolidates all theories and accounts for the activation of the muscle as the final common event in the onset of labour. It incorporates some aspects of other theories into a unified concept of how the myometrium contracts as a syncytium during labour to produce forceful contractions. Thus, in most species, changes in oestrogens and progesterones lead to the formation of junctions. In humans, the control of the junctions is unknown but they appear during labour (Garfield & Hayashi, 1981; Sakai *et al.*, 1992*c*). Once the junctions appear, the uterus is able to respond to oxytocin, prostaglandins and other stimulants. The gap junction theory, therefore, demonstrates how hormones convert the uterus into an active organ. Antiprogesterones also effectively increase gap junctions and induce labour in all animals tested including guinea-pigs, which like humans fail to demonstrate an obvious control by progesterone at term or to increased responsiveness to oxytocin (Chwalisz *et al.*, 1991). Therefore, it is possible that progesterone controls the onset of the appearance of gap junctions in all species. The mechanism of the regulation by progesterone remains obscure in humans.

Model for control of labour

All previous models of events which initiate or control labour neither define obligatory steps nor do they adequately explain the role of contractile agonists

---

Preparatory process – Genomic mechanisms
(↑↓ **Protein synthesis**)

↑ Properties favour contractions*   * ↑ Gap junctions

   • Phasic*   ↑ Ion channels

   • Forceful*   ↑ (Ca^{2+}, Na^+, K^+)

   • Coordinated*   ↑ Ion pumps

   • Frequent*   ↑↓ Transduction mechanism

↑ Properties foster stimulation*   (cAMP, cGMP, IP_3)

↓ Properties support inhibition*   ↑ Stimulation receptors
                                    (Oxytocin, alpha,
                                    endothelin, PG_s)

                                ↓ Inhibitory receptors
                                  ($ß_2$, PG_s)

Fig. 22. Genomic events involved in the preparatory process during conversion of myometrial activity and initiation of labour. Note that an increase in myometrial gap junctions (*) produces conditions which favour contraction and stimulation, and decreases properties which support inhibition.

or inhibitors. No model describes reversibility which is important in treatment of labour problems. Labour is not simply the transition from inactive muscle to an active muscle by the addition of a contractile stimulant or the withdrawal of an inhibitor. Rather, successful labour is achieved through a series of stages, with some possibly irreversible steps.

Csapo (1981) suggested that the uterus goes through a conversion process leading to an active organ. Similarly, investigations with antiprogesterones by Elger *et al.* (1990) have indicated that the uterus goes through a conditioning step prior to labour. Our work with gap junctions and nitric oxide (see above) demonstrates that the conditioning step outlined by Csapo and Elger is an essential preparatory process, possibly irreversible and independent of other stages (Fig. 21). The preparatory process is followed by others which depend upon the preparation but are reversible.

We propose that the preparatory process is controlled by genomic mechanisms and involves the increase or decrease of specific proteins that control the force and frequency of phasic contractions of labour and receptors for stimulation or inhibition (Fig. 22). The changes in proteins that are part of the preparatory process consists of an increase in gap junctions and channels (Mironneau, 1990), ion pumps (Khan *et al.*, 1992), systems for myofilament interaction, IP_3

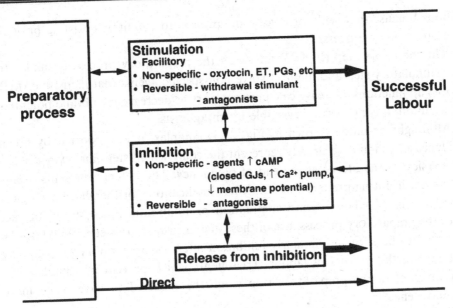

Fig. 23. Secondary stages controlling steps between preparatory process and successful labour. See text for details.

transduction mechanisms (Harbon *et al.*, 1990), and receptors for oxytocin (Soloff *et al.*, 1979; Garfield & Beier, 1989), stimulatory prostaglandins and alpha receptors for noradrenaline (Kawarabayashi & Osa, 1976). A decrease in proteins which favour relaxation include the cGMP effector system (see above) and a decline in inhibitory receptors.

The preparatory process is achieved (Step 1, Fig. 21) in most animals with the withdrawal of progesterone and the rise in oestrogens which accompanies or precedes the induction of new proteins or the decrease in others. This process is stimulated by oestrogens or increases in oestrogen/progesterone ratios. However, there may be several pathways that lead to the preparatory process in humans or other animals. In humans, the preparatory process may occur more slowly and involve stretch, prostaglandins, IL-1, oxytocin, fetal ischaemia, steroid hormones and other substances.

Once the preparatory process is complete successful labour may proceed without any additional assistance or any other inhibitory phase (the direct route, Step 2, Fig. 21). However, at this point (stimulatory stage) oxytocin and other agonists (prostaglandins, endothelins, etc.) stimulate contractility to accelerate labour (Fig. 23). Thus, these agents may be facilitatory rather than essential. The process is non-specific and can be achieved through the use of almost any agonist. This step is also reversible by the application of antagonists or the withdrawal of the stimulant. But antagonists or withdrawal of stimulants will not prevent labour because they will not reverse the process to conditions existing prior to the preparatory process.

The inhibitory step (Fig. 23) following the preparatory process is similar to the stimulatory step and might involve non-specific agents that increase cAMP, close gap junctions, increase calcium transport or decrease membrane potential. In addition, this process is reversible by antagonists.

Although the model shown in Fig. 21 is complex, it is supported by much evidence and should accurately represent the complicated steps and stages of the conversion of the uterus at the end of pregnancy. The model represents events which occur during pre-term labour. It has implications for the pharmacological management of labour, either stimulation or inhibition. Since stimulants act after the preparatory process, use of these agents prior to this step would not be expected to be effective. Similarly inhibition after the preparatory process may not reverse the process of labour. Treatments which prevent or stimulate the development of the preparatory step would be expected to have much more dramatic effects.

References

Abe, Y. (1967). Cable properties of smooth muscle. *Journal of Physiology London*, 1968.

Bedford, C. A., Challis, J. R. G., Harrison, F. Q. & Heap, R. B. (1972). The role of oestrogens and progesterone in the onset of parturition in various species. *Journal of Reproduction and Fertility*, **16**, 1.

Bergman, R. A. (1968). Uterine smooth muscle fibers in castrate and oestrogen treated rats. *Journal of Cell Biology*, **36**, 639–48.

Beyer, E. C., Kistler, J., Paul, D. L. & Goodenough, D. A. (1989). Antisera directed against connexin 43 peptides react with a 43-kD protein localized to gap junctions in myocardium and other tissues. *Journal of Cell Biology*, **108**, 595.

Blennerhassett, M. G. & Garfield, R. E. (1991). Effect of gap junction number and permeability on intercellular coupling in rat myometrium. *American Journal of Physiology*, **261** (Cell Physiology) C1001.

Bozler, E. (1938). Electrical stimulation and conduction of excitation in smooth muscle. *American Journal of Physiology*, **122**, 616–23.

Bozler, E. (1941). Influence of estrone on the electric characteristics and motility of uterine muscle. *Endocrinology*, **29**, 225–7.

Broderick, R. & Broderick, K. A. (1990). Ultrastructure and calcium stores in the myometrium. In *Uterine Function Molecular and Cellular Aspects*. Ed. M. E. Carsten and J.D. Miller, pp. 1–33, Plenum Press, New York.

Carsten, M. E. (1968). Regulation of myometrial composition, growth and activity. In *Biology of Gestation Vol. 1. The Maternal Organism*. Ed. N. S. Asssli, pp. 355–425, Academic Press, NY.

Chwalisz, K., Fahrenholz, F., Hackenberg, M., Garfield, R. E. & Elger, W. (1991). The progesterone antagonist onaprostone increases the effectiveness of oxytocin to produce delivery without changing the myometrial oxytocin receptor concentrations. *American Journal of Obstetrics and Gyneocology*, **165**, 1760.

Cole, W. C., Garfield, R. E. & Kirkaldy, J. S. (1985). Gap junctions and direct intercellular communication between rat uterine smooth muscle cells. *American Journal of Physiology*, **249**, C20.

Cole, W. C. & Garfield, R. E. (1986). Evidence for physiological regulation of gap junction permeability. *American Journal of Physiology*, **251**, C411.

Csapo, A. I. (1961). Defense mechanism of pregnancy. In *Progesterone and the Defense Mechanism of Pregnancy*. Ciba Foundation Study Group No. 9. Ed. G. E. W. Wolstenholme and M. P. Cameron, Churchill, London.

Csapo, A. I. (1962). Smooth muscle as a contractile unit. *Physiology Review*, **5**, 7–33.

Csapo, A. I. (1981). Force of labour. In *Principles and Practice of Obstetrics and Perinatology*. Ed. L. Iffy and H. A. Kamientzky, pp. 761–99, John Wiley and Sons, NY.

Dahl, G., Azarnia, R. & Werner, R. (1980). *De novo* construction of cell-to-cell channels. *In Vitro*, **16**, 1068.

Demianczuk, N., Towell, M. E. & Garfield, R. E. (1984). Myometrial electrophysiological activity and gap junctions in the pregnant rabbit. *American Journal of Obstetrics and Gynecology*, **149**, 485.

Diamond, J. (1983). Lack of correlation between cyclic GMP elevation and relaxation of nonvascular smooth muscle by nitroglycerin, nitroprusside, hydroxylamine and sodium azide. *Journal of Pharmacological Experimental Therapy*, **225**, 422.

Edman, K. A. P. & Schild, H. O. (1962). The need for calcium in the contractile responses induced by acetylcholine and potassium in the rat uterus. *Journal of Physiology*, **161**, 424.

Elger, W., Chwalisz, K., Fahnrich, M. *et al.* (1990). Studies on labor conditioning and labor inducing effects of antiprogesterones in animal models. In *Uterine Contractility: Mechanisms of Control*. Ed. R. E. Garfield, pp. 153–76, Serono Symposium, USA.

Finn, C. A. & Porter, D. G. (1975). *The Uterus*. Elek Science, London.

Furchgott, R. F. & Vanhoutte, P. M. (1989). Endothelium derived relaxing and contracting factor. *FASEB Journal*, **3**, 2007.

Gabella, G. (1981). Structure of smooth muscle. In *Smooth Muscle: An Assessment of Current Knowledge*, ed. E. Bulbring, A. F. Brading, A. W. Jones & T. Tomita, pp. 1–46, Edward Arnold, London.

Garfield, R. E. (1984). Myometrial ultrastructure and uterine contractility. Uterine Contractility. Ed S. Bottari, J. P. Thomas, A. Vokaer, R. Vokaer, pp. 81–109, Mason, New York.

Garfield, R. E., Sims, S. & Daniel, E. E. (1977). Gap junctions: their presence and necessity in myometrium during gestation. *Science NY*, **198**, 958.

Garfield, R. E., Sims, S. M., Kannan, M. S. & Daniel, E. E. (1978). Possible role of gap junctions in activation of myometrium during parturition. *American Journal of Physiology*, **235**, C168.

Garfield, R. E., Rabideau, S., Challis, J. R. G. & Daniel, E. E. (1979). Hormonal control of gap junction formation in sheep myometrium during parturition. *Biology of Reproduction*, **21**, 999.

Garfield, R. E., Kannan, M. S. & Daniel, E. E. (1980). Gap junction formation in myometrium: control by estrogens, progesterone and prostaglandins. *American Journal of Physiology*, **238**, C81 (*Cell Physiology* **7**).

Garfield, R. E., Merrett, D. & Grover, A. K. (1980). Gap junction formation and regulation in myometrium. *American Journal of Physiology*, **239**, C217 (*Cell Physiology* 8).

Garfield, R. E. & Hayashi, R. H. (1981). Appearance of gap junctions in the myometrium of women during labor. *American Journal of Obstetrics and Gynecology*, **140**, 254.

Garfield, R. E., Puri, C. P. & Csapo, A. I. (1972). Endocrine structural and functional changes in the uterus during premature labor. *American Journal of Obstetrics and Gynecology*, **142**, 21.

Garfield, R. E., Daniel, E. E., Dukes, M. & Fitzgerald, J. D. (1982). Changes in gap junctions in myometrium of guinea pig at parturition and abortion. *Canadian Journal of Physiology and Pharmacology*, **60**, 335–41.

Garfield, R. E. & Somlyo, A. P. (1985). Structure of smooth muscle. In *Calcium and Contractility*. Ed. A. K. Grover and E. E. Daniel, pp. 1–36, The Human Press.

Garfield, R. E., Gasc, J. M. & Baulieu, E. E. (1987). Effects of the antiprogesterone RU 486 on preterm birth in the rat. *American Journal of Obstetrics and Gynecology*, **157**, 1281.

Garfield, R. E., Blennerhassett, M. G. & Miller, S. M. (1988). Control of myometrial contractility: role and regulation of gap junctions. *Oxford Review in Reproductive Biology*, **10**, 436.

Garfield, R. E. & Beier, S. (1989). Increased myometrial responsiveness to oxytocin during term and preterm labor. *American Journal of Obstetrics and Gynecology*, **161**, 454.

Garfield, R. E. & Hertzgerg, E. L. (1990). Cell-to-cell coupling in the myometrium: Emil Bozler's prediction. In *Frontiers in Smooth Muscle Research*. Ed. N. Sperelakis and J. D. Wood, p. 673, Wiley-Liss, New York.

Grover, A. K. (1986). Role of cellular membranes in calcium-mobilization of uterine smooth muscle. In *The Physiology and Biochemistry of the Uterus in Pregnancy and Labor*. Ed. G. Huszar, pp. 93–107, CRC Press.

Grover, A. K., Kwan, C. Y., Crankshaw, J., Crankshaw, D. J., Garfield, R. E. & Daniel, E. E. (1980). Characteristics of calcium transport and binding by rat myometrium plasma membrane subfractions. *American Journal of Physiology*, **239**, C66–C74.

Harbon, S. *et al.* (1990). Multiple regulation of the generation of inositol phosphates and cAMP in myometrium. In *Serono Symoposia, Uterine Contractility*. Ed. R. E. Garfield, pp. 123.

Hendrix, M. E., Lomneth, C. S., Wilfinger, W. W., Hertzberg, E. L., Mao, S. J. T., Chen, L. & Larsen, W. J. (1992). Quantitative immunoassay of total cellular gap junction protein connexin32 during liver regeneration using antibodies specific to the COOH-terminus. *Tissue and Cell*, **24**, 61–73.

Ignarro, L. J. & Kadowitz, P. J. (1985). The pharmacological and physiological role of cyclic GMP in vascular smooth muscle relaxation. *Annual Review of Pharmacology and Toxicology*, **25**, 171.

Izumi, H., Ichihara, J., Uchiumi, Y. & Shirakawa, K. (1990). Gestational changes in mechanical properties of skinned muscle tissues of human myometrium. *American Journal of Obstetrics and Gynecology*, **163**, 638.

Izumi, H., Yallampalli, C. & Garfield, R. E. (1993). Gestational changes in Larginine induced relaxation of pregnant rat and human myometrial smooth muscle. *American Journal of Obstetrics and Gynecology*, **169**, 1327–37.

Kanter, H. L., Safitz, J. & Beyer, E. C. (1992). Cardiac myocytes express multiple gap junction proteins. *Circulation Research*, **70**, 438–44.

Kao, C. V. (1977). Electrophysiological properties of the uterine smooth muscle. In *Biology of the Uterus*. Ed. R. M. Wynn, pp. 423–84, Plenum Press, New York.

Kao, C. Y. (1989). Electrophysiological properties of uterine smooth muscle. In *Biology of the Uterus*. 2nd edn. Eds R. M. Wynn and W. P. Jollie, p. 403, Plenum Press, New York.

Kawarabayashi, T. & Osa, T. (1976). Comparative investigations of alpha- and beta-effects on the longitudinal and circular muscles of the pregnant rat myometrium. *Japan Journal of Physiology*, **26**, 403.

Khan, I., Tabb, T., Garfield, R. E. & Grover, A. K. (1992). Ca pump messenger RNA expression in pregnant rat uterus. *Biochemistry International*, **27**, 189–96.

Kuriyama, H. (1961). Recent studies on the electrophysiology of the uterus. *Progesterone and the Defence Mechanism of Pregnancy*. pp. 51–70, Ciba Foundation Study Group. Boston Little.

Li, C. C. & Rand, M. J. (1991). Evidence that part of the NANC relaxant response of guinea-pig trachea to electrical field stimulation is mediated by nitric oxide. *British Journal of Pharmacology*, **102**, 91.

Liggins, G. C., Kennedy, P. C. & Holm, L. W. (1967). Failure of initiation of parturition after electro-coagulation of the pituitary of the fetal lamb. *American Journal of Obstetrics and Gynecology*, **98**, 1080.

Liggins, G. C. (1979). Initiation of parturition. *British Medical Bulletin*, **35**, 145.

Lodge, S. & Sproat, J. E. (1981). Resting membrane potentials of pacemaker and nonpacemaker areas in rat uterus. *Life Science*, **28**, 2251.

MacKenzie, L. W. & Garfield, R. E. (1985). Hormonal control of gap junctions in the myometrium. *American Journal of Physiology*, **248**, C296–308.

Marshall, J. M. (1962). Regulation of activity in uterine smooth muscle. *Physiology Reviews*, **42**, 213.

Matlib, M. A., Crankshaw, J., Garfield, R. E., Crankshaw, D. J., Kwan, C. Y., Branda, L. & Daniel, E. E. (1979). Characterization of membrane fractions and isolation of plasma membrane from rat myometrium. *Journal Biological Chemistry*, **254**, 1834–40.

Miller, S. M., Garfield, R. E. & Daniel, E. E. (1989). Improved propagation in myometrium associated with gap junctions during parturition. *American Journal of Physiology*, **256**, C130 (*Cell Physiology* **25**).

Mironneau, J. (1990). Electrical signals and uterine contractility: ion channels and excitation–contraction coupling in myometrium. *Serono Symposia, Uterine Contractility*. Ed. R. E. Garfield, p. 9.

Moncada, S., Palmer, R. M. G. & Higgs, E. A. (1991). Nitric oxide: physiology, pathophysiology and pharmacology. *Pharmacological Reviews*, **43**, 109.

Osa, T. & Katase, T. (1975). Physiological comparison of the longitudinal and circular muscles of the pregnant rat uterus. *Japan Journal of Physiology*, **25**, 153–64.

Peracchia, C. (1980). Structural correlates of gap junction permeation. *International Review of Cytology*, **66**, 81.

Pickard, R. S., Powell, P. H. & Zar, M. A. (1991). The effect of inhibitors of nitric oxide biosynthesis and cyclic GMP formation on nerve-evoked relaxation of human covernosal smooth muscle. *British Journal of Pharmacology*, **104**, 55.

Puri, C. P. & Garfield, R. E. (1982). Changes in hormone levels and gap junctions in the rat uterus during pregnancy and parturition. *Biology of Reproduction*, **27**, 967.

Reynolds, S. R. M. (1949). *Physiology of the Uterus*, 2nd edn. P.B. Hoeber Inc., NY.

Riemer, R. K. & Roberts, J. M. (1986). Endocrine modulation of myometrial response. In *The Physiology and Biochemistry of the Uterus in Pregnancy and Labor*. Ed G. Huszar, p. 53, CRC Press, Boca Raton, FL.

Risek, B., Guthrie, S., Kumar, N. & Gilula, N. B. (1990). Modulation of gap junction transcript and protein expression during pregnancy in the rat. *Journal of Cell Biology*, **110**, 269.

Ross, R. & Klebanoff, S. J. (1967). Fine structural changes in uterine smooth muscle and fibroblasts in response to estrogen. *Journal of Cell Biology*, **32**, 155–67.

Saez, J. C., Berthoud, V. M., Moreno, A. P. & Spray, D. C. (1993). Gap junctions: multiplicity of controls in differentiated and undifferentiated cells and possible functional implications. *Advances in Second Messenger and Phosphoprotein Research*, **27**, 163–98.

Sakai, N., Blennerhassett, M. G. & Garfield, R. E. (1992a). Effects of antiprogesterones on myometrial cell-to-cell coupling in pregnant guinea pigs. *Biology of Reproduction*, **46**, 358.

Sakai, N., Blennerhassett, M. G. & Garfield, R. E. (1992b). Intracellular cyclic AMP concentration modulates gap junction permeability in parturient rat myometrium. *Canadian Journal of Physiology and Pharmacology*, **70**, 358.

Sakai, N., Tabb, T. & Garfield, R. E. (1992c). Modulation of cell-to-cell coupling between myometrial cells of the human uterus during pregnancy. *American Journal of Obstetrics and Gynecology*, **167**, 2, 472.

Sakai, N., Tabb, T. & Garfield, R. E. (1992d). Studies of connexin 43 and cell-to-cell coupling in cultured human myometrial cells. *American Journal of Obstetrics and Gynecology*, **167**, 5, 1267.

Sanders, K. M. & Ward, S. M. (1992). Nitric oxide as a mediator of nonadrenergic noncholinergic neurotransmission. *American Journal of Physiology*, **262**, G379.

Savineau, J. P., Mironneau, J. & Mironneay, C. (1988). Contractile properties of chemically skinned fibers from pregnant rat myometrium: existence of an internal Ca-store. *Pflügers Archives*, **411**, 296–303.

Sims, S. M., Daniel, E. E. & Garfield, R. E. (1982). Improved electrical coupling in uterine smooth muscle is associated with increased numbers of gap junctions at parturition. *Journal of General Physiology*, **80**, 353.

Singer, S. J. & Nicholson, G. L. (1972). The fluid mosaic model of the structure of cell membranes. *Science*, **175**, 720–31.

Somlyo, A. V. (1980). Ultrastructure of vascular smooth muscle. In *Handbook of Physiology. The Cardiovascular System*. Vol. 2, ed. D. F. Bohr, A. P. Somlyo & H. V. Sparks, American Physiological Society, Bethesda, MD. pp. 33–67.

Soloff, M. S., Alexandrova, M. & Fernstrom, M. J. (1979). Oxytocin receptors: triggers for parturition and lactation. *Science, NY*, **204**, 1313.

Spray, D. C. & Bennett, M. V. L. (1985). Physiology and pharmacology of gap junctions. *American Journal of Physiology*, **47**, 281.

Tabb, T., Thilander, G., Grover, A., Hertzberg, E. & Garfield, R. E. (1992). An immunochemical and immunocytologic study of the increase in myometrial gap junctions (and connexin 43) in rats and humans during pregnancy. *American Journal of Obstetrics and Gynecology*, **167**, 559–67.

Thorbert, G. (1979). Regional changes in structure and function of adrenergic nerves in guinea-pig uterus during pregnancy. *Acta Obstetrica et Gynecologica Scandinavica Suppl.* **79**. 5–32.

Thorburn, G. D. & Challis, J. R. G. (1979). Endocrine control of parturition. *Physiology Review*, **59**, 863–918.

Verhoeff, A., Garfield, R. E., Ramondt, J. & Wallenburg, H. (1985). Myometrial activity related to gap junction area in periparturient and ovariectomized, estrogen-treated sheep. *Acta Physiologica Hungarica*, **66**, 539.

Wang, H. Z., Li, J., Lemanski, L. F. & Veenstra, R. D. (1992). Gating of mammalian cardiac gap junction channels by transjunctional voltage. *Biophysics Journal*, **63**, 139.

Yallampalli, C. & Garfield, R. E. (1993). Inhibition of nitric oxide synthesis produces signs similar to preeclampsia. *American Journal of Obstetrics and Gynecology*, **169**, 1316–20.

Yallampalli, C., Garfield, R. E. & Byam-Smith, M. (1993). Nitric oxide inhibits uterine contractility during pregnancy but not during delivery. *Endocrinology*, **133**, 1899–902.

Yallampalli, C., Izumi, H., Byam-Smith, M. & Garfield, R. E. (1994a). An L-arginine: nitric oxide system exists in the uterus and inhibits contractility during pregnancy. *American Journal of Obstetrics and Gynecology*, **170**, 175–85.

Yallampalli, C., Byam-Smith, M., Nelson, S. O. & Garfield, R. E. (1994b). Steroid hormones modulate the production of nitric oxide and cGMP in the rat uterus. *Endocrinology*, **134**. 1971–4.

5

Cell biology of the endometrium: histology, cell types and menstrual changes

M. A. WARREN, T. C. LI AND L. D. KLENTZERIS

The uterus consists of three parts: 1. the perimetrium (or serosa), a mesothelium of simple squamous cells plus a thin layer of aereolar tissue, 2. the myometrium, consisting of three layers of smooth muscle cells and associated connective tissue fibres and matrix. It is the thickest layer measuring 10–15 mm (Robertson, 1984), 3. the endometrium, a complex layer which lies nearest to the uterine lumen and undergoes a series of cyclical changes in both structure and function in response to endocrinological events.

The most commonly cited description of the cyclic changes in the endometrium is that of Noyes, Hertig & Rock (1950). More recently, the cyclical changes in the histology of the endometrium have been correlated with the surge of luteinizing hormone (LH), which occurs about 16 hours before ovulation (designated by LH + 0). Using the LH peak as a reference point for dating histological specimens, rather than other reference points such as onset of next menstrual period or basal body temperature, gives an improvement in both accuracy and precision of dating (Li et al., 1987). These improvements are essential for the study of a tissue such as the endometrium which undergoes rapid, sequential changes. Dockery and Rogers (1989) enumerated a series of factors which can influence apparent variability in the assessment of endometrial structure. These included adequate dating of the specimen, definition of normality, sampling and methods of analysis. By accounting for such variability, the study of timed cellular events, which are the essence of normal endometrial function and successful pregnancy, is much enhanced (Johannisson et al., 1987; Dockery et al., 1988a).

The endometrium is made up of stroma (or lamina propria) which blends with the myometrium, a basal layer and a decidual layer (the functionalis). It contains epithelial, connective, vascular and lymphoid cells as well as connective tissue fibres and matrix.

Epithelial cells of the endometrium

It is convenient, for purposes of description, to separate glandular from luminal cells. Endometrial glands extend through the full depth of the endometrium (4–5 mm thick at its maximum), from the lumen of the uterus to the myometrium. The basal part of the glands lies in the basal layer, which is retained at menses, and is the source of the re-epithelialization which occurs after cessation of menstrual flow (Ferneczy, 1976). The basal cells change little throughout the cycle. It is generally believed that the rest of the gland (in the functionalis) is lost every month during the non-pregnant reproductive life of an individual. An alternative view suggests that most of the endometrium is conserved and re-epithelialization occurs only in regions of localized damage (Wilborn & Flowers, 1984).

Gland formation begins soon after menstruation ends, and in this early proliferative phase mitoses are common. Unlike tubular glands in the intestine, where mitoses are restricted to basal areas of gland, in the endometrium mitoses occur throughout the gland. Gland cell mitoses are less common in the post-ovulatory secretory phase. The term secretory may be something of a misnomer since it has been pointed out that the *volume* of endometrial glandular transudation and secretion increases during the proliferative phase and reaches a peak around the time of ovulation (Johannisson, 1985). It is likely that these events are hormonally directed; for example, in ovariectomized rats oestradiol causes increased uterine blood flow and capillary permeability, both of which are likely to increase secretory potential (Clark & Markeverich, 1981).

Fluid reduction in the uterine cavity begins after ovulation and may be the result of water resorption following sodium uptake across the endometrium. However, pinocytosis via irregular protrusions (pinopods) of endometrial cells is a factor in some species (Edwards, 1980). Fluid removal reduces the size of the uterine lumen, and thus apposes blastocyst and endometrium, thereby causing the first mechanical contact between blastocyst and endometrium (Johannisson, 1985). Just as the cells themselves vary, the volume, viscosity and concentration of uterine secretions change throughout the cycle (Beier, 1974). It is clear that these cells deserve detailed consideration.

Light microscopy

Endometrial glands are made up of tall columnar cells arranged as a simple epithelium (Fig. 1). They have large round or oval nuclei with their long axis oriented along that of the cell. Significant morphological changes are seen to correlate with the ovarian cycle. Glandular mitoses decrease from about 23 per 1000 cells on day LH−3 to about 7 per 1000 cells on day LH+3, after which

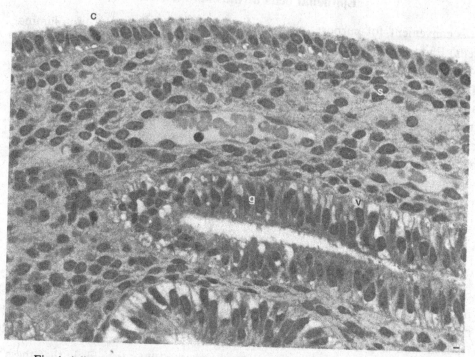

Fig. 1. A light micrograph of a JB4 resin-embedded section of early luteal phase
endometrium stained with acid Fuchsin and Toluidine Blue. Luminal epithelium
with cilia (c), stromal cells (s) and glandular epithelium (g) are present. Some
secretory vacuoles (v) are also visible. Scale bar = 4 μm.

it virtually ceases (Johannisson *et al.*, 1982). The diameter of glandular lumina
increases from about 50 μm on day LH + 0 to 100 μm on day LH + 8 and shows
a significant ($P < 0.01$) correlation with oestradiol levels (Johannisson, 1985).
Scanning electron microscopy shows changes consistent with these observations
(Hafez & Ludwig, 1977).

Although gland cell height and nuclear volume show little variation during
the early secretory phase the proportion of cell made up of nucleus is reduced
significantly (Johannisson, 1985; Dockery *et al.*, 1988a). This is largely due to the
rapid accumulation of secretory material in sub-nuclear vacuoles after ovulation.
On about day LH + 3, basal accumulation of secretory material causes the
nucleus, which is usually in a basal position, to be pushed upwards to the centre
of the cell. Since this happens at slightly different times in adjacent cells the nuclei
appear to be stratified (pseudo-stratification, Noyes *et al.*, 1950). The contents of
the basal vacuole are transported to the cell apex where they are released into
the lumen, at which time (day LH + 6) the nucleus returns to its basal position.

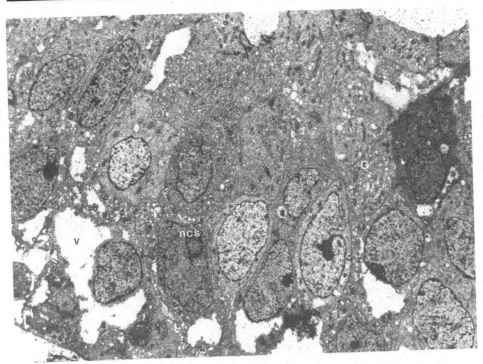

Fig. 2. Electron micrograph of glandular epithelium at day LH+6 showing secretory vacuolar spaces (v), Golgi apparatus (G) and a nuclear channel system (ncs). Scale bar = 0.6 μm.

Although glycogen is a major constituent of the secretion other components are present; for example the D9B1 epitope, which has been studied by Smith *et al.* (1989) using semi-quantitative immunohistochemical methods.

By light microscopy, the nucleus is seen to be relatively small and round in the early proliferative phase, large and oval mid-cycle, and contracted and irregular with inconspicuous nucleoli by the end of the cycle (Gordon, 1974; Cornillie, Lauweryns & Brosens, 1985). More detailed cellular changes may be observed at the electron microscopical level.

Electron microscopy

Glandular cells have all of the ultrastructural machinery that would be expected of a secretory cell. In addition they possess three features which are unique to endometrial glandular cells. These three structures ('giant' mitochondria, glycogen deposits and nuclear channel systems (ncs)) are collectively known as the triad and are seen only in the early secretory phase (Figs. 2 and 3).

Several descriptions of the ultrastructure of gland cells have been reported (e.g.

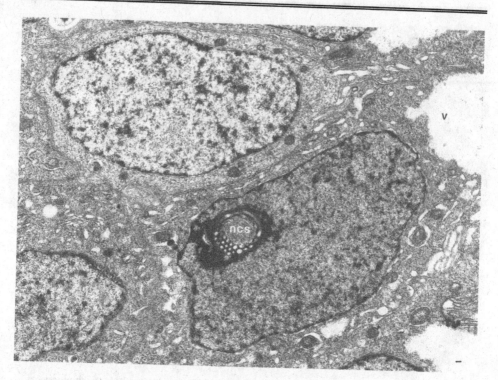

Fig. 3. Electron micrograph showing glandular cell nuclei at day LH+6. The curved tubular nuclear channel system is clearly visible (ncs). Secretory vacuolar spaces (v) are also seen. Scale bar = 200 nm.

Kohorn *et al.*, 1972; More *et al.*, 1974; Hafez & Ludwig, 1977; Cornillie *et al.*, 1985; Dockery *et al.*, 1988*b*; Dockery & Rogers, 1989), although that of Dockery & Rogers seems to be the most systematic having used carefully timed and sampled biopsies from a relatively large group of normal fertile volunteers. As may be expected of an epithelium actively involved in secretion and absorption, the apical surface has many microvilli. These are long and slender in the early proliferative phase and increase in height in relation to the rise in oestrogen levels (Cornillie *et al.*, 1985). Around the time of implantation, at least in the rat, microvilli become irregular and show fundamental changes in plasma membrane molecular dynamics which are essential for implantation (Murphy & Turner, 1991). By day LH+10 the microvilli have become blunted, possibly related to apocrine desquamation into the lumen (Armstrong *et al.*, 1973).

At the time of ovulation the nucleus is a large, euchromatic structure with the oval profile and prominent nucleolus typical of a cell actively involved in transcription (Fig. 2). The nuclear membrane is unremarkable, being made up of a double membrane each leaf of which is about 7 nm thick and of similar construction to the plasmalemma. The perinuclear space, the cavity between the double membrane, is about 20–40 nm wide and is continuous with the cavity in the endoplasmic reticulum.

By day LH +3, some cells contain a nuclear channel system (Fig. 3). This remarkable structure is apparently composed of a complex, possible double, tubular structure which is continuous with the inner nuclear membrane (Luginbuhl, 1968; More *et al.*, 1974). The lumen of the tubules is about 500–600 nm in diameter and is thought to be continuous with the perinuclear space (Terzakis, 1965). Nuclear channel systems have been reported variously to be spherical, ellipsoidal and hollow (Terzakis, 1965; More & McSeveney, 1980). Some nuclei have profiles of more than one ncs, but it is unclear whether this represents several ncs or one which is branched. Terzakis (1965) suggested that a ncs is a channel by which recently synthesized mRNA is passed rapidly from the nucleus to the cytoplasm.

Kohorn, Rice & Gordon (1970) have reported that the 17-β-position on the D-ring of progesterone is essential for ncs formation. Although progesterone is essential for their formation, ncs do not (at least *in vitro*) appear to be a requirement for secretion; their role may, however, be related to implantation (Luginbuhl, 1968). Since their regression is rarely seen by electron microscopy it is thought to be a very rapid process. The incidence of ncs in glandular cells declines from day LH+6. *In vivo* and *in vitro* exogenous oestrogen can cause dissolution of ncs in glandular epithelial cells (Gordon *et al.*, 1973; Dehou *et al.*, 1987).

The cytoplasm of glandular cells around the time of ovulation contains both free and bound ribosomes, mitochondria and Golgi apparatus. Apart from the presence of a few, apparently randomly situated areas of (presumed) glycogen deposits the cells are entirely as would be predicted for a synthetic cell. There is no obvious organelle polarity and the cells all look very similar (Dockery *et al.*, 1988*b*).

By day LH+3 the cells have become more variable in appearance, some cells being more advanced than others. Large areas of the basal cytoplasm appear as empty spaces. By using a cytochemical technique to identify carbohydrate macromolecules (glycogen and glycogen-rich material; Rambourg, Hernandez & LeBlond, 1969) Dockery *et al.* (1988*b*) have demonstrated that these apparently empty spaces contain glycogen. Lipid-like vacuoles are often found scattered within and around the glycogen.

At about this time, giant mitochrondria become prominent. Unlike normal-sized mitochondria, which are about 0.2 μm in diameter, long, thread-like and oriented to the long axis of the cell, giant mitochondria may be measured in micrometers. They are large, complex organelles with many branches and usually having tubular cristae (a feature seen in other tissues related to steroid hormones).

Giant mitochondria can often be seen in close proximity to coils of rough (or semi-rough) endoplasmic reticulum which envelop them (Cavazos *et al.*, 1967; Dockery *et al.*, 1988*b*). Serial sectioning and reconstruction of giant mitochondria has shown them to be localized swellings of the normal-sized variety thought to be the result of progesterone action on mitochondrial DNA (Coaker, Downie & More, 1982). Human chorionic gonadotrophin has been reported to further expand mitochrondria (Ancla, Belaisch & De Brux, 1969). By day LH + 10, giant mitochondria are rare and are thought to have involuted; mitochondrial profiles have been reported in autophagocytic granules (Armstrong *et al.*, 1973). The function of these organelles is unknown, but is likely to be related to the massive energy demands of the cells at this time and the steroid-directed synthesis of glycoprotein (More *et al.*, 1980; Dockery & Rogers, 1989).

Ribosome number increases throughout the proliferative phase in order to meet the requirement of cell synthesis. By day LH + 4, bound ribosomes are well developed and already in close proximity to mitochondria (Cavazos *et al.*, 1967). They continue to increase well into the secretory phase.

The Golgi apparatus is relatively poorly developed in the early proliferative phase, but increases markedly until it reaches maximum activity around day LH + 5 (just before the time when implantation would occur). Stacks of Golgi cisternae can be seen initially in the apical cytoplasm where, on day LH + 3, they lie parallel to the apical surface just above the nucleus (Wynn, 1977). Over the next few days they come to lie parallel to the long axis of the cell (Dockery & Rogers, 1989). Around day LH + 6 the Golgi cisternae become notably dilated, presumably an indication of increased activity (Fig. 2). The Golgi system decreases in size and activity towards menstruation, and the cisternae close (Verma, 1983).

These changes in the Golgi apparatus reflect the progression of secretions, such as the D9B1 epitope mentioned earlier (Smith *et al.*, 1989), from the basal to the apical parts of the cell where it is finally released across the apical plasmalemma into the gland lumen. It seems likely that the massive increase in smooth endoplasmic reticulum during the time of translocation of secretory material (maximal about day LH + 6) is the cellular mechanism responsible for its mobilization (Dockery *et al.*, 1988*b*). The relationship between D9B1 (a monoclonal antibody which binds to peptide-associated sialylated oligosaccharide) and the Golgi apparatus (where glycosylation occurs) remains unclear since Golgi have not been reported in basal locations (Smith *et al.*, 1989).

It is clear from the description above that substantial changes in the cell membrane occur during the early secretory phase. Large changes are also seen in the plasmalemma at this time, probably in consequence of the exo- and endocytosis occurring at the apical surface. Increasing complexity of the basal lateral cell membranes has also been reported at about the time when the secretions pass into the gland lumen (Davie, Hopwood & Levison, 1977; Cornillie *et al.*, 1985; Dockery *et al.*, 1988*b*). Functionally these changes may reflect membrane redistribution due to secretion and water absorption, involution and increased lateral cell adhesion, amongst others (Davie *et al.*, 1977; Cornillie *et al.*, 1985; Dockery *et al.*, 1988*b*). Increased epithelial–stromal interaction has been reported in the early secretory phase, evidenced by an increased density of gap junctions between epithelial cells and epithelial projections through the basement membrane (Roberts, Walker & Lavia, 1988).

It is likely that further study of the cellular processes of gland formation and cell behaviour will provide important information on implantation and early development. The use of *in vitro* models which produce glands very similar to those seen *in vivo* (e.g. Rinehart, Lyn-Cook & Kaufmann, 1988; Hill & Warren, unpublished observations) may prove invaluable.

Although much emphasis has been given to secretory cells, ciliated cells form a significant proportion of the endometrial epithelium. Hafez & Ludwig (1977) describe two types of ciliated cell; those with typical motile cilia (seen in the endometria of all mammals) and a much rarer cell with a single, apparently non-motile, cilium found in the connective tissue of the uterus of hamsters and rats under certain hormonal conditions. The functional significance of the 'solitary' ciliated cells remains unclear, but they may be related to mitosis (Hafez & Ludwig, 1977).

In the gland cilia beat upwards, with cilia on the luminal epithelium appearing to beat towards the vagina (Edwards, 1980). Ciliated cells are reduced in chronic endometriosis and following menopause (Ludwig & Metzger, 1976). Cilia density increases rapidly in the proliferative phase and their number seems to be correlated with levels of oestrogen.

Luminal epithelial cells also possess ciliated and secretory cells which, basically, are similar to those seen in glands. However, the cyclical changes expressed by luminal cells is much less dramatic than that of glandular cells (Cornillie *et al.*, 1985) probably because they have fewer receptors than those in glands. Although ncs and glycogen deposits have been reported in luminal cells, giant mitochondria have not (Dockery & Rogers, 1989). Generally morphological changes in luminal cells lag behind those of gland cells, although they produce glycogen a few days earlier than gland cells (Johannisson, 1985).

There is relatively little published information on the luminal epithelium, with some notable exceptions (for example, Ferneczy, 1977; Martel, Frydman & Glissant, 1987; Murphy, Rogers & Leetoh, 1987). Generally, these have not used LH-dated biopsies. The relative lack of information on the luminal cells seems surprising since it is the first site of mechanical contact between the blastocyst and mother; clearly it is an area ripe for further investigation.

Stroma

Although there is relatively little published information on stromal tissue, it undergoes changes which are probably as dramatic and well coordinated as those seen in the epithelium.

In the early proliferative phase stromal cells are similar to undifferentiated fibroblasts (Verma, 1983) (Fig. 1). *In vitro*, Holinka & Gurpide (1987) have shown that the proliferative potential of human stromal cells is substantially greater than that of most other adult tissues, with 30% of specimens exhibiting fifty or more doublings. Stromal cells undergo their sequence of morphological changes apparently independently of epithelial cells, although they also play a key role in successful pregnancy (More *et al.*, 1974).

Light microscopy

Stromal mitoses range from about 2 per 1000 cells on day LH−10 to a peak of about 10 per 1000 cells around ovulation (Johannisson, 1985). This declines to almost nothing on day LH+6 and shows a second peak just before menstruation (Noyes *et al.*, 1950). Other cellular changes include infiltration by leukocytes (from about day LH+10 through to the end of menses), increased stromal cell nuclear diameter between days LH +2 and LH +8, increased stromal cell density from days LH+2 to LH+6, stromal oedema (maximal about day LH+8) and the formation of pre-decidual cells from about day LH+9 onwards (Noyes *et al.*, 1950; Dockery *et al.*, 1990). Granulocytes have been reported to differentiate from stromal cells in the second half of the secretory phase (Dallenbach-Hellweg, 1987), although Bulmer, Hollings & Ritson (1987) have shown them to be derived from bone marrow.

Electron microscopy

Ultrastructurally (Fig. 4) stromal cells have large, pale nuclei with little cytoplasm and are typically spindle-shaped. They are involved in the production and remodelling of the extracellular matrix including synthesis and removal of collagen fibrils (Cornillie *et al.*, 1985). They become more fibroblast-like during the proliferative phase. The increased activity results in cells which are larger, with more protein-synthesizing machinery, and a nucleus with more euchromatin and more prominent nucleoli than at earlier stages. Stromal mitochondria are small and round with short cristae, although they do elongate during the early secretory phase (Wienkie *et al.*, 1968). More *et al.* (1974) noted that mitochondria become surrounded by whorls of rough endoplasmic reticulum in the secretory phase

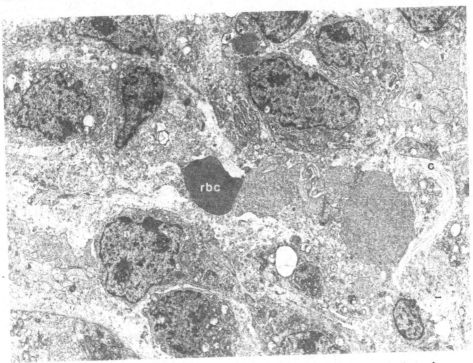

Fig. 4. Stromal cells seen under the electron microscope typically have irregular nuclei (n). Collagen fibrils (c) and red blood cells (rbc) are also common. Scale bar = 400 nm.

and that simple membrane thickening occurs between stromal cells. Desmosomes have also been seen between adjacent cells and stromal cells form a continuous network with processes which are preferentially oriented with luminal, but not glandular, epithelium; this orientation may be related to patterns of cell communication.

The Golgi apparatus of stromal cells is poorly developed in the early proliferative phase, but becomes prominent later in the secretory phase. Cytoplasmic vacuoles and granules show a similar pattern. Glycogen is commonly found in stromal cell cytoplasm in the mid-secretory phase (Wienke *et al.*, 1968). However, More *et al.* (1974) suggest glycogen may be produced independently of hormonal influences since maturing fibroblasts accumulate glycogen *in vitro* without hormonal supplement.

In the second half of the secretory phase decidual-like changes occur in the stroma. Decidualization only occurs in pregnancy or following continued exogenous oestrogen administration, but similar changes may be seen from about day LH + 9 and are usually called 'pre-decidual' (Johnannisson, 1985). Decidual cells are first seen around spiral arteries, then deep in the epithelium. Their function is unclear. Since they contain glycogen a nutritional role seems likely, but they may also act as a mechanical and immunological barrier in response to pregnancy. They have been reported to produce decidual prolactin, but the function of this molecule is also uncertain (Johannisson, 1985).

Two components of the stroma which deserve separate mention are blood vessels and cells of the immune system (see next section), although there is surprisingly little published on either.

Blood vessels proliferate in response to the thickening endometrium and there is an increase in capillary luminal size towards the end of the secretory phase (Sheppard & Bonnar, 1980). Blood vessel luminal diameter increases further and there is increased branching after implantation. Increased vascular permeability in the mid-secretory phase may be a cause of stromal oedema (Cornillie *et al.*, 1985). The precise sequence of events involved in the loss of part or all of the endometrium remains unclear; however, the collapse or spasmic contraction of spiral arteries, leading to 'blanching' of the overlying tissue is clearly a major factor (see later and Dockery & Rogers, 1989 for further discussion of this topic).

Endometrial leukocytes

The immunological mechanisms for successful implantation include the presence of immunosuppressive factors at the fetal–maternal interface, alteration of maternal endometrial lymphocyte populations and production of maternal blocking antibodies against antigens of the semiallogeneic fetus (Houwert-de-Jong, Bruinse & Termijteleu, 1990). Various of these immune implantation mechanisms have been proposed as functions of local endometrial leukocyte populations (Clark, 1990).

The endometrium hosts a wide spectrum of immunocompetent cells the detailed characterization of which has become feasible with the development of monoclonal antibodies reactive with leukocyte surface antigens (Morris *et al.*, 1985; Kamat & Isaackson, 1987). T-lymphocytes, macrophages and endometrial granulated lymphocytes constitute the main leukocytic population of the endometrium (Table 1).

T-lymphocytes

Morris *et al.* (1985) reported that during both the proliferative and secretory phases endometrial T-lymphocytes (CD3 + cells) showed three different patterns of distribution: intra-epithelial, interstitial and lymphoid aggregates in the zona basalis. In all three areas, the majority of CD3 + cells were CD8 + (T suppressor/ cytotoxic) and the ratio between CD8 + and CD4 + (T helper/inducer) cells was

Table 1. *Main leukocyte subsets in human endometrium and their proposed function*

Cell type	Phenotype	Proposed function
Granulated lymphocytes	CD56+, CD38+, CD2±, CD3−, CD16−	Control of trophoblast invasion, transforming growth factor production
T-lymphocytes	CD3+, CD8+	Immunosuppression, promote proliferation of placental cells
Macrophages	CD68+, CD14+ Class II MHC+	Immunosuppression, antigen presentation

approximately 4:1. Other investigators (Bulmer *et al.*, 1991) reported that CD3[+] cells accounted for approximately 40% of the cells reactive with an antibody against the leukocyte common antigen (CD 45) during proliferative and early secretory phases; 65% of T lymphocytes were CD8+ cells. The predominance of CD8[+] (T suppressor/cytotoxic) leukocytic subset among CD3+ cells has also been reported by Marshall and Jones (1988).

However all the studies which have reported characterization of leukocyte subpopulations in the endometrium have a number of inadequacies:

(a) They lack precise chronological dating of the endometrium and therefore interpretation of the reported changes in relation to implantation and early placental development is difficult. All the investigators have used the last menstrual period for chronological dating of the biopsy. None have dated biopsies from the luteinizing hormone (LH) surge, a procedure which significantly improves the precision of measurements made on endometrial structure (Li *et al.*, 1987).

(b) Some of the studies have either examined heterogeneous groups, including fertile, infertile and women with irregular menses (Kamat & Isaakson, 1987), or their normal subjects have not been well defined.

In a recent study (Klentzeris *et al.*, 1991) endometrial leukocyte subpopulations were characterized using precisely timed endometrial biopsies and a well-defined group of normal fertile women. Endometrial biopsies obtained 4, 7, 10 and 13 days following the LH surge were examined and image analysis was used to quantitate the leukocytes. T-lymphocytes (CD3+ cells) increased significantly from day LH+4 to day LH+7 and this increase was due to a significant rise in the number of T suppressor/cytotoxic (CD8+) cells. In the peri-implantation phase (LH+7), 22% of endometrial stromal leukocytes were CD8+ cells and only 8% were CD4 + cells. The ratio between T suppressor/cytotoxic and T helper/inducer (CD8 + /CD4 +) cells was 2.8 at all stages of the luteal phase.

Daya *et al.* (1985) reported the presence of two types of suppressor cells in non-pregnant human endometrium and decidua, but immunocytochemical characterization was not performed. The activity of a large hormone-dependent, non-granulated cell subsides gradually during the luteal phase, and during pregnancy is replaced by a small trophoblast-dependent granulated suppressor cell (Daya *et al.*, 1987). These large suppressor cells could be T suppressor lymphocytes which have been reported to express the progesterone receptor in the peripheral circulation during pregnancy (Szekeres-Bartho *et al.*, 1983). In the mouse large hormone dependent suppressor cells bear markers of suppressor T cells.

The functional contribution of endometrial T-lymphocytes to successful implantation and placental development is still unclear. Both immunosuppression and immunostimulation have been attributed to T-lymphocytes in endometrium and decidua.

Immunosuppression

The hypothesis has been put forward that local immunosuppression prevents sensitization of the maternal immune system to paternal alloantigens expressed by the fetus. Beauman & Hoversland (1988) induced abortion in mice with a monoclonal antibody which bound molecules produced by T suppressor lymphocytes. Ribbing *et al.* (1988) showed that, in the mouse peri-implantation phase, T cell suppressor factors (TsF) levels, detected by ELISA, in the uterus and the regional lymph nodes draining the uterus were increased by 15-fold and 100-fold over background, respectively. It was concluded that T cell suppressor factors are particularly important at the time of implantation. After stimulation with progesterone, CD8 + cells from healthy pregnant women secrete a 34 kDa molecule which inhibits natural killer cytolytic activity (Szekeres-Bartho *et al.*, 1989). Dietl *et al.* (1990) proposed 'functional inactivation' of maternal T cells migrating into human decidua. Intradecidual T cells expressed CD3 but lacked surface expression of α/β or c/d heterodimers. In contrast peripheral blood CD3 + cells of the same patients had normal expression of α/β or c/d T cell receptor heterodimers.

Immunostimulation

The principle of immunotrophism is that recognition of fetal cell surface antigens by maternal endometrial immunocompetent cells results in secretion of factors that promote the growth of placental tissue (Wegmann, 1988). Athanassakis *et al.* (1987) suggested that, in the mouse, maternal T cells stimulated by fetally derived placental antigens secreted granulocyte-macrophage-colony stimulating factor (GM-CSF) and interleukin-3 (IL-3) which subsequently induced proliferation of placental cells. They reported that elimination of maternal T cells during pregnancy resulted in reduction of the proliferative activity of the placenta. However, the immunostimulation or immunotrophic theory has come under criticism (Clark, 1989).

B-lymphocytes

In contrast to T cells, only 2–3% of the leukocytes (CD45 + cells) in the endometrium of normal fertile women are B-lymphocytes (CD22 + cells). B-lymphocytes have been observed either isolated in the stroma or forming part of lymphoid aggregates. In a quantitative study of precisely timed luteal phase endometrial biopsies, there was no significant change in the number of B cells from day LH + 4 to day LH + 13 (Klentzeris *et al.*, 1991). Bulmer, Lunny & Hagin (1988) reported that occasional B-cells were present in lymphoid aggregates of the zona basalis, and that their concentration did not change during the menstrual cycle. Other investigators have also reported a deficiency of B-cells in human endometrium (King *et al.*, 1989a). Hence the role of B-lymphocytes in the reproductive performance of normal fertile women is likely to be insignificant. The lack of β-cells and plasma cells contrasts with other mucoid sites such as the gastrointestinal tract or even the cervix.

Endometrial granulated lymphocytes (eGLs)

Granular endometrial stromal cells (Körnchenzellen, also termed 'K' cells) are present in both pregnant and non-pregnant human endometrium. They are scanty in proliferative endometrium but become prominent in the late secretory phase and early pregnancy. After the first trimester of pregnancy the number of granulated decidual cells decline and they are virtually absent at term. The cells have a round, reniform or oval densely stained nucleus, often eccentric in position and their cytoplasm contains a variable number of acidophilic and phloxinophilic granules. The origin and function of these cells remain controversial.

Early views on endometrial granulated lymphocytes

Granular cells in human endometrium were initially considered to be derived from endometrial stromal cells. Dallenbach-Hellweg (1987) suggested that the granular cells originate from undifferentiated stromal cells which develop under progestogenic influence during the second half of the secretory phase. She also termed these cells 'endometrial granulocytes'. A number of investigators have confirmed that endometrial granulocytes have many structural and functional similarities with granulated metrial gland cells (GMG) of the rat and mouse.

Ultrastructural studies have suggested that the cytoplasmic granules of endometrial stromal granulocytes develop within preformed sacculi which probably represent dilated cisternae of the endoplasmic reticulum or Golgi complex. Relaxin was identified as the main component of the granules in human endometrial granulocytes and in rat granulated metrial gland cells, using an immunofluorescence technique and a polyclonal antibody to relaxin (Dallenbach-Hellweg *et al.*, 1965). However, a negative result was achieved when the polyclonal antibody was tested with positive controls (Dallenbach-Hellweg *et al.*, 1965). Also Larkin (1974) presented conclusive evidence that rat metrial gland cells were neither a source nor a storage site of biologically active relaxin.

Modern views on endometrial granulated lymphocytes

Electron microscopic studies of rat and mouse metrial gland cells suggested that endometrial granulocytes originate from lymphocyte precursors through a series of differentiation stages. Peel *et al.*, (1983) presented evidence from rat–mouse chimeras that the granulated metrial gland cells of the mouse uterus are derived from bone marrow-derived precursors. Mitchell and Peel (1984) noted that granulated metrial gland cells express the leukocyte common antigens. Bulmer and Sunderland (1983) reported that the endometrial granulocytes in the early human placental bed originate from the bone marrow. Bulmer *et al.* (1987) later provided a detailed antigenic profile for the endometrial granulated lymphocytes. They observed that eGLs are granulated cells which have an unusual antigenic phenotype: CD45+, CD56+, CD3−, CD2±, CD38+, CD7±, CD4−, CD8−, CD16−, CD57− and belong to the group of 'large granular lymphocytes'. King *et al.* (1989a) reported that, at the time of implantation, the majority of endometrial leukocytes were CD56+, CD16−, CD2+, CD3−, HLA DR− and morphologically similar to large granular lymphocytes. There is now little doubt that the eGLs are migrating cells of bone marrow origin within the group of large granular lymphocytes.

Cyclic variation and kinetic pattern

A number of studies have indicated that eGLs form a small proportion of the endometrial leukocytes in the proliferative phase of the menstrual cycle (Marshall

& Jones, 1988; Bulmer *et al.*, 1988; King *et al.*, 1989*a*). However, their stromal concentration increases rapidly and dramatically during the mid and late luteal phase. Bulmer *et al.* (1991) reported that CD56+, CD38+, CD2±, CD3− cells constitute 57% and 80% of endometrial stromal leukocytes during the late secretory phase and early pregnancy respectively. Klentzeris *et al.* (1991) noted that the stromal concentration of endometrial granulated lymphocytes (CD56+, CD38+ cells) increased significantly from day LH+7 to day LH+10 and from day LH+10 to day LH+13. At day LH+13, approximately 55% of stromal leukocytes were granulated lymphocytes. Although CD56+, CD38+ cells were identified throughout the stroma, they tended to aggregate around glands and spiral arteries.

The kinetics and differentiation of endometrial granulated lymphocytes have raised some questions. For example, it is not clear whether fully differentiated eGLs enter the endometrium directly from blood or whether the cells differentiate *in situ* from bone marrow-derived precursors. Two recent studies support the latter explanation for the dramatic increase in eGLs numbers in the late luteal phase.

Pace *et al.* (1989) using Ki 67 as a marker of proliferation found that the mitotic activity of eGLs increased from late proliferative (25%) to late secretory phase (93%). Klentzeris *et al.* (1991) used morphometric techniques to assess the volume fraction of endometrium occupied by the nuclei of eGLs and programmed digitization to measure the changes of nuclear diameters of these cells from day LH+4 to day LH+13. The volume fraction of the eGL nuclei did not change significantly from day LH+4 to day LH+13. In contrast, the nuclear axial ratio (AxR=maximum/minimum nuclear diameter) demonstrated a significant decrease from day LH+7 to day LH+10 and from day LH+10 to day LH+13. The combination of these two findings suggests *in situ* proliferation of eGLs, which could explain the significant increase in CD56+, CD38+ cells noted from day LH+7 to day LH+13 in frozen sections.

Endometrial granulated lymphocytes may play an immunological role in the early stages of the embryo-maternal dialogue. The immuno-suppressive activity of murine decidua has been associated with a small granulated non-T non-B lymphoid cell which inhibits activation of T helper/inducer (CD4+) cells by blocking the activity of interleukin-2. The blocking effect appears to be mediated by secretion of a transforming growth factor-B2 (TGF-B2) (Clark *et al.*, 1990). The same mechanism of action has been proposed for a population of small suppressor cells which have been detected in first trimester human decidua (Daya *et al.*, 1987). This common mode of action, in combination with the structural and phenotypic similarities between non-T non-B granulated suppressor cells in murine decidua and eGLs, has led to speculation that eGLs in human decidua may have an immunosuppressive role. However, many other cell types in human decidua and endometrium, including macrophages, decidualized stromal cells and epithelial cells have also been implicated as suppressor cells.

Endometrial granulated lymphocytes express the natural killer cell antigen CD56. King *et al.* (1989*b*) extracted lymphocytes from first trimester human decidua and observed that eGLs showed natural killer activity against K562 cells. Other investigators have also reported non-MHC restricted cytotoxicity by eGLs.

It has been suggested that the lytic activity of eGLs may be directed towards control of trophoblast invasion. However, natural killer activity against embryonic tissue is rather unlikely since first trimester cytotrophoblast resists lysis by natural killer cells. Control of trophoblast invasion remains a possible contribution of eGLs to successful implantation and early pregnancy development. Their action *in vivo* is probably mediated via secreted cytokines.

Macrophages

Macrophages (CD14+ and CD68+ cells) constitute a significant proportion of endometrial leukocytes. In proliferative endometrium macrophages account for 33% of bone marrow derived leukocytes (CD45+ cells) (Bulmer *et al.*, 1991). In secretory phase endometrium, the number of CD68+ cells increases significantly from day LH+10 to day LH+13 (Klentzeris *et al.*, 1991) and this observation is in agreement with reports from other investigators (Kamat & Isaackson, 1989; Bulmer *et al.*, 1991). The cells are located primarily around glands, dispersed in the stroma and occasionally between surface and glandular epithelial cells.

The macrophages may play several roles in the embryo–maternal dialogue:

1. Immunosuppression

Lala *et al.* (1986) suggested that macrophages can suppress the activation of lymphocytes and the subsequent generation of functional killer cells. This function may be related to prostaglandin E_2 which is secreted by the macrophages.

2. Antigen presentation

Antigen presenting capacity has been demonstrated in human and murine decidua. In the mouse this capacity has been attributed to class II major histocompatibility complex-positive macrophages.

3. Cytokines

Macrophages synthesize and secrete a wide spectrum of cytokines including tumour necrosis factor (TNF), granulocyte-colony stimulating factor (G-CSF), macrophage-colony stimulating factor (M-CSF), and granulocyte-macrophage-colony stimulating factor (GM-CSF). Placental receptors have been described for these molecules. Some of the functions of macrophages may be mediated via cytokines. Non-specific defence against infection and phagocytosis of tissue debris are two further roles proposed for the endometrial macrophages.

Natural killer cells

The antigenic phenotype of the majority of natural killer (NK) cells is CD56+, CD16+ (Knapp *et al.*, 1989). Nagler *et al.* (1989) identified and characterized three subpopulations of CD56+ peripheral blood NK cells based on the surface expression of CD16 molecules. The $CD16^{bright}$ subset accounted for 10% to 15% of peripheral blood lymphocytes, whereas the $CD16^{dim}$ and $CD16^{negative}$ subset accounted for less than 1% of the peripheral blood lymphocytes. The $CD16^{dim}$ and $CD16^{bright}$ were large granular lymphocytes with potent NK activity. In contrast, $CD16^{negative}$ cells were agranular and did not function as NK cells. In endometrium, although the CD56+ cells comprise more than 50% of the leukocytes, CD16+ cells have not been identified or account for a very small proportion of stromal leukocytes. In a quantitative study, Bulmer *et al.*, (1991) reported that CD16+ cells constituted only 3.4% of stromal leukocytes in the proliferative phase; Klentzeris *et al.* (1991) noted that CD16+ cells comprised 2% of the bone marrow derived cells in secretory endometrium and showed no significant change from day LH + 4 to day LH + 13.

The effect of exogenous hormone treatment on the morphology of the endometrium

The response of the endometrium to exogenous hormone treatment varies according to a number of factors:

1 Which class of hormone or hormone combination (e.g. oestrogen, progestogen or oestrogen–progestogen combination) has been given.
2 Of a particular class of hormone administered, which type has been used (e.g. whether natural or synthetic and, if synthetic, which particular one and what potency).
3 Dose: whether the hormone has been given in a single or multiple doses; if multiple, what has been the daily dose and the total duration of treatment.

4 The time of the menstrual cycle in which the treatment begins. This will govern
   the state of the endometrium prior to the hormonal treatment.
5 Bioavailability: including the route of administration, e.g. whether oral,
   intramuscular, vaginal or transdermal; and the formulation, e.g. whether in
   tablet or microcrystalline form.
6 Biological variation in individual response.

Oestrogen

Oestrogen administration in the follicular phase

Oestrogen given in sufficient dose in the follicular phase inhibits ovulation and
abolishes the luteal phase. Proliferation of glands and stroma is stimulated.
Prolonged use may produce cystic glandular hyperplasia, adenomatous glandular
hyperplasia, and atypical hyperplasia (Abell, 1975; Hendrickson & Kempson,
1980).

Oestrogen administration in the luteal phase

Relatively high doses of oestrogen given in the early luteal phase may act as a
form of postcoital contraception. Haspels, Linthorst & Kicoric (1977) in a study
of five healthy volunteers examined the effect of intramuscular administration of
oestrogens (12.5 mg of oestradiol benzoate and 10 mg oestradiol phenylpropionate)
in the early luteal phase; if the oestrogens were given on day LH + 4 or after, no
change in endometrial histology was noted. However, if the oestrogens were given
on days LH + 1 to LH + 3, the endometrium demonstrated 'dissociated secretory'
changes or secretory endometrium with pronounced epithelial proliferation.

Progestogens

The changes elicited by most progestogens are similar, and consist of a variable
degree of secretory response in the glands followed by suppression of glandular
proliferation and secretion, and suppressed stromal proliferation commonly
followed by a decidual reaction (Abell, 1975).

Continuous high doses of progestogens

Continuous high dose progestogen therapy is used in the treatment of hyperplastic
endometrial lesions or endometriosis. The initial responses are suppression of
glandular proliferation, an incomplete glandular secretory response, and stromal

oedema. These are soon followed by the characteristic changes of glandular atrophy with diffuse decidual change in the stroma typical of long-term high dose progestogen treatment (Abell, 1975; Haines & Taylor, 1975). The decidua may persist for weeks after cessation of treatment and may be shed as an endometrial cast.

Continuous low dose of progestogen

Continuous low dose progestogen administration is used as the 'minipill' for contraception. The endometrium becomes thin with a compact stroma, sparse glands and an absence of stromal oedema (Moghissi, Syner & McBride, 1973). Norgestrel in particular may have an additional effect on endometrial blood vessels showing many well developed arterioles and dilated sinusoids, which may account for the higher incidence of breakthrough bleeding with this progestogen (Graham & Fraser, 1982).

Cyclical treatment with progestogen

Cyclical treatment with progestogens, from days 5 to 25 of the menstrual cycle, has been studied by Borushek *et al.* (1963) and Flowers (1964). The initial response consists of a lack of epithelial proliferation with glands which are hypoplastic and tubular. Between days 7 and 12, there is spotty, incomplete vacuolation of epithelium and marked stromal oedema. The vessels may be prominent and congested. Later changes depend on the dose of progestogen administered. Historically, when a 19-nor steroid progestogen was initially used, the dose administered was high and the stroma underwent a diffuse decidual transformation that could not be distinguished from the decidual reaction of pregnancy. Today, the dose of 19-nor steroid is considerably reduced and a decidual reaction is not observed, or is patchy or poorly formed. Progestogens with an acetate radical produce either no decidual response, or a patchy and ill-developed decidual reaction (Abell, 1975).

Cyclical treatment with low dose progestogen for contraceptive purposes is associated with a hypoplastic endometrium, similar to that of a resting endometrium.

Progestogen treatment in the luteal phase

Both natural progesterone and synthetic progestogens such as dydrogesterone have been used to treat retarded endometrial development in the luteal phase, and as a form of 'luteal support' in women undergoing *in vitro* fertilization and embryo transfer, especially if follicle stimulation is achieved with gonadotrophin (Sharma *et al.*, 1990; Jones, 1985). However, we have recently observed that a single, large dose (100 mg) of progesterone administered intramuscularly in the early luteal phase did not advance development in normally developing endometrium (Li, Dockery & Cooke, 1991). Similarly, endometrial morphology in artificial cycles treated with standard doses or high doses (5 times standard) of progesterone are similar, suggesting that supraphysiological doses of progesterone do not advance endometrial development (Li *et al.*, 1992).

Oestrogen-progestogen combinations

Combined oral contraceptive pill

In general, women on oral contraceptives may show early secretory activity in endometrial glands but secretory changes typical of the mid and late luteal phase do not develop. Instead, during the last week of the cycle the glands become atrophic, small and tubular with a lining of flattened cuboidal epithelium. Variable pre-decidual and vascular changes may be seen in the stroma. This atrophic gland appearance and the decidual change may increase in subsequent treatment cycles (Haines & Taylor, 1975).

Sequential pill

In the sequential pill, oestrogen is usually started on day 5 of the menstrual cycle for 14 days, followed by an oestrogen–progestogen combination for five or six days. The oestrogen inhibits ovulation and stimulates the proliferation of glands and stroma. About two days after progestogen has been added there is secretory vacuolation similar to an early luteal phase. However, it does not progress beyond this stage. Similarly, the stroma does not progress to pre-decidual changes as in the combined oral contraceptive pill. Often, the glandular epithelium retains a secretory pattern with prominent vacuolation until a withdrawal bleeding occurs (Ober, 1966).

Oestrogen–progestogen combination administered in mid-cycle or early luteal phase as postcoital contraception

Ling *et al.*, (1979) studied the effect of 0.1 mg of ethinyloestradiol and 1 mg of DL-norgestrel given at the predicted time of ovulation, on two occasions, 12 hours apart. They found significant asynchrony in the development of glandular and stromal endometrial components: the glands appeared to lag from two to six days behind the stroma in maturation. Similar findings were obtained by Yuzpe *et al.* (1974) using a single dose of the same combination of hormones.

Menstruation

When implantation fails to take place, corpus luteum function declines and menstruation ensues. Menstruation can be regarded as the shedding of the functional layer of the endometrium which has failed to achieve its primary function (implantation), so that the tissue can prepare itself for implantation in the next cycle.

Mechanism of menstruation

The current theories of endometrial shedding and haemostasis have been reviewed by Christiens, Sixma & Haspels (1985) and Smith *et al.* (1985). With the onset of luteolysis at approximately three days prior to menstruation, the progesterone level falls. As a result, lysosomes in the endometrium become unstable and release phospholipase, which in turn acts on phospholipids to produce arachidonic acid (precursor of prostaglandin), and eventually leading to the synthesis of increasing amounts of prostaglandins. The prostaglandin $F_{2\alpha}$ so produced constricts the spiral arterioles supplying the superficial layers of the endometrium, causing ischaemia and necrosis of that layer. The increased coiling and constriction of spiral arterioles is thought to be an important factor in the haemostasis of menstrual bleeding. On the other hand, straight arteries which supply the basal endometrium are not affected by prostaglandins, and the basal endometrium is unaffected by menstruation.

Morphological changes during menstruation

Many of the changes in the endometrium prior to the onset of the menstruation are consequent upon the vascular changes of the spiral arterioles. An early feature is the appearance of stromal haemorrhage and increased number of stromal granulocytes. The functional layer undergoes shrinkage, and its constituent glands and stroma fragment and crumble. Finally, menstruation ensues with the shedding of the degenerated functional layer.

Menstruation may be artificially induced by the administration of a progesterone receptor antagonist, mifepristone (RU486). In a recent study, we compared endometrial histology of spontaneously occurring menstruation with that induced by mifepristone (Li *et al.*, 1990). The results are shown in Table 2.

Table 2. *Comparison of histological features of endometrium taken from women whose menstruation was induced by mifepristone to those occurring spontaneously*

	Induced menstruation ($n = 13$)	Spontaneous menstruation ($n = 8$)	Wilcoxon rank sum test
1. Number of mitoses per 1000 gland cells	0	0	n.s.
2. Gland cell height (μm)	13.9–31.2 (median 21.3)	13.2–20.9 (median 17.9)	$P < 0.05$
3. Amount of secretion in gland lumen (score 0–3)	0–2 (median 0.5)	1–3 (median 2)	$P < 0.01$
4. Volume fraction of gland occupied by gland cell	74.5–92.5 (median 85.7)	57.3–81.3 (median 68.0)	$P < 0.01$
5. Volume fraction of endometrium occupied by gland	16.0–43.8 (median 31.0)	12.4–39.3 (median 22.8)	n.s.
6. Volume fraction of gland cell occupied by nucleus	19.2–26.2 (median 22.8)	14.7–26.1 (median 19.5)	$P < 0.05$
7. Number of supranuclear secretory vacuoles per 100 gland cells	0–44 (median 0)	0–25 (median 0)	n.s.
8. Number of subnuclear secretory vacuoles per 100 gland cells	0–36 (median 1)	0–41 (median 0)	n.s.
9. Amount of pseudostratification of gland cells (score 0–3)	0–2 (median 1.0)	0	$p < 0.01$
10. Number of apoptotic bodies per 1000 gland cells	0–74 (median 30)	3–40 (median 12)	n.s.
11. Number of mitoses per 1000 stromal cells	0–3.0 (median 1.0)	0–3.3 (median 1.2)	n.s.
12. Amount of stromal oedema (score 0–3)	0	0–1.0 (median 0)	n.s.
13. Amount of pre-decidual reaction (score 0–3)	0–1.0 (median 0.5)	2.5–3.0 (median 3.0)	$p < 0.001$
14. Amount of leukocytic infiltration in stroma (score 0–3)	0–2.0 (median 1.0)	2.5–3.0 (median 2.5)	$p < 0.001$
15. Amount of extravasation in stroma (score 0–3)	0.5–3.0 (median 2.0)	0–3.0 (median 2.0)	n.s.

First published in *Obstetrics and Gynecology* (1990).
n.s.: not significant.

Several histological features were found to be similar in both types of menstruation. These included the amount of glandular mitotic activity, secretory vacuoles, apoptotic bodies and the volume fraction of endometrium occupied by glands; and in the stroma, the amount of mitotic activity, oedema and extravasion.

Of more interest were those histological features of the endometrium which were found to differ between the two types of menstruation. When compared to menstruation occurring spontaneously, that induced by mifepristone was associated with an increase in gland cell height, a reduced amount of secretory material in the gland lumen, an increase in the volume fraction of gland occupied by gland cells, an increase in the volume fraction of gland cell occupied by nucleus, an increase in the amount of pseudostratification of gland cells, a reduced amount of stromal predecidual reaction and a reduced amount of leukocytic infiltration in the stroma. The first five of these are related to the secretory activity of the gland. With a reduction in the secretory activity of the gland cells, the absolute volume of cell cytoplasm is reduced so that the volume fraction of gland cell occupied by the nucleus is increased. With a diminished amount of secretory material present in the gland lumen, the gland is less distended and becomes partially collapsed; hence gland cells are more closely packed and appear taller as well as more pseudostratified. At the same time the volume fraction of gland occupied by gland cells is increased.

Normal menstruation is associated with a characteristic level of glandular secretory activity, stromal pre-decidual reaction and leukocytic infiltration. The observation that menstruation can be induced in endometrium with significantly reduced levels of these features suggests that they are not essential for the initiation of menstruation.

Induction of menstruation by mifepristone may or may not be followed by bleeding around the expected time of menstruation for that cycle (Li *et al.*, 1988*a*; Garzo *et al.*, 1988; Swahn *et al.*, 1988). The reason for this second episode of bleeding is unknown, although preliminary evidence suggests menstrual induction by mifepristone may not necessarily be associated with endometrial shedding. If endometrial shedding does not occur, further menstrual bleeding will occur; if endometrial shedding has already occurred, no further bleeding will result (Li *et al.*, 1988*b*). Endometrial histology in women who had bled once was associated with a more marked predecidual reaction than in those who had bled twice (Li *et al.*, 1990).

In the pre-decidual reaction the stromal cells become plump, due both to the enlargement of nuclei and an increase of finely granular cytoplasm. The presence of a large amount of glycogen and fat in these cells suggests that they may have a nutritive role for the implanting blastocyst. In addition, these cells have been thought to play a role in 'restraining the invasiveness of the conceptus' (Johnson

& Everitt, 1984) and to offer immunoprotection for the implanting blastocyst by producing a protein with immunosuppressive activity (Bolton *et al.*, 1987; Pockley *et al.*, 1988). Current observations suggest that the pre-decidual reaction, although not essential for the initiation of menstrual bleeding, may be closely related to shedding of the endometrium during menstruation.

Pre-decidualization or decidualization of the stroma in the human endometrium is associated with loss of interstitial collagen type VI, which is normally present in the form of a network of microfibrils that connect the larger fibrils of the major collagen types (Aplin, Charlton & Ayad, 1988). It is possible that pre-decidual change in the stroma is accompanied by loss of type VI collagen-containing microfibrils which, in turn, loosen the stroma and facilitate shedding.

Acknowledgements

We would like to thank Mrs C. Pigott for skilled technical assistance and the Secretarial staff of the Department of Biomedical Science for typing the manuscript.

References

Abell, M. R. (1975). Endometrial biopsy: normal and abnormal diagnostic characteristics. In *Gynaecological Endocrinology*. Ed. J. J. Gold, pp. 156–90, Harper & Row, New York.

Ancla, M., Belaisch, J. & De Brux, J. (1969). Action of chorionic gonadotrophin on cellular structures in the human endometrium in the secretory phase. *Journal of Reproduction and Fertility*, **19**, 291–7.

Aplin, J. D., Charlton, A. K. & Ayad, S. (1988). An immunohistochemical study of human endometrial extracellular matrix during the menstrual cycle and first trimester of pregnancy. *Cell Tissue Research*, **253**, 231–40.

Armstrong, E. M., More, I. A. R., McSeveney, D. & Chatifield, W. R. (1973). Reappraisal of the ultrastructure of the human endometrial glandular cell. *Journal of Obstetrics and Gynaecology of the British Commonwealth*, **80**, 446–60.

Athanassakis, I., Bleackley, R. C., Paetkan, V., Guilbert, L., Barr, P. J., Wegmann, T. G. (1987). The immunostimulatory effect of T cells and T cell lymphokines on murine fetally derived placental cells. *Journal of Immunology*, **1**, 37–44.

Beauman, K. D. & Hoversland, R. C. (1988). Induction of abortion in mice with a monoclonal antibody specific for suppressor T-lymphocyte molecules. *Journal of Reproduction and Fertility*, **82**, 691–6.

Beier, H. M. (1974). Oviductal and uterine fluids. *Journal of Reproduction and Fertility*, **37**, 221–37.

Bolton, A. E., Pockley, A. G., Clough, K. J. *et al.* (1987). Identification of placental protein 14 as an immunosuppressive factor in human reproduction. *Lancet*, **i**, 593–5.

Borushek, S., Abell, M. R., Smith, L. & Gold, J. J. (1963). The effects of Provest on the endometrium. *International Journal of Fertility*, **8**, 605–18.

Bulmer, J. N. & Sunderland, C. A. (1983). Bone marrow origin of endometrial granulocytes in the early human placental bed. *Journal of Reproductive Immunology*, **5**, 383–7.

Bulmer, J. N., Hollings, D. & Ritson, A. (1987). Immunocytochemical evidence that endometrial stromal granulocytes are granulated lymphocytes. *Journal of Pathology*, **153**, 281–8.

Bulmer, J. N., Lunny, D. P. & Hagin, S. V. (1988). Immunohistochemical characterization of stromal leukocytes in non-pregnant human endometrium. *American Journal of Reproductive Immunology and Microbiology*, **17**, 83–90.

Bulmer, J. N., Morrison, L., Longfellow, M., Ritson, A. & Pace, D. (1991). Granulated lymphocytes in human endometrium histochemical and immunohistochemical studies. *Human Reproduction*, **6**, 791–8.

Cavazos, F., Green, J. A., Hall, D. G. & Lucas, F. V. (1967). Ultrastructure of the human endometrial glandular cell during the menstrual cycle. *American Journal of Obstetrics and Gynecology*, **99**, 833–54.

Christiens, G. C. M. L., Sixma, J. J. & Haspels, A. A. (1985). Vascular and haemostatic changes in menstrual endometrium. In *Mechanism of Menstrual Bleeding. Serono Symposia Publications*. ed. D. T. Band and E. A. Michie, pp. 27–34, Raven Press, New York.

Clark, D. A. (1989). Cytokines and pregnancy. In *Current Opinion in Immunology*. ed. I. Roitt, vol. 1, pp. 1141–7, Alden Press, London.

Clark, D. A. (1990). Paraimmunology in the decidua. *American Journal of Reproductive Immunology*, **24**, 37–9.

Clark, D. A., Flanders, K. C., Banwatt, D. K. *et al.* (1990). Murine pregnancy decidua produces a unique immunosuppressive molecule related to transforming growth factor beta-2. *Journal of Immunology*, **144**, 3008–14.

Clark, J. H. & Markeverich, B. M. (1981). Relationship between Type I and Type II estradiol binding sites and estrogen induced responses. *Journal of Steroid Biochemistry*, **15**, 49–54.

Coaker, T., Downie, T. & More, I. A. R. (1982). Complex giant mitochondria in the endometrial glandular cell: serial sectioning, high voltage electron microscopy and three-dimensional reconstruction studies. *Journal of Ultrastructural Research*, **78**, 283–91.

Cornillie, F. J., Lauweryns, J. M. & Brosens, I. A. (1985). Normal human endometrium. *Gynecological and Obstetric Investigations*, **20**, 113–29.

Dallenbach-Hellweg, G., Battista, K. V. & Dallenbach, F. D. (1965). Immunohistological and histochemical localization of relaxin in the metrial gland of the pregnant rat. *American Journal of Anatomy*, **117**, 433–50.

Dallenbach-Hellweg, G. (1987). The normal histology of the endometrium. In *Histopathology of the Endometrium*. ed. G. Dallenbach-Hallweg, 5th edn, pp. 25–92, Springer-Verlag, Berlin.

Davie, R., Hopwood, D. & Levison, D. A. (1977). Intercelluar spaces and cell junctions in endometrial glands, their possible role in menstruation. *British Journal of Obstetrics and Gynaecology*, **84**, 467–76.

Daya, S., Clark, D. A., Devlin & C. & Zarell, Z. (1985). Preliminary characterization of two types of suppressor cells in the human uterus. *Fertility and Sterility*, **44**, 778–85.

Daya, S., Rosenthall, K. L. & Clark, D. A. (1987). Immunosuppressor factors(s) produced by decidua-associated suppressor cells: a proposed mechanism for fetal allograft survival. *American Journal of Obstetrics and Gynecology*, **156**, 344–9.

Dehou, M. F., Lejeune, B., Airjis, C. & Leroy, F. (1987). Endometrial morphology in stimulated *in vitro* fertilisation cycles and after steroid replacement therapy in cases of primary ovarian failure. *Fertility and Sterility*, **48**, 995–1000.

Dietl, J., Horny, H. P., Ruck, P. *et al.* (1990). Intradecidual T lymphocytes lack immunohistochemically detectable T-cell receptors. *American Journal of Reproductive Immunology*, **24**, 33–6.

Dockery, P., Li, T. C., Rogers, A. W., Cooke, I. D., Lenton, E. A. & Warren, M. A. (1988*a*). An examination of the variation in timed endometrial biopsies. *Human Reproduction*, **3**, 715–20.

Dockery, P., Li, T. C., Rogers, A. W., Cooke, I. D. & Lenton, E. A. (1988*b*). The ultrastructure of the glandular epithelium in the timed endometrial biopsy. *Human Reproduction*, **3**, 826–34.

Dockery, P. & Rogers, A. W. (1989). The effects of steroids on the fine structure of the endometrium. *Baillière's Clinical Obstetrics and Gynaecology*, **3**, 227–48.

Dockery, P., Warren, M. A., Li, T. C., Rogers, A. W., Cooke, I. D. & Mundy, J. (1990). A morphometric study of the human endometrial stroma during the peri-implantation period. *Human Reproduction*, **5**, 112–16.

Edwards, R. G. (1980). *Conception in the Human Female*. Academic Press, London.

Ferneczy, A. (1977). Surface ultrastructural response of the human uterine lining to hormonal environment. A scanning microscopic study. *Journal of Clinical Endocrinology and Metabolism*, **21**, 566–72.

Ferneczy, A. (1976). Studies on the cytodynamics of human endometrial regeneration. I Scanning electron microscopy. *American Journal of Obstetrics and Gynecology*, **124**, 64–74.

Flowers, C. E. Jr. (1964). Effects of a new low-dosage form of norethynodrelmestranol: clinical evaluation and endometrial biopsy study. *Journal of American Medical Association*, **188**, 1115–20.

Garzo, V. G., Liu, J., Ulmann, A., Baulieu, E. & Yen, S. S. C. (1988). Effects of an antiprogesterone (RU486) on the hypothalamic–hypophysial–ovarian–endometrial axis during the luteal phase of the menstrual cycle. *Journal of Clinical Endocrinology Metabolism*, **66**, 508–17.

Gordon, M., Kohorn, E. I., Gore, B. Z. & Rice, S. I. (1973). Effect of postovulatory oestrogens on the fine structure of the epithelial cells in the human endometrium. *Journal of Reproduction and Fertility*, **34**, 375–8.

Gordon, M. (1974). Cyclic changes in the fine structure of the epithelial cells of the human endometrium. *International Reviews in Cytology*, **42**, 127–72.

Graham, S. & Fraser, I. S. (1982). The progesterone-only mini-pill. *Contraception*, **26**, 373–88.

Haines, M. & Taylor, C. W. (1975). *Gynaecological Pathology*. 2nd edn, pp. 130–157, Churchill Livingstone, Edinburgh.

Hafez, E. S. E. & Ludwig, H. (1977). Scanning electron microscopy of the endometrium. In *Biology of the Uterus*. Ed. R. M. Wynn, pp. 309–40, Plenum Press, New York and London.

Haspels, A. A., Linthorst, G. A. & Kicoric, P. M. (1977). Effect of postovulatory administration of a 'morning-after' injection on corpus luteum function and endometrium. *Contraception*, **15**, 105–12.

Hendricksson, M. R. & Kempson, R. L. (1980). Iatrogenic endometrial patterns. In *Surgical Pathology of the Uterine Corpus*. pp. 264–84, WB Saunders, Philadelphia.

Holinka, C. F. & Gurpide, E. (1987). Proliferative potential and polymorphism of human endometrial stromal cells. *Gynecological Endocrinology*, **1**, 71–81.

Houwert-Dejong, M. H., Bruinse, H. W. & Termijteleh, A. (1990). The immunology of normal pregnancy and recurrent abortion. In *Early Pregnancy Failure*. Ed. H. J. Huisjes and T. Lind, pp. 27–38. Churchill Livingstone, Edinburgh.

Johannisson, E., Parker, R. A., Landgren, B.-M. & Diczfalusy, E. (1982). Morphometric analysis of the human endometrium in relation to peripheral hormone levels. *Fertility and Sterility*, **38**, 564–71.

Johannisson, E. (1985). Cyclical changes in endometrial morphology. In *Clinical Reproductive Endocrinology*. pp. 128–64, Ed. R. P. Shearman, Churchill Livingstone, Edinburgh.

Johannisson, E., Landgren, B.-M., Rohr, H. P. & Diczfalusy, E. (1987). Endometrial morphology and peripheral hormone levels in women with regular menstrual cycles. *Fertility and Sterility*, **48**, 401–8.

Johnson, M. & Everitt, B. (1984). Implantation and the establishment of the placenta. In *Essential Reproduction*. 2nd edn. pp. 215–42, Blackwell Scientific Publications, Oxford.

Jones, G. S. (1985). The role of luteal support in a programme for *in vitro* fertilization. In *Implantation of the Human Embryo*. Ed. R. G. Edwards, J. M. Purdy and P. C. Steptoe, pp. 285–97, Academic Press, London.

Kamat, B. R. & Isaackson, P. G. (1987). The immunocytochemical distribution of leukocytic subpopulation in human endometrium. *American Journal of Pathology*, **127**, 66–73.

King, A., Birkby, C. & Loke, Y. W. (1989*b*). Early human decidual cells exhibit NK activity against the K562 cell line but not against first trimester trophoblast. *Cell Immunology*, **118**, 337–44.

King, A., Wellings, V., Gardner, L. & Loke, Y. W. (1989*a*). Immunocytochemical characterization of the unusual large granular lymphocytes in human endometrium throughout the menstrual cycle. *Human Immunology*, **24**, 195–205.

Klentzeris, L. D., Bulmer, J. N., Warren, A. M., Morrison, L., Li, T. C. & Cooke, I. D. (1992). Endometrial lymphoid tissue in the timed endometrial biopsy: Morphometric and immunohistochemical aspects. *American Journal of Obstetrics and Gynecology*, **167**(3), 667–74.

Kohorn, E. I., Rice, S. I. & Gordon, M. (1970). *In vitro* production of nucleolar channel system by progesterone in human endometrium. *Nature (London)*, **228**, 671–2.

Kohorn, E. I., Rice, S. I., Hemperly, S. & Gordon, M. (1972). The relation of the structure of progestational steroids to nucleolar differentiation in human endometrium. *Journal of Clinical Endocrine Metabolism*, **34**, 257–64.

Knapp, W., Rieber, P., Dorken, B., Schmidt, R. E., Stein, H. & Borne, A. E. (1989). Towards a better definition of human leukocyte surface molecules. *Immunology Today*, **10**, 253–8.

Lala, P. K., Kearns, M., Parhar, R. S., Scodras, J. & Johnson, S. (1986). Immunological role of the cellular constitutes of the decidua in the maintenance of semiallogenic pregnancy. *Annals of NY Academy of Sciences*, **476**, 183–205.

Larkin, L. H. & Flickinger, C. J. (1969). Ultrastructure of the metrial gland cell in the pregnant rat. *American Journal of Anatomy*, **126**, 337–54.

Li, T. C., Rogers, A. W., Lenton, E. A., Dockery, P. & Cooke, I. D. (1987). A comparison between two methods of chronological dating of human endometrial biopsies during the luteal phase and their correlation with histological dating. *Fertility and Sterility*, **48**, 928–32.

Li, T. C., Dockery, P., Thomas, P., Rogers, A. W., Lenton, E. A. & Cooke, I. D. (1988*a*). The effects of progesterone receptor blockade in the luteal phase of normal fertile women. *Fertility and Sterility,* **50,** 732–42.

Li, T. C., Lenton, E. A., Dockery, P., Rogers, A. W. & Cooke, I. D. (1988*b*). Why does RU486 fail to prevent implantation despite success in inducing menstruation? *Contraception,* **38,** 401–6.

Li, T. C., Dockery, P., Rogers, A. W. & Cooke, I. D. (1990). Histological and clinical features of menstruation induced by antiprogestin RU486 as compared to menstruation occurring spontaneously. *Journal of Obstetrics and Gynecology,* **10,** 411–14.

Li, T. C., Dockery, P. & Cooke, I. D. (1991). Effect of exogenous progesterone administration on the morphology of normally developing endometrium in the pre-implantation period. *Human Reproduction,* **6,** 641–4.

Li, T. C., Warren, M. A., Dockery, P., Ramsewak, S. S., Lenton, E. A. & Cooke, I. D. (1992). Endometrial response in artificial cycles: a prospective, randomized study comparing three different progesterone doses. *British Journal of Obstetrics and Gynaecology,* **99,** 319–24.

Ling, W. Y., Robichaud, A., Zayid, I., Wrixon, W. & MacLeod, S. C. (1979). Mode of action of dl-norgestrel and ethinylestradiol combination in postcoital contraception. *Fertility and Sterility,* **32,** 297–302.

Ludwig, H. & Metzger, H. (1976). *The Human Female Reproductive Tract: A Scanning Electron Microscopic Atlas.* pp. 1–247, Springer-Verlag, Berlin.

Luginbuhl, W. H. (1968). Electron microscopic studies of the effects of tissue culture on human endometrium. *American Journal of Obstetrics and Gynecology,* **102,** 192–201.

Marshall, R. J. & Jones, D. B. (1988). An immunohistochemical study of lymphoid tissue in human endometrium. *Journal of Gynecological Pathology,* **7,** 225–35.

Martel, D., Frydman, R. & Glissant, M. (1987). Scanning electron microscopy of postovulatory human endometrium in spontaneous cycles and cycles stimulated by hormone treatment. *Journal of Endocrinology,* **114,** 319–24.

Mitchell, B. S. & Peel, S. (1984). Identification of cells bearing leukocyte surface antigens in metrial gland tissue from rat: at different gestational ages, strains or parities. *Immunology,* **53,** 63–8.

Moghissi, K. S., Syner, F. N. & McBride, L. C. (1973). Contraceptive mechanism of microdose norethindrone. *Obstretrics and Gynecology,* **41,** 585–90.

More, I. A. R., Armstrong, E. M., McSeveney, D. & Chatfield, W. R. (1974). The morphogenesis and fate of the nucleolar channel system in the human endometrial glandular cell. *Journal of Ultrastructural Research,* **47,** 74–85.

More, I. A. R. & McSeveney, D. (1980). The three-dimensional structure of the nucleolar channel system in the endometrial glandular cell: serial sectioning and high voltage electron microscopic studies. *Journal of Anatomy,* **130,** 673–82.

Morris, H., Edwards, J., Tiltman, A. & Emms, M. (1985). Endometrial lymphoid tissue: an immunological study. *Journal of Clinical Pathology,* **38,** 644–52.

Murphy, C. R., Rogers, A. W. & Leeton, J. (1987). Surface ultrastructure of uterine epithelial cells in women with premature ovarian failure following steroid hormone replacement. *Acta Anatomica,* **130,** 348–50.

Murphy, C. R. & Turner, V. F. (1991). Glycocalyx carbohydrates of uterine epithelial cells increase during early pregnancy in the rat. *Journal of Anatomy,* **177,** 109–15.

Nagler, A., Lanier, L. L., Cwirla, S. & Phillips, J. H. (1989). Comparative studies of human FCRIII positive and negative natural killer cells. *Journal of Immunology*, **143**, 3183–91.

Noyes, R. W., Hertig, A. T. & Rock, J. (1950). Dating the endometrial biopsy. *Fertility and Sterility*, **1**, 3–25.

Ober, W. B. (1966). Synthetic progestogen-oestrogen preparations and endometrial morphology. *Journal of Clinical Pathology*, **19**, 138–47.

Pace, D., Morrison, L. & Bulmer, J. N. (1989). Proliferative activity in endometrial stromal granulocytes through the menstrual cycle and early pregnancy. *Journal of Clinical Pathology*, **42**, 35–9.

Peel, S., Stewart, J. J. & Bulmer, D. (1983). Experimental evidence for the bone marrow origin of granulated metrial gland cells of the mouse uterus. *Cell Tissue Research*, **33**, 647–56.

Pockley, A. G., Mowles, E. A., Stoker, R. J., Westwood, O. M. R., Chapman, M. G. & Bolton, A. E. (1988). Suppression of *in vitro* lymphocyte reactivity to phytohemagglutinin by placental protein 14. *Journal of Reproductive Immunology*, **13**, 31–9.

Rambourg, A., Harnandez, W. & LeBlond, C. P. (1969). Detection of complex carbohydrates in the Golgi apparatus of rat cells. *Journal of Cell Biology*, **40**, 395–414.

Ribbing, S. L., Hoverland, R. C. & Beauman, K. D. (1988). T cell suppressor factors play an integral role in preventing fetal rejection. *Journal of Reproductive Immunology*, **14**, 83–95.

Renechart, C. A. *et al.* (1988). *In vitro Cell Developmental Biology*, **24**, 1037–41.

Roberts, D. K., Walker, N. J. & Lavia, L. A. (1988). Ultrastructural evidence of stromal epithelial interactions in the human endometrial cycle. *American Journal of Obstetrics and Gynecology*, **158**, 854–61.

Robertson, W. B. (1984). A reappraisal of the endometrium in infertility. *Clinical Obstetrics and Gynaecology*, **11**, 209–26.

Rinehard, C. A., Lyn-Cook, B. D. & Kaufman, D. G. (1988). Gland formation from human endometrial epithelial cells *in vitro*. *In vitro Cell Developmental Biology*, **24**, 1037–41.

Sharma, V., Whitehead, M., Mason, B. *et al.* (1990). Influence of superovulation on endometrial and embryonic development. *Fertility and Sterility*, **53**, 822–9.

Sheppard, B. L. & Bonnar, J. (1980). The development of vessels of the endometrium during the menstrual cycle. In *Endometrial Bleeding and Steroidal Contraception*. Ed. E. Diczfalusy, I. S. Fraser and F. T. G. Webb, pp. 65–77, Pitman Press, Bath, England.

Smith, R. A., Seif, M. W., Rogers, A. W., Li, T. C., Dockery, P., Cooke, I. D. & Aplin, J. D. (1989). The endometrial cycle: the expression of a secretory component correlated with the luteinizing hormone peak. *Human Reproduction*, **4**, 236–42.

Smith, S. K., Abel, M. H., Kelly, R. W., Lumsden, M. A. & Baird, D. T. (1985). Uterine prostaglandins and excessive menstruation. In *Mechanisms of Menstrual Bleeding*. *Serono Symposia Publications*. Ed. D. T. Baird and E. A. Michie, pp. 241–52, Raven Press, New York.

Swahn, M. L., Johannisson, E., Daniore, V., de la Torre, B. & Bygdeman, M. (1988). The effect of RU486 administered during the proliferative and secretory phase of the cycle on the bleeding pattern, hormonal parameters and the endometrium. *Human Reproduction*, **3**, 915–21.

Szekeres-Bartho, J., Csernus, V., Hadnagy, I. & Pasca, A. S. (1983). Immuno-suppressive effect of serum progesterone during pregnancy depends on the progesterone binding capacity of the lymphocytes. *Journal of Reproductive Immunology,* **5,** 81–8.

Szekeres-Bartho, J., Autray, B., Debre, P., Andreu, G., Denver, L. & Chaouat, G. (1989). Immunoregulatory effects of a suppressor factor from healthy pregnant women's lymphocytes after progesterone induction. *Cell Immunology,* **122,** 281–94.

Terzakis, J. A. (1965). The nucleolar channel system of human endometrium. *Journal of Cell Biology,* **27,** 293–304.

Verma, V. (1983). Ultrastructural changes in human endometrium at different phases of the menstrual cycle and their functional significance. *Gynecological and Obstetric Investigations,* **15,** 193–212.

Wegmann, T. G. (1988). Maternal T cells promote placental trophoblast growth and prevent spontaneous abortion. *Immunology Letters,* **17,** 297–302.

Wienke, E. C., Cavazos, F., Hall, D. G. & Lucas, F. V. (1968). Ultrastructure of the human endometrial stromal cell during the menstrual cycle. *American Journal of Obstetrics and Gynecology,* **102,** 65–77.

Wynn, R. M. (1977). Histology and ultrastructures of the human endometrium. In *Biology of the Uterus.* pp. 308–30, Plenum Press, New York and London.

Wilborn, W. H. & Flowers, C. E. (1984). Cellular mechanisms for endometrial conservation during menstrual bleeding. *Seminars in Reproductive Endocrinology,* **2,** 307–42.

Yuzpe, A. A., Thurlow, H. J., Rarazy, I. & Leyshon, J. I. (1974). Postcoital contraception – a pilot study. *Journal of Reproductive Medicine,* **13,** 53–8.

6

Products of endometrial differentiation

J. D. APLIN

Introduction

Precisely timed changes occur in the histoarchitecture of human endometrium under the influence of steroid hormones during the menstrual cycle (Noyes *et al.*, 1950; Dallenbach-Hellweg, 1981; Li *et al.*, 1987; Dockery *et al.*, 1988; Buckley & Fox, 1989). Interest has grown in the control of gene expression in the target tissue by steroid hormones, the contribution of non-steroidal signalling molecules, the contribution of cellular interactions within the tissue and the biochemical basis of the structural changes engendered (Aplin, 1989). Ultimately, the aim of biochemical analysis in endometrium must be to elucidate the function of the tissue in relation to pregnancy (Bell, 1990), including preimplantation interaction with the embryo and corpus luteum, control of implantation (Denker, 1990; Glasser *et al.*, 1991), and postimplantational support of the conceptus (Aplin, 1991*a*). Since the demonstration in rodent endometrium of a 1-day period of receptivity to embryo implantation (for review see Psychoyos, 1986; Glasser *et al.*, 1991), criteria have been sought that might be used to define and detect a receptive state in women. This aim, yet to be fulfilled, would have the practical benefit of defining appropriate treatment regimens in assisted fertility programmes, and resolving uncertainty in the diagnosis of infertility associated with defective implantation.

Histology provides a convenient frame of reference for a review of endometrial biochemistry, since the location of a molecule is of paramount importance in relation to its function. Epithelial secretions are relevant to gamete transport and peri-implantational events; the stromal compartment is particularly important in the first few weeks of pregnancy when placental morphogenesis is occurring. At this time haemochorial contact is incomplete but access of trophoblast to the maternal vascular compartment is of critical importance from the earliest phases of implantation (Aplin, 1991*a*). Thus knowledge of the pattern of hormonal regulation and spatio-temporal distribution of a molecule may aid in identifying its function.

Another requirement of the tissue is to act as host to immune cells and components which guard against infection. Changes in the consistency of cervical mucus, which in much of the cycle provides a barrier to infection of the upper tract, give rise to changing immunological demands on the endometrium. Later, menstruation presents the possibility of direct access of pathogenic organisms to the stroma and vasculature. In pregnancy, the system is required to tolerate the fetal allograft while continuing to combat infection.

These multiple functional requirements often give rise to uncertainty in interpretation of biochemical data: does a given cytokine function in relation to the immune or the reproductive function of the tissue? If the latter, is the molecule carrying an autocrine (addressed to the endometrium) or paracrine (addressed to the embryo) signal? How are multiple functions combined within the epithelial secretory repertoire? Such considerations can complicate design of experiments which already present great ethical and practical problems. *In vitro* models of early implantational events are becoming available and will assume increasing importance. Comparative studies of endometrium in animals, especially those in which implantation is interstitial, will continue to be valuable (Glasser *et al.*, 1991). Although the focus of this review will be on human endometrium and its preparation for pregnancy, data from other species will be considered where relevant.

Signalling molecules

The ovarian steroid hormones oestrogen (E) and progesterone (P) are necessary for reproductive function. Advances in molecular genetics have led to increased understanding of steroid receptors and the mechanisms whereby transcriptional activation of target genes occurs (Beato, 1989). Indeed, the identification within genomic sequences of sites for the binding of steroid hormone–receptor complexes now provides a means of *de novo* identification of activated products. A second potentially powerful approach to identifying steroid-activated products involves the use of subtraction libraries of cDNA made from endometrium exposed to different steroid regimens (Misrahi, Atger & Milgrom, 1987).

The distribution of E and P receptors (ER, PR) has been studied intensively in endometrial cell populations (Press *et al.*, 1984; Bergeron *et al.*, 1988; Glasser *et al.*, 1991). ER levels are high in both epithelium and stroma in the proliferative phase and induce transcription of the PR (Savouret *et al.*, 1991). Thus E stimulates proliferation as well as preparing the tissue to respond to P. By the late proliferative phase PR levels are high in the epithelium, with lower levels in the stroma. High levels of PR occur in both tissue compartments in the early secretory phase. At this time ER is still present in the epithelium but decreases in the stroma, suggesting that continuing oestrogenic stimulation may not be necessary for stromal PR expression. The PR concentration declines in the epithelium from mid to late secretory phase, but high levels continue to be detectable in the stroma. Receptor studies also provide a rationale for different responses to steroids seen in the superficial (functional) and basal parts of the tissue (Bergeron *et al.*, 1988; Padykula, 1989); thus, for example, ER is apparent in both epithelium and stroma of the basalis in the late secretory phase, presumably in readiness for post-menstrual regeneration.

It is perhaps surprising to discover that growth factors/cytokines also seem to play a role in endometrial differentiation. However, an increasing body of evidence (Brigstock *et al.*, 1989; Tabibzadeh, 1991; Findlay & Salamonsen, 1991) points to this conclusion. Thus, for example, EGF is a potent mitogen in the endometrium of ovariectomized mice, and antibody to EGF inhibits this effect (Nelson *et al.*, 1991). Synthesis and secretion of lactoferrin, normally a response to oestrogen (see below), also occurs in response to EGF (Nelson *et al.*, 1991). EGF binding sites have been demonstrated in human endometrium in both stromal and epithelial compartments (Chegini, Rao & Sanfilippo, 1986) and EGF itself is detectable immunocytochemically (Hofmann *et al.*, 1991). Furthermore, EGF can promote trophoblast differentiation (for review see Aplin, 1991a). CSF-1 is produced in murine endometrial epithelium and acts on its receptor (*c-fms*) in the placenta (Pollard, 1990); in the human, both CSF-1 and *c-fms* are present in endometrium, levels of the growth factor increasing in the secretory phase (Kauma *et al.*, 1991). Insulin-like growth factors may play an important role in utero-placental function in several species (for review see Fazleabas, Bell & Verhage, 1991a). Other factors detected in animals including PDGF, acidic and basic FGF, TGFα and β and IL-6 have also been suggested as local regulators in the human endometrium and conceptus (Findlay & Salamonsen, 1991; Tabibzadeh, 1991; Giudice, 1994). The principle is well established, through studies of the interferon-like molecule ovine trophoblast protein-1, that embryo-derived signals can influence endometrial metabolism (Vallet *et al.*, 1987).

Growth factors can act as intermediaries in the uterine response to steroids as well as in paracrine interactions with the placenta. This may be relevant to the fact that direct steroid hormone-receptor-mediated activation of transcription (Beato, 1989) cannot apply to all gene products. The kinetics of the response vary enormously. Some progesterone-activated products (e.g. secretory mucin) increase within 1–2 days of exposure to the hormone, while others (e.g. α2-PEG) may take as long as a week and do not correlate with expression of steroid receptors. Much remains to be discovered about the mechanism whereby certain genes (e.g. for stromal cell laminin) are activated in a cell- and tissue-specific manner.

Epithelial products

High molecular weight secretory glycoconjugates in women

Uterine fluid contains a mixture of plasma-derived components and endometrial secretions, many of the latter deriving from the apical secretory activity of glandular and luminal epithelial cells. This provides the environment into which sperm migrate, and that of the peri-implantation embryo. There is some evidence in animals to support the concept that uterine fluid provides an advantageous environment for the embryo (Fischer *et al.*, 1990). The composition in pregnancy is also of interest because embryos produce signals for the endometrium or corpus luteum (Vallet *et al.*, 1987; Sharif *et al.*, 1989; Thatcher *et al.*, 1989).

The epithelial secretions are carbohydrate-rich and can be monitored histologically by staining with PAS or lectins (Aplin, 1991*b*). Glycan biosynthesis and epithelial secretory activity are present in the proliferative phase. On exposure to P, a rapid increase occurs in the biosynthetic capacity of the epithelium, with the appearance of subnuclear masses of glycogen, enlarged mitochondria, the nuclear channel system, very prominent Golgi stacks and large numbers of secretory vesicles in the apical cytoplasm (Dockery *et al.*, 1988). This gives rise to a greatly increased secretory output including glycogen, which originates in the cytoplasm and appears to escape from cells by an apocrine route, and secretory glycoconjugates, which are presumably transferred from Golgi to secretory vesicles and thence to the lumen by exocytosis.

Mucins are quantitatively significant in the secretory process. The polymorphic epithelial mucin (MUC-1) is present in epithelial cells, and, to a restricted extent, in gland secretions in the proliferative phase; there is an increase in the secretory phase (Aplin & Graham, unpublished observations). The MUC-1 gene has been cloned (Gendler *et al.*, 1990) and the deduced amino acid sequence (Fig. 1) features a large central domain of up to 80 tandem repeat cassettes of 20 amino acids, the VNTR (variable number tandem repeat) region. Variations in the number of repeats account for the polymorphism, individuals inheriting different alleles from each parent. As a result, the polypeptide can vary in size from 120–250 kDa. However, MUC-1 is known as a 'small mucin' to distinguish it from larger molecules such as cervical mucin.

Near the C-terminus of MUC-1 is a *trans*-membrane sequence, followed by a short hydrophilic cytoplasmic domain. This molecule exists in a membrane-spanning form as well as a secretory form, the latter perhaps released as a result of proteolytic trimming. Immunolocalization studies reveal a dense array of mucin epitopes in close association with the apical cell surface of both glandular and luminal epithelial cells in endometrium (Seif *et al.*, 1989*a*; Campbell *et al.*, 1988; Hey *et al.*, 1994; and c.f. Fig. 2).

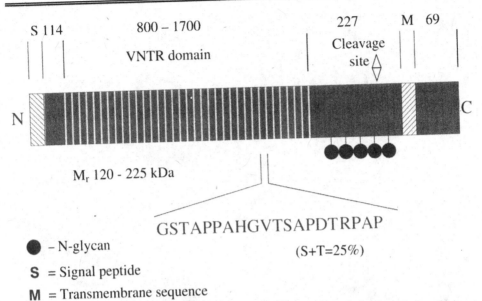

Fig. 1. Diagrammatic view of the core protein sequence of the human polymorphic epithelial mucin (MUC-1). (Based on Gendler *et al.*, 1990.) 'Cleavage site' indicates a postulated site of proteolytic conversion into a non-membrane-anchored form of the molecule.

The VNTR contains 5 serine or threonine residues with multiple O-glycosylation. In addition there are five potential N-glycosylation sites C-terminal to the VNTR, and the same domain contains a serine/glycine-rich sequence that may bear the addition of O-linked glycosaminoglycan. The addition of carbohydrate may increase the Mr to as much as 400 kDa, with considerable microheterogeneity. MUC-1 is expressed in numerous epithelial tissues, and the pattern of glycosylation varies, with tissue and pathology. Glycosylation in the endometrium varies with the stage of the cycle; indeed certain terminal sugar structures can be used as very sensitive indices of differentiation (Aplin, 1991*b*).

Probing of the endometrium with a range of lectins (for review see Aplin, 1991*b*) shows a large variety of glycans in the epithelium and its associated secretions. A general increase of secretory glycans follows the appearance of a greatly enlarged secretory apparatus under the influence of progesterone (Dockery *et al.*, 1988), but many structures are conserved in all phases of the cycle. Thus, for example, terminal sialylation as detected by the lectins from *Sambucus nigra* (α2-6-linkage) or Maackia amurensis (α2-3-linkage) is detectable in gland cells in the proliferative phase and to an increased extent in the secretory phase. Interestingly, however, the sialoglycan epitopes detected by monoclonal antibodies B72.3 (NeuAcα2-6GalNAc; Thor *et al.*, 1987; Hanisch *et al.*, 1989; Soisson *et al.*, 1989) and D9B1 (sialokeratan sulphate; Smith *et al.*, 1989; Hoadley, Seif & Aplin, 1990; Fig. 2) are

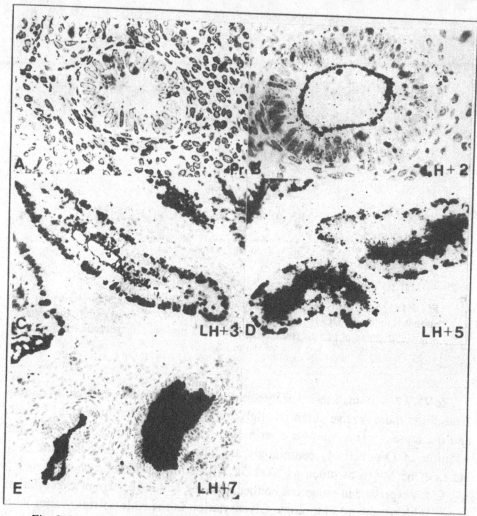

Fig. 2. Immunoperoxidase localisation of sialokeratan sulphate in endometrial gland cells using the monoclonal antibody D9B1: A proliferative phase, B 2 days after the LH peak (LH + 2), C LH + 3, D LH + 5, E LH + 7. The section shown in A has stronger counterstaining to reveal an unstained gland and surrounding stroma. In B a rim of immunopositivity is detected at the apical surface of the glandular epithelium. One day later C heavy immunodeposits have accumulated in the gland cell bases and there are positive vesicular structures in the apical cytoplasm. During the following 2 days, the material is secreted into the gland lumens, with continuing production in the cells D. By 7 days after the LH peak, secretions are maximal, but production is halted E. (Reproduced with permission from Smith *et al.*, 1989.)

specific to the secretory phase. Both are associated with the small mucin fraction, as is the keratan sulphate epitope recognized by antibody 5D4 (for review see Aplin, 1991*b*). The D9B1 epitope is dependent on P for its production but not secretion (Graham *et al.*, 1991). Taken together, this suggests that two processes affect MUC-1 as secretory endometrium differentiates: an increase in production of the polypeptide (probably controlled at the transcriptional level by progesterone; Lancaster *et al.*, 1991; Hey *et al.*, 1994) and specific changes in the pattern of Golgi-associated terminal glycosylation.

Production of the sialoepitope recognized by D9B1 has been examined in relation to the luteinizing hormone peak in normal cycles (Smith *et al.*, 1989) and shown to be at a maximum at the expected time of implantation (Fig. 2). Luminal epithelial cells have a dense apical glycocalyx (Jansen *et al.*, 1985; Campbell *et al.*, 1988) and changes in charge density or sugar composition could be related to implantation (Jansen *et al.*, 1985; Anderson *et al.*, 1986; Johannisson, 1991). Indeed, in the mouse the blood group H type I structure (Galβ1-3[Fucα1-2]GlcNAc) may be involved in blastocyst attachment (Kimber, Lindenberg & Lundblad, 1988; Kimber & Lindenberg, 1990; Lindenberg *et al.*, 1988). This is interesting in the light of the involvement of cell surface glycan in the interaction of platelets and neutrophils with the vascular endothelium at sites of injury and inflammation (Brandley, Swiedler & Robbins, 1990). There is also evidence that small mucins or their glycan structures (Singhal, Fohn & Hakomori, 1991) can fulfil immune adjuvant roles.

Endometrial secretions also contain a larger mucin molecule ($M_r > 2 \times 10^6$) with features in common with other mucins such as that found in respiratory secretions (Aplin and Sheehan, unpublished). This molecule is sialylated and sulphated (van Kooij *et al.*, 1982), but little structural characterization has been attempted.

High molecular weight secretory glycoconjugates in other species

Verhage and coworkers (Murray *et al.*, 1985; Murray, Verhage & Jaffe, 1986; Verhage *et al.*, 1988) have identified a secretory glycoprotein in cats that shows features reminiscent of MUC-1 including polymorphism, high M_r (330 kDa) and an apical secretory pathway. This product, however, is stimulated by oestrogen and inhibited by progesterone, and it has been suggested that it may play a role in sperm transport or capacitation. Pregnant ewes also produce a group of high molecular weight basic proteins that have been associated with an immunosuppressive function (Hansen *et al.*, 1987a).

Cell culture experiments indicate the presence of a range of polyanionic glycoconjugates amongst the apical secretions of endometrial epithelial cells in various species. Glasser and coworkers have established conditions for the propagation of rodent (Glasser *et al.*, 1988) and rabbit (Glasser *et al.*, 1991; Mani, Carson & Glasser, 1992) epithelial cells, and they have shown that, after the cells reach confluence on a porous substrate, normal polarization occurs enabling an analysis of both apical and basal secretions. As expected, nutrient uptake is largely from the cell base. Amongst the apical secretions of rabbit epithelial cells is found a sialosulphomucin of $M_r > 230$ kDa, i.e. in the small mucin range (Mani *et al.*, 1992). However, unlike MUC-1, this product lacks lactosaminoglycan. The secretion was reduced 3-fold by E or P treatment. In addition, the rabbit cells secrete hyaluronan from their apical surface, and this process may be stimulated up to 1.5-fold by either steroid. Sulphation by endometrial microsomes is increased in rabbits after treatment with oestrogen and diminished after progesterone (Isemura, Munakata & Yosizawa, 1981; Munakata, Isemura & Yosizawa, 1985).

In cultured polarized rat epithelial cells (Carson *et al.*, 1988) the major apical secretory glycans are keratan sulphate (sulphated lactosaminoglycan) and heparan sulphate, each conjugated to its own core protein. Production of each is stimulated by E. In mice, lactosaminoglycans are also present in epithelial secretions, and Babiarz & Hathaway (1988) have demonstrated that terminal modifications including fucosylation and sialylation occur under hormonal control.

Other human epithelial products

A major secretory product of late secretory phase endometrial epithelial cells is a homodimeric glycoprotein of 56 kDa (for review see Bell, 1986) called variously pregnancy-associated endometrial $\alpha 2$-globulin ($\alpha 2$-PEG), placental protein 14 (a misnomer) and progestogen-associated endometrial protein. Data from cDNA sequencing predicts a polypeptide of 18 787 Da (180 residues containing an 18 residue signal peptide) with three potential N-glycosylation sites and four cysteine residues. The amino acid sequence is highly homologous to the β-lactoglobulins, including conservation of the cysteines (Julkunen, Seppala & Janne, 1988*a*). However, the mRNA has been detected only in secretory endometrium, decidua and seminal plasma, and the human glycoprotein, unlike its homologues in other species, is not found in milk. Analysis of endometrial cDNA species by PCR amplification using primers from the non-coding 3′ and 5′ regions of $\alpha 2$-PEG has shown that complex alternative splicing of pre-mRNA can occur, two products of which contain deletions that would give rise to shorter forms of the polypeptide (Garde, Bell & Eperon, 1991). However, there is as yet no evidence that such forms are produced.

Production of $\alpha 2$-PEG begins in the mid-secretory phase (6 days after the LH peak) and increases in the late secretory phase, when very high concentrations (1 mg . ml^{-1}) can be found in uterine fluid. Significant amounts of the mRNA can still be detected on day 3 of the proliferative phase, but by day 6 the mRNA is undetectable and protein is confined to a few basal glands (Waites *et al.*, 1988*a*; Julkunen *et al.*, 1990). Thus regulation of production is not a straightforward result of the action of P on gland cell receptors.

In the first trimester synthesis continues to increase and PP14 levels in maternal serum reach maximum levels during weeks 8–10 (Bell, 1986). High concentrations are found in amniotic fluid (Bell, 1986). Although no function has been identified for α2-PEG, it is possible that it may act as a binding protein for ligand transport to the fetus in early pregnancy.

An important feature of the immunological function of the endometrium is the presence in gland secretions of IgA, which is transferred by epithelial cells from the surrounding interstitium. This process is mediated by complexation of IgA with secretory component (SC); the complex then binds to receptors on the basal cell surface which mediate transfer to the apical compartment. SC is detectable by immunohistochemistry in basal glands through the cycle, while in the functional layer a cycle-dependent variation is observed with low levels of expression in proliferative and early secretory phase, and elevated levels in mid- and late secretory phase (Suzuki *et al.*, 1984). This behaviour is in keeping with the need to maintain a protective function in the peri-implantation phase of pregnancy.

The 27 kDa human heat shock protein (hsp27) is also a cyclically-regulated product. Hsp27 is oestrogen-stimulated in mammary carcinoma cells. In the late proliferative phase it appears in the glandular epithelium of the endometrium, while in the luminal epithelium appearance is delayed until the mid-secretory phase (Ciocca *et al.*, 1983). Decidual stromal cells also express hsp27, which has strong homologies to the low molecular weight heat shock proteins of *Drosophila* and the mammalian α-crystallins (Fuqua, Blum-Salingaros & McGuire, 1989).

Secretory glycoproteins in other species

Endometrial secretory products have been isolated in species with both interstitial and non-interstitial implantation. In the latter, uterine fluid plays a vital role in providing nutrients to the conceptus (Roberts & Bazer, 1988; Aplin, 1989). It is possible that certain functional parallels may exist notwithstanding the divergence of placental anatomy. Thus endometrial secretions play an important nutritional role for the conceptus in epitheliochorial (non-invasive) placentation as, for example, in the pig, sheep, cow and horse. A similar function may occur transiently in the pre-haemochorial phases of pregnancy in women. It is also possible that regulated proteolysis is required in the uterine environment in non-invasive as well as invasive types of implantation. Furthermore, the immunological function of uterine fluid is retained across species.

Uteroferrin (Simmen, Baumbach & Roberts, 1988) is a progesterone-dependent secretory product of porcine endometrial epithelium. As with human α2-PEG, prolonged exposure to progesterone is required to achieve maximal biosynthesis. Uteroferrin transports iron to the developing fetus. A glycoprotein of the same family, lactotransferrin, is an oestrogen-induced secretory product of murine endometrial epithelial cells (Teng *et al.*, 1989). The human homologue is also detectable in the uterus. Functions may include iron transport and bacteriocidal activity.

Uteroglobin is a progesterone-induced secretory protein of rabbit endometrial epithelium (Cato & Beato, 1985). It is thought to bind progesterone, but the functional significance of this is unknown.

The major progesterone-responsive basic glycoproteins secreted into the sheep uterus are members of the serpin superfamily of serine protease inhibitors (Ing & Roberts, 1989). These are two closely related products of 55 and 57 kDa with strong sequence similarities to primate α1-antitrypsin and α1-antichymotrypsin; indeed α1-antitrypsin has been detected in uterine fluid in women (Fazleabas, Khan-Dawood & Dawood, 1987). However, no protease inhibitory activity has yet been demonstrated for the sheep uterine milk serpins. Pig endometrial secretions also contain a progesterone-dependent plasmin/trypsin protease inhibitor (Fazleabas *et al.*, 1985) and antileukoproteinase, an inhibitor of the serine proteases cathepsin G and elastase (Farmer, Fliss & Simmen, 1990).

A cat endometrial secretory product, also progesterone-dependent, has been cloned and sequenced and found to be homologous to the cysteine protease cathepsin L (Jaffe *et al.*, 1989; Li *et al.*, 1990). This protein has collagenolytic and elastolytic activities. Placentation in cats is endotheliochorial, and this maternal protease may be required for penetration of the endometrium. In rabbits there is protease activity at implantation (Denker, 1982), and in the human trophoblast-derived protease activity is clearly important in placental morphogenesis (for review see Aplin, 1991*a*). In rats, prothrombin enters the uterus and is activated as part of the transudation of plasma proteins in response to oestrogen (Henrikson *et al.*, 1990). Thrombin may play a role, possibly as a mitogen, in the tissue response to steroidal stimulation.

An important oestrogen-stimulated secretory product in the uterine epithelium of the rat is the glycoprotein complement component C3 which comprises two subunits of 115 and 65 kDa (Brown *et al.*, 1990). C3 is a member of the α2 macroglobulin family. Biosynthesis of C3 *in vivo* is blocked at transcription by progesterone. Whether the presence of C3 reflects complement-mediated target cell killing and opsonization in the uterine lumen, or a reproduction-associated function, is unknown.

Biochemistry of stromal differentiation

The endometrial stroma fulfils three main functions: 'autocrine' support of the differentiating epithelium; paracrine support for the implanting conceptus; and provision of a physical environment within which the conceptus can gain access to the maternal vascular supply.

Endometrial epithelial cells in culture lose the ability to respond to either the mitogenic or differentiative effects of steroids. By analogy with other steroid-dependent tissues such as the breast (Haslam & Counterman, 1991) it is probable that the proliferative and secretory phase stroma provides signals for epithelial differentiation. This is also consistent with observations that epithelial differentiation in embryos is dependent on mesenchyme (Cunha *et al.*, 1985). In rodents, the same process later occurs in reverse: the epithelium releases a substance, possibly a prostaglandin, that stimulates the onset of decidualization at the implantation site (Glasser *et al.*, 1991). In women, by contrast, decidual differentiation occurs spontaneously in late secretory phase stromal cells in non-conception cycles. Human stromal cells in culture also differentiate when stimulated with progesterone (Bell *et al.*, 1991), suggesting that there is no need for an epithelial signal to the stroma unless it were acting to inhibit this process from occurring too early. Biochemical attributes of the late secretory phase stroma are of considerable clinical interest and are much better characterized than those of the early cycle. One aim of research in this area is to utilise biochemical methods to analyse early events (i.e. those occurring in advance of overt decidual change) in the preparation of the stroma for pregnancy.

Soluble secretions

A major progesterone-dependent product of the primate endometrial stromal cell is an insulin-like growth factor binding protein (IGF-BP1), also known as α1-PEG and PP12 (Waites *et al.*, 1988b; Julkunen *et al.*, 1988b). This is a single subunit protein (25 kDa) that appears in endometrial stromal cells in the mid-secretory phase, becoming increasingly abundant in the late secretory phase. Five different phosphorylated isoforms are produced, and progestogen increases the level of phosphorylation (Frost & Tseng, 1991). Expression of IGFBP-1 occurs primarily, but not exclusively, in morphologically differentiated stromal cells (Waites *et al.*, 1988b). Small amounts of IGFBP-1 are also detected in epithelial cells in the mid-secretory phase (Waites *et al.*, 1988b). In the baboon the epithelium is a major site of production, synthesis occurring locally in stromal cells at the implantation site from day 25 of pregnancy (Fazleabas *et al.*, 1991a). These observations provide circumstantial evidence of a paracrine interaction with the conceptus (see Bell, this volume). An association of the stromal product with extracellular matrix has been observed (Waites, James & Bell, 1989), and it is notable that it contains the RGD sequence which is associated with integrin-mediated cell adhesion (Julkunen *et al.*, 1988b). The molecule may compete with cell surface receptors for binding of IGFs (Rutanen, Pekonen & Makinen, 1988).

Two other members of the family, IGFBP-2 (31 kDa with one RGD motif) and IGFBP-3 (29 kDa and larger glycoforms) have also been reported in human

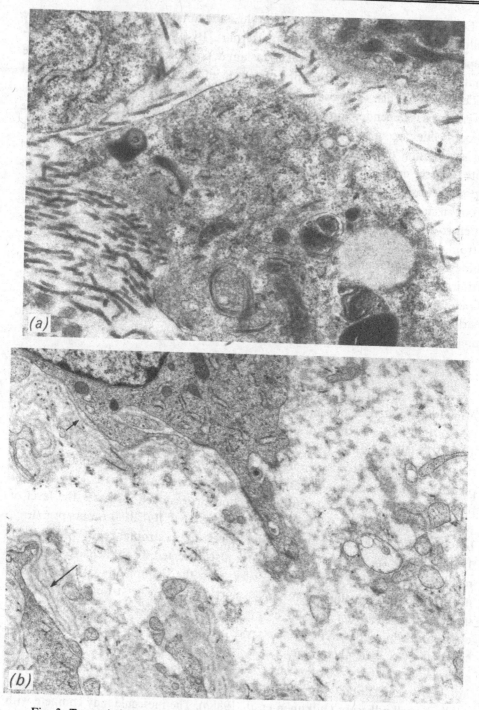

Fig. 3. Transmission electron micrographs of endometrial stroma in (a) early secretory phase and (b) late first trimester of pregnancy. Note the bundle of aligned uniform diameter collagen fibrils closely associated with the stromal cell membrane

endometrium (Giudice *et al.*, 1991). Both are detectable in proliferative phase extracts, and both increase in the secretory phase. In cultured stromal cells, secretion of IGFBP-2 and IGFBP-3 is stimulated by E and P treatment. They are also secreted by an endometrial adenocarcinoma cell line, Hec-1A. Curiously, no IGFBP-1 was detected by Giudice *et al.* (1991) in stromal cell culture medium even after treatment with E and P.

Another candidate for paracrine interaction with the embryo is prolactin (PRL), a progesterone-dependent secretory product of the late secretory phase endometrial stroma (for review see Bell, 1986; Aplin, 1989). Human myometrium also produces PRL (Gellerson *et al.*, 1991). PRL, like IGFBP-1, is found in amniotic fluid into which it is assumed to diffuse via the chorioamnion. Although uterine PRL is identical to its pituitary-derived counterpart, the corresponding mRNAs differ as a result of the use of two different transcriptional start sites (DiMattia *et al.*, 1990). The result of this is that uterine PRL is under the control of a different promoter region and shows a completely different pattern of control of expression.

Stromal extracellular matrix (ECM)

The proliferative and early secretory phase ECM is dense and fibrillar with many intercellular spaces containing bundles of 20 or 30 uniform diameter banded collagen fibrils (Aplin & Jones, 1989; Fig. 3(*a*)). Collagen types I, III, and V are present, together with the microfibrillar collagen type VI (Fig. 4(*a*)), which surrounds and forms non-covalent interconnections between the large fibril bundles and structures such as glands, nerves and vessels (Aplin, Charlton & Ayad, 1988; for review see Aplin, 1989). Tenascin is restricted to the periglandular stroma (Vollmer *et al.*, 1990).

In contrast, decidual stroma contains a radically remodelled ECM in which few bundles of striated collagen are present (Fig. 3(*b*)); instead, single fibrils are found which vary in diameter and which run anisotropically through the tissue. Thus there is a decrease in the overall concentration of fibrillar collagen, and type VI collagen is lost except from the walls of vessels (Fig. 4(*b*)). Meanwhile the decidual cells become encapsulated in a basal lamina containing collagen type IV, laminin and heparan sulphate proteoglycan (Aplin *et al.*, 1988; Aplin, 1989; Aplin & Jones, 1989; Fig. 3(*b*)). Fibronectin persists from proliferative phase to decidual stroma, but along with the major collagens it undergoes alterations

Caption for fig. 3 (*cont.*).
in (*a*). The decidual extracellular matrix (*b*) contains amorphous material and few fibrils or bundles. Note the cell processes and pericellular basement membrane material (arrows) which are not seen in (*a*). (Adapted with permission from Aplin & Jones, 1989.)

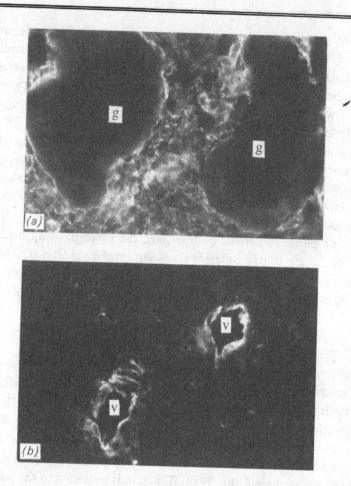

Fig. 4. Immunofluorescence of type VI collagen in proliferative phase endometrium (*a*) and late first trimester decidua (*b*). Two glands (g, lumens) are shown in (*a*) with a fibrillar pattern of staining in the periglandular stroma and surrounding vessels. This immunoreactivity disappears in pregnancy (*b*), leaving only the vessel-associated staining (v, vessel lumens). (Adapted with permission from Aplin & Jones, 1989.)

in distribution in parallel with the change in interstitial architecture (Aplin & Jones, 1989).

Little is known about the mechanism of this remodelling process (Aplin, 1990). However, it is clear that late secretory phase endometrial stroma exhibits aspects of decidual ECM: for example, some cells have a partial or complete basal lamina (Faber *et al.*, 1986; Aplin *et al.*, 1988). In the mid-secretory phase there is the stromal oedema familiar to the histologist (Dockery *et al.*, 1990), and this is correlated with local breakdown of collagen VI (Aplin *et al.*, 1988) and the disappearance of periglandular tenascin (Vollmer *et al.*, 1990). Even in the early secretory phase, preparation for decidualization is detectable since cytoplasmic and pericellular deposits of laminin are seen by immunohistochemistry in the stromal cells (Faber *et al.*, 1986). There are strong similarities between rodent and human stroma in their patterns of ECM remodelling in preparation for pregnancy (Aplin, 1989; Glasser *et al.*, 1991; Mulholland *et al.*, 1992).

Immune and vascular cells

Two important aspects of endometrial stromal function are the bone marrow-derived cells and the vasculature. Relatively little is known of the biochemistry of the cell populations. The type of bone marrow-derived cells in the stroma varies during the menstrual cycle: levels of T cells and macrophages remain constant while increasing numbers of large granular lymphocytes populate the stroma in the late secretory phase or first trimester decidua (Starkey, Clover & Rees, 1991). Mast cells are also present (Drudy, Sheppard & Bonnar, 1991). In addition to their function in defence against pathogens, these cells could play a role in intercellular signalling or tissue remodelling.

The endometrial vasculature provides a striking example of non-pathological angiogenesis, supplies humoral signals to and from the tissue and provides the implanting embryo with access to maternal nutrients. Angiogenic stimuli are present, though they have not been widely studied (Rogers *et al.*, 1992; Charnock-Jones *et al.*, 1993). Steroid hormones influence the blood vessels (Akerlund, 1991) and advanced muscularization of small arteries has been observed in artificially stimulated cycles (Seif *et al.*, 1992). Hyaluronan (HA) degradation products have been implicated as angiogenic agents (West *et al.*, 1985) and HA has been detected in rabbit (Mani *et al.*, 1992), mouse (Carson, Dutt & Tang, 1987) and pig (Ashworth, Fliss & Bazer, 1990) uterus. Polypeptide growth factors have also been implicated in this process (discussed by Guidice, 1994). The vascular differentiation that occurs during (pseudo) decidualization (Buckley & Fox, 1989) has not been investigated at a molecular level.

There is much interest in the possible role of platelet activating factor (PAF) in pregnancy (O'Neill, 1991). PAF is produced by blastocysts of several species and bone marrow-derived cells. It is also present in endometrial stromal cells in culture where it is regulated by P (Alecozay *et al.*, 1989). PAF may be responsible for a mild thrombocytopenia in the first week of pregnancy in women; its reproductive function is unclear, though it may act as an autocrine growth factor for the embryo (O'Neill, 1991).

Assessment and pathology: the biochemistry of defective endometrial differentiation

Biochemical markers are now available for endometrium in different parts of the secretory phase (Bell, 1990). Components that have been timed in relation to ovulation include the small mucin-associated sialoglycans D9B1 (Smith *et al.*, 1989; Fig. 2) and B72.3 (Thor *et al.*, 1987; our unpublished results) which appear in the glandular epithelium 2–3 days after the LH peak and reach maximal levels in the peri-implantation phase of the cycle. Alpha2-PEG (Waites *et al.*, 1988*a*) appears in the mid secretory phase, but is primarily a late-secretory phase marker of gland cell activity. The functional significance of these components is unknown, but it seems likely that early post-ovulatory assessment of the target tissue response to ovarian stimulation would provide a valuable tool in assisted reproduction. Ultimately, biochemical methods might define the receptive phase of the tissue. Switching on of hormonally activated gene products might be detected some days in advance of the receptive phase. For example, immunohistochemistry can be used at days LH+3 to LH+5 to predict the likely production of the D9B1 sialoglycan at day LH+7 (Smith *et al.*, 1989).

This information is already providing new insights into endometrial responses in infertility investigations and in assisted reproduction. Fazleabas *et al.* (1991*b*) have confirmed earlier findings that high doses of clomiphene citrate decrease production of α2-PEG in luteal phase endometrium. In endometrium with glandular-stromal asynchrony, decreased production was also observed. Manners (1990) has shown atypical patterns of endometrial protein (decreased α2-PEG, increased hsp27) in stimulated cycles, and in one-third of the patients the histological findings were normal. Several studies (Seif, Aplin & Buckley, 1989*b*; Seif *et al.*, 1989*c*; 1992; Graham *et al.*, 1990, 1991; Critchley *et al.*, 1991) indicate that late steps in glycosylation of secretory mucins including sialylation and sulphation are sensitive indices of epithelial differentiation (Aplin, 1991*b*). In patients with unexplained infertility, glycosylation of secretory mucin was found to be reduced compared to a normal fertile group (Graham *et al.*, 1990; Klentzeris *et al.*, 1991). Indeed, secretory phase endometrium considered histologically normal often demonstrates abnormalities of glycosylation. These promising observations suggest that biochemical indices of differentiation will provide useful diagnostic information in future clinical applications.

Acknowledgements

I am grateful to Dr Ros Graham for Fig. 2 and Dr Carolyn Jones for Fig. 3 and to Dr Mourad Seif and Dr Steve Campbell for constructive criticism.

References

Akerlund, M. (1991). Functions of blood vessels relative to implantation. *Clinical Obstetrics and Gynaecology*, **5.1**, 15–23.

Alecozay, A. A., Casslen, B. G., Riehl, R. M. *et al.* (1989). Platelet-activating factor in human luteal phase endometrium. *Biology of Reproduction*, **41**, 578–86.

Anderson, T. L., Olson, G. E. & Hoffman, L. H. (1986). Stage-specific alterations in the apical membrane glycoproteins of endometrial epithelial cells related to implantation in rabbits. *Biology of Reproduction*, **34**, 701–20.

Aplin, J. D., Charlton, A. K. & Ayad, S. (1988). An immunohistochemical study of human endometrial extracellular matrix during the menstrual cycle and first trimester of pregnancy. *Cell Tissue Research*, **253**, 235–40.

Aplin, J. D. (1989). Cellular biochemistry of the endometrium. In *Biology of the Uterus*. Ed. R. M. Wynn and W. P. Jollie, pp. 89–129, Plenum Press, New York.

Aplin, J. D. & Jones, C. J. P. (1989). Extracellular matrix in endometrium and decidua. In *Placenta as a Model and Source*. Ed. O. Genbacev, A. Klopper and R. Beaconsfield, pp. 115–128, Plenum Press, New York.

Aplin, J. D. (1991*a*). Implantation, trophoblast differentiation and haemochorial placentation: mechanistic evidence *in vivo* and *in vitro*. *Journal of Cell Science*, **99**, 681–92.

Aplin, J. D. (1991*b*). Glycans as biochemical markers of human endometrial secretory differentiation. *Journal of Reproduction and Fertility*, **91**, 525–41.

Ashworth, C. J., Fliss, M. F. V. & Bazer, F. W. (1990). Evidence for steroid control of a putative angiogenic factor in the porcine uterus. *Journal of Endocrinology*, **125**, 15–19.

Babiarz, B. S. & Hathaway, H. J. (1988). Hormonal control of the expression of antibody-defined lactosaminoglycans in the mouse uterus. *Biology of Reproduction*, **39**, 699–706.

Beato, M. (1989). Gene regulation by steroid hormones. *Cell*, **56**, 335–44.

Bell, S. C. (1986). Secretory endometrial and decidual proteins: studies and clinical significance of a maternally derived group of pregnancy-associated serum proteins. *Human Reproduction*, **1**, 129–43.

Bell, S. C. (1990). Assessment of endometrial differentiation and function. *British Medical Bulletin*, **46**, 720–32.

Bell, S. C., Jackson, J. A., Ashmore, J., Zhu, H. H. & Tseng, L. (1991). Regulation of insulin-like growth factor binding protein 1 synthesis and secretion by progestin and relaxin in long term cultures of endometrial stromal cells. *Journal of Clinical Endocrinology Metabolism*, **72**, 1014–24.

Bergeron, C., Ferenczy, A., Toft, D. O., Schneider, W. & Shyamala, G. (1988). Immunocytochemical study of progesterone receptors in the human endometrium during the menstrual cycle. *Laboratory Investigations*, **59**, 862–9.

Brandley, B. K., Swiedler, S. J. & Robbins, P. W. (1990). Carbohydrate ligands of the LEC cell adhesion molecules. *Cell*, **63**, 861–3.

Brown, E. O., Sundstrom, S. A., Komm, B. S., Zheng, YI., Teuscher, C. & Lyttle, C. R. (1990). Progesterone regulation of estradiol-induced rat uterine secretory protein, complement C3′. *Biology of Reproduction*, **42**, 713–19.

Buckley, C. H. & Fox, H. (1989). *Biopsy Pathology of the Endometrium*. Chapman and Hall Medical, London.

Campbell, S., Seif, M. W., Aplin, J. D., Richmond, S. J., Haynes, P. & Allen, T. D. (1988). Expression of a secretory product by microvillous and ciliated cells of the human endometrial epithelium *in vivo* and *in vitro*. *Human Reproduction*, **3**, 927–34.

Carson, D. D., Dutt, A. & Tang, J. P. (1987). Glycoconjugate synthesis during early pregnancy: hyaluronate synthesis and function. *Developmental Biology*, **120**, 228–35.

Carson, D. D., Tang, J. Y., Julian, J. & Glasser, S. R. (1988). Vectorial secretion of proteoglycans by polarised rat uterine epithelial cells. *Journal of Cell Biology*, **107**, 2425–34.

Cato, A. C. B. & Beato, M. (1985). The hormonal regulation of uteroglobin gene expression. *Anticancer Research*, **5**, 65–72.

Charnock-Jones, D. S., Sharkey, A. M., Rajput-Williams, J. *et al.* (1993). Identification and localization of alternately spliced mrNAs for VEGF in human uterus. *Biology of Reproduction*, **48**, 1120–8.

Chegini, N., Rao, Ch. V. & Sanfilippo, J. (1986). Binding of ^{125}I-epidermal growth factor in human uterus. *Cell Tissue Research*, **246**, 543–8.

Ciocca, D. R., Asch, R. H., Adams, D. J. & McGuire, W. L. (1983). Evidence for modulation of a 24 K protein in human endometrium during the menstrual cycle. *Journal of Clinical Endocrinological Metabolism*, **57**, 496–9.

Critchley, H. O. D., Buckley, C. H., Anderson, D. C., Aplin, J. D. & Seif, M. W. (1991). Secretory differentiation of endometrium after steroid replacement in women with premature ovarian failure. *Journal of Obsetetrics and Gynaecology*, **11**, 161.

Cunha, G. R., Bigsby, R. M., Cooke, P. S. & Sugimura, Y. (1985). Stromal-epithelial interactions in adult organs. *Cell Differentiation*, **17**, 137–48.

Dallenbach-Hellweg, G. (1981). Histopathology of the Endometrium. Springer Verlag, Berlin.

Denker, H.-W. (1982). Proteases of the blastocyst and of the uterus. In *Proteins and Steroids in Early Pregnancy*. Ed. H. M. Beier and P. Karlson, pp. 183–208, Springer-Verlag, Berlin.

Denker, H.-W. (1990). Trophoblast-endometrial interactions at embryo implantation: a cell biological paradox. In *Trophoblast Invasion and Endometrial Receptivity: Novel. Aspects of the Cell Biology of Embryo Implantation*. Ed. H.-W. Denker and J. D. Aplin. *Trophoblast Research*, **4**, 3–29.

DiMattia, G. E., Gellersen, B., Duckworth, M. L. & Friesen, H. G. (1990). Human prolactin gene expression: the use of an alternative non-coding exon in decidua and the IM-9-P3 lymphoblast cell line. *Journal of Biological Chemistry*, **256**, 16412–21.

Dockery, P., Li, T. C., Rogers, A. W., Cooke, I. D. & Lenton, E. A. (1988). The ultrastructure of the glandular epithelium in the timed endometrial biopsy. *Human Reproduction*, **3**, 826–34.

Dockery, P., Warren, A., Li, T. C., Rogers, A. W., Cooke, I. D. & Mundy, J. (1990). A morphometric study of the human endometrial stroma during the preimplantation period. *Human Reproduction*, **5**, 494–8.

Drudy, L., Sheppard, B. L. & Bonnar, J. (1991). The ultrastructure of mast cells in the uterus throughout the normal menstrual cycle and the post menopause. *Journal of Anatomy*, **175**, 51–63.

Faber, M., Wewer, U. M., Berthelsen, J. G., Liotta, L. A. & Albrechtsen, R. (1986). Laminin production by human endometrial stromal cells relates to the cyclic and pathological state of the endometrium. *American Journal of Pathology*, **124**, 384–91.

Farmer, S. J., Fliss, A. E. & Simmen, R. C. M. (1990). Complementary DNA clonic and regulation of expression of the messenger RNA encoding a pregnancy-associated porcine uterine protein related to human antileukoproteinase. *Molecular Endocrinology*, **4**, 1095–104.

Fazleabas, A. T., Bazer, F. W., Hansen, P. J., Geisbert, R. D. & Roberts, R. M. (1985). Differential patterns of secretory protein localization within the pig uterine endometrium. *Endocrinology*, **116**, 240–5.

Fazleabas, A. T., Khan-Dawood, F. S. & Dawood, M. Y. (1987). Protein, progesterone and protease inhibitors in uterine and peritoneal fluids of women with endometriosis. *Fertility and Sterility*, **47**, 218–24.

Fazleabas, A. T., Bell, S. C. & Verhage, H. G. (1991a). Insulin-like growth factor binding proteins: a paradigm for conceptus-maternal interactions in the primate. In *Uterine and Embryonic Factors in Early Pregnancy*. Ed. J. F. Strauss III and C. R. Lyttle, pp. 157–165, Plenum Press, New York.

Fazleabas, A. T., Yeko, T. R., Donnelly, K. M., Dawood, M. Y. & Bell, S. C. (1991b). Effect of clomiphene citrate on the synthesis and release of the human β-lactoglobulin homologue, pregnancy associated endometrial α2-globulin, by the uterine endometrium. *Human Reproduction*, **6**, 783–90.

Findlay, J. K. & Salamonsen, L. A. (1991). Paracrine regulation of implantation and uterine function. *Baillière's Clinical Obstetrics and Gynaecology*, **5**, 117–31.

Fischer, B., Jung, T., Hegele-Hartung, C. & Beier, H. M. (1990). Development of preimplantation rabbit embryos in uterine flushing-supplemented culture media. *Molecular Reproductive Development*, **27**, 216–23.

Frost, R. A. & Tseng, L. (1991). Insulin-like growth factor-binding protein-1 is phosphorylated by cultured human endometrial stromal cells and multiple protein kinases *in vitro*. *Journal of Biological Chemistry*, **266**, 18082–8.

Fuqua, S. A., Blum-Salingaros, M. & McGuire, W. L. (1989). Induction of the progesterone-regulated 24k protein by heat shock. *Cancer Research*, **49**, 4126–9.

Garde, J., Bell, S. C. & Eperon, I. C. (1991). Multiple forms of mRNA encoding human pregnancy-associated endometrial α_2-globulin, a β-lactoglobulin homologue. *Proceedings of the National Academy of Sciences, USA*, **88**, 2456–60.

Gellerson, B., Bonhoff, A., Hunt, N. & Bohnet, H. G. (1991). Decidual-type prolactin expression by the human myometrium. *Endocrinology*, **129**, 158–68.

Gendler, S. J., Lancaster, C. A., Taylor-Papadimitriou, J. *et al.* (1990). Molecular cloning and expression of human tumour-associated polymorphic epithelial mucin. *Journal of Biological Chemistry*, **265**, 15286–93.

Giudice, L. C. (1994). Growth factors and growth modulators in human uterine endometrium: their potential relevance to reproductive medicine. *Fertility and Sterility*, **61**, 1–17.

Giudice, L. C., Milkowski, D. A., Lamson, G., Rosenfeld, R. G. & Irwin, J. C. (1991). Insulin-like growth factor binding proteins in human endometrium: steroid-dependent messenger ribonucleic acid expression and protein synthesis. *Journal of Clinical Endocrinology Metabolism*, **72**, 779–87.

Glasser, S. R., Julian, J., Decker, G. L., Tang, J. Y. & Carson, D. D. (1988). Development of morphological and functional polarity in primary cultures of immature rat uterine epithelial cells. *Journal of Cell Biology*, **107**, 2409–23.

Glasser, S. R., Mulholland, J., Mani, S. K., Julian, J., Munir, M. I., Lampelo, S. & Soares, M. J. (1991). Blastocyst–endometrial relationships: reciprocal interactions between uterine epithelial and stromal cells and blastocysts. *Trophoblast Research*, **5**, 229–80.

Graham, R. A., Aplin, J. D., Seif, M. W., Li, T.-C., Cooke, I. D., Dockery, P. & Rogers, A. W. (1990). An endometrial factor in unexplained infertility. *British Medical Journal*, **300**, 1428–31.

Graham, R. A., Li, T.-C., Seif, M. W., Aplin, J. D. & Cooke, I. D. (1991). The effects of the antiprogesterone RU486 (Mifepristone) on an endometrial secretory glycan: an immunocytochemical study. *Fertility and Sterility*, **55**, 1132–6.

Hanisch, F.-G., Uhlenbruck, G., Egge, H. & Peter-Katalinic, J. (1989). A B72.3 second generation monoclonal antibody (CC49) defines the mucin-carried carbohydrate epitope Galβ1-3 (NeuAcα2-6) GalNAc. *Biological Chemistry Hoppe-Seyler*, **370**, 21–6.

Haslam, S. Z. & Counterman, L. J. (1991). Mammary stroma modulates hormonal responsiveness of mammary epithelium *in vivo* in the mouse. *Endocrinology*, **129**, 2017–23.

Henrikson, K. P., Jazin, E. E., Greenwood, J. A. & Dickerman, H. W. (1990). Prothrombin levels are increased in the estrogen-treated immature rat uterus. *Endocrinology*, **126**, 167–75.

Hoadley, M. E., Seif, M. W. & Aplin, J. D. (1990). Menstrual cycle-dependent expression of keratan sulphate in human endometrium. *Biochemical Journal*, **266**, 757–63.

Hofmann, G. E., Scott, R. T., Bergh, P. A. & Deligdisch, L. (1991). Immunohistochemical localization of epidermal growth factor in human endometrium, decidua and placenta. *Journal of Clinical Endocrinology Metabolism*, **73**, 882–7.

Hey, N. A., Graham, R. A., Seif, M. W. & Aplin, J. D. (1994). The polymorphic epithelial mucin MUC1 in human endometrium is regulated with maximal expression in the implantation phase. *Journal of Clinical Endocrinology Metabolism*, **78**, 337–42.

Ing, N. H. & Roberts, R. M. (1989). The major protesterone-modulated proteins secreted into the sheep uterus are members of the serpin superfamily of serine protease inhibitors. *Journal of Biological Chemistry*, **264**, 3372–9.

Isemura, M., Munakata, H. & Yosizawa, Z. (1981). Hormonal effects on the sulfation of sulfated glycoprotein in a particulate fraction of the endometrium of rabbitserum. *Journal of Biochemistry*, **89**, 1815–19.

Jaffe, R. C., Donnelly, K. M., Mavrogianis, P. A. & Verhage, H. G. (1989). Molecular cloning and characterization of a progesterone-dependent cat endometrial secretory protein complementary deoxyribonucleic acid. *Molecular Endocrinology*, **3**, 1807–14.

Jansen, R. P., Turner, M., Johannisson, E., Landgren, B.-M. & Diczfalusy, E. (1985). Cyclic changes in human endometrial surface glycoproteins: a quantitative histochemical study. *Fertility and Sterility*, **44**, 85–91.

Johannisson, E. (1991). Morphological and histochemical factors related to implantation. *Baillière's Clinical Obstetrics and Gynaecology*, **5**, 191–209.

Julkunen, M., Seppala, M. & Janne, O. A. (1988a). Complete amino acid sequence of human placental protein 14: a progesterone-regulated uterine protein homologous to β-lactoglobulins. *Proceedings of the National Academy of Sciences, USA*, **85**, 8845–9.

Julkunen, M., Koistinen, R., Aalto-Setala, K., Seppala, M., Janne, O. A. & Kontula, K. (1988b). Primary structure of human insulin-like growth factor-binding protein/placental protein 12 and tissue-specific expression of its mRNA. *FEBS Letters*, **236**, 295–302.

Julkunen, M., Koistinen, R., Suikkari, A.-M., Seppala, M. & Janne, O. A. (1990). Identification by hybridization histochemistry of human endometrial cells expressing mRNAs encoding a uterine β-lactoglobulin homologue and insulin-like growth factor-binding protein-1. *Molecular Endocrinology*, **4**, 700–7.

Kauma, S. W., Aukerman, S. L., Eierman, D. & Turner, T. (1991). Colony-stimulating factor-1 and *c-fms* expression in human endometrial tissues and placenta during the menstrual cycle and early pregnancy. *Journal of Clinical Endocrinology Metabolism*, **73**, 746–51.

Kimber, S. J., Lindenberg, S. & Lundblad, A. (1988). Distribution of some Galβ1-3(4)GlcNAc related carbohydrate antigens on the mouse uterine epithelium in relation to the peri-implantational period. *Journal of Reproductive Immunology*, **12**,

297–313.

Kimer, S. J. & Lindenberg, S. (1990). Hormonal control of a carbohydrate epitope involved in implantation in mice. *Journal of Reproduction and Fertility*, **89**, 13–21.

Klentzeris, L. D., Bulmer, J. N., Li, T. C., Morrison, L., Warren, A. & Cooke, I. D. (1991). Lectin binding of endometrium in women with unexplained infertility. *Fertility and Sterility*, **56**, 660–7.

Lancaster, C. A , Peat, N., Duhig, T., Wilson, D., Taylor-Papadimitiou, J. & Gendler, S. J. (1991). Structure and expression of the human polymorphic epithelial mucin gene: an expressed VNTR unit. *Biochemical Biophysical Research Communications*, **173**, 1019–29.

Li, T. C., Rogers, A. W., Lenton, E. A., Dockery, P. Cooke, I. D. (1987). A comparison between two methods of chronologically dating human endometrial biopsies during the luteal phase and their correlation with histologic dating. *Fertility and Sterility*, **48**, 928–32.

Li, W. G., Jaffe, R. C., Fazleabas, A. T. & Verhage, H. G. (1990). Progesterone-dependent cathepsin L proteolytic activity in cat uterus flushings. *Biology of Reproduction*, **44**, 625–31.

Lindenberg, S., Sundberg, K., Kimber, S. J. & Lundblad, A. (1988). The milk oligosaccharide, lacto-N-fucopentaose I, inhibits attachment of mouse blastocysts on endometrial monolayers. *Journal of Reproduction and Fertility*, **83**, 149–58.

Mani, S. K., Carson, D. D. & Glasser, S. R. (1992). Steroid hormones differentially modulate glycoconjugate synthesis and vectorial secretion by polarized uterine epithelial cells *in vitro. Endocrinology*, **130**, 240–8.

Manners, C. V. (1990). Endometrial assessment in a group of infertile women on stimulated cycles for IVF; immunohistochemical findings. *Human Reproduction*, **5**, 128–32.

Maudelonde, T. & Rochefort, H. (1987). A 51K progestin-regulated protein secreted by human endometrial cells in primary culture. *Journal of Clinical Endocrinology Metabolism*, **64**, 1294–301.

Misrahi, M., Atger, M. & Milgrom, E. (1987). A novel progesterone-induced messenger RNA in rabbit and human endometria. Cloning and sequence analysis of the complementary DNA. *Biochemistry*, **26**, 3975–82.

Mulholland, J., Aplin, J. D., Ayad, S., Hong, L. & Glasser, S. R. (1992). Loss of collagen type VI from rat endometrial stroma during decidualisation. *Biology of Reproduction*, **46**, 1136–43.

Munakata, H., Isemura, M. & Yosizawa, Z. (1985). Enzymatic sulfation of exogenous high molecular weight glycopeptides by microsomal fraction of the rabbit uterine endometrium. *Journal of Biological Chemistry*, **260**, 6851–6.

Murray, M. K., Verhage, H. G., Buhi, W. C. & Jaffe, R. C. (1985). The detection and purification of a cat uterine secretory protein that is estrogen dependent (CUOED). *Biology of Reproduction*, **32**, 1219–27.

Murray, M. K., Verhage, H. G. & Jaffe, R. C. (1986). Quantification of an estrogen-dependent cat uterine protein (CUOED) in uterine flushings of estrogen- and progesterone-treated ovariectomized cats by radioimmunoassay. *Biology of Reproduction*, **35**, 531–6.

Nelson, K. G., Takahashi, T., Bossert, N. L., Walmer, D. K. & McLachlan, J. A. (1991). Epidermal growth factor replaces estrogen in the stimulation of female genital-tract growth and differentiation. *Proceedings of the National Academy of Sciences, USA*, **88**, 21–5.

Noyes, R. W., Hertig, A. T. & Rock, J. (1950). Dating the endometrial biopsy. *Fertility and Sterility*, **1**, 3–25.

O'Neill, C. (1991). A consideration of the factors which influence and control the viability and developmental potential of the preimplantation embryo. *Baillière's Clinical Obstetrics and Gynaecology*, **5**, 159–78.

Padykula, H. (1989). Regeneration in the primate uterus: the role of stem cells. In *Biology of the Uterus*, eds R. M. Wynn and W. P. Jollie, pp. 279–288, Plenum, New York.

Pollard, J. W. (1990). Regulation of polypeptide growth factor synthesis and growth factor-related gene expression in the rat and mouse uterus before and after implantation. *Journal of Reproduction and Fertility*, **88**, 721–31.

Press, M. F., Nousek-Goebl, N., King, W. J., Herbst, A. L. & Greene, G. L. (1984). Immunohistochemical assessment of estrogen receptor distribution in the human endometrium throughout the menstrual cycle. *Laboratory Investigation*, **51**, 495–9.

Psychoyos, A. (1986). Uterine receptivity for nidation. *Annals of the NY Academy of Sciences*, **476**, 36–9.

Roberts, R. M. & Bazer, F. (1988). The function of uterine secretions. *Journal of Reproduction and Fertility*, **82**, 875–92.

Rogers, P. A. W., Abberton, K. M. & Susil, B. (1992). Endothelial cell migratory signal produced by human endometrium during the menstrual cycle. *Human Reproduction*, **7**, 1061–6.

Rutanen, E.-M., Pekonen, F. & Makinen, T. (1988). Soluble 34k binding protein inhibits the binding of IGF-1 to its receptors in human secretory phase endometrium: evidence for autocrine/paracrine regulation of growth factor action. *Journal of Clinical Endocrinology Metabolism*, **66**, 173–80.

Savourat, J. F., Bailly, A., Misrahi, M., Rauch, C., Redeuilh, G., Chauchereau, A. & Milgrom, E. (1991). Characterisation of the hormone responsive element involved in the regulation of the progesterone receptor gene. *EMBO Journal*, **10**, 1875–83.

Seif, M. W., Aplin, J. D., Foden, L. J., Tindall, V. R. (1989a). A novel approach for monitoring the endometrial cycle and detecting ovulation. *American Journal of Obstetrics and Gynecology*, **160**, 357–62.

Seif, M. W., Aplin, J. D. & Buckley, C. H. (1989b). Luteal phase defect: the possibility of an immunohistochemical analysis. *Fertility and Sterility*, **51**, 273–9.

Seif, M. W., Aplin, J. D., Awad, H. & Wells, D. (1989c). The effect of the intrauterine contraceptive device on endometrial secretory function. An immunohistochemical study. *Contraception*, **40**, 81–9.

Seif, M. W., Pearson, M., Ibrahim, Z. H. Z. *et al.* (1992). Endometrium in IVF cycles: morphological and functional differentiation in the implantation phase. *Human Reproduction*, **7**, 6–11.

Sharif, S. F., Francis, H., Keisler, D. H. & Roberts, R. M. (1989). Correlation between the release of ovine trophoblast protein-1 by the conceptus and the production of polypeptides by the maternal endometrium of ewes. *Journal of Reproduction and Fertility*, **85**, 471–6.

Simmen, R. C. M., Baumbach, G. A. & Roberts, R. M. (1988). Molecular cloning and temporal expression during pregnancy of the messenger ribonucleic acid encoding uteroferrin, a progesterone-induced uterine secretory protein. *Molecular Endocrinology*, **2**, 253–62.

Singhal, A., Fohn, M. & Hakomori, S. (1991). Induction of Tn antigen-mediated cellular immune response for active immunotherapy in mice. *Cancer Research*, **51**, 1406–11.

Smith, R. A., Seif, M. W., Rogers, A. W. *et al.* (1989). The endometrial cycle: the expression of a secretory component correlated with the luteinising hormone peak. *Human*

Reproduction, **4**, 236–42.

Soisson, A. P., Berchuck, A., Lessey, B. A. *et al.* (1989). Immunohistochemical expression of TAG-72 in normal and malignant endometrium: correlation of antigen expression with estrogen receptor and progesterone receptor levels. *American Journal of Obstetrics and Gynecology*, **161**, 1258–63.

Starkey, P. M., Clover, L. M. & Rees, M. C. P. (1991). Variation during the menstrual cycle of immune cell populations in human endometrium. *European Journal of Obstetrics, Gynecology and Reproduction Biology*, **39**, 203–7.

Suzuki, M., Ogawa, M., Tamada, T., Nagura, H. & Watanabe, K. (1984). Immunohistochemical localization of secretory component and IgA in the human endometrium in relation to the menstrual cycle. *Acta Histochemica Cytochemica*, **17**, 223–9.

Tabibzadeh, S. (1991). Human endometrium: an active site of cytokine production and action. *Endocrine Review*, **12**, 272–90.

Teng, C. T., Pentecost, B. T., Chen, Y. H., Newbold, R. R., Eddy, E. M. & McLachlan, J. A. (1989). Lactotransferrin gene expression in the mouse uterus and mammary gland. *Endocrinology*, **124**, 992–9.

Thatcher, W. W., Hansen, P. J., Gross, T. S., Helmer, S. D., Plante, C. & Bazer, F. W. (1989). Antiluteolytic effects of bovine trophobast protein-1. *Journal of Reproduction Fertility Suppl.* 1, **37**, 91–9.

Thor, A., Viglione, M. J., Muraro, R., Ohuchi, N., Schlom, J. & Gorstein, F. (1987). Monoclonal antibody B72.3 reactivity with human endometrium: a study of normal and malignant tissues. *International Journal of Gynecological Pathology*, **6**, 235–47.

Vallet, J. L., Bazer, F. W. & Roberts, R. M. (1987). The effect of ovine trophoblast protein-one on endometrial protein secretion and cyclic nucleotides. *Biology of Reproduction*, **37**, 1307–16.

Van Kooij, R. J., Roelofs, H. J. M., Kathman, G. A. M. & Kramer, M. F. (1982). Synthesis of a mucous glycoprotein in the human uterus. *European Journal of Obstetrics Gynecology and Reproductive Biology*, **14**, 191–7.

Verhage, H. G., Fazleabas, A. T., Mavrogianis, P. A. & Jaffe, R. C. (1988). Detection and quantification of CUPED, an estrogen-dependent uterine protein, in uterine fluid and endometrial tissue of estrous and pregnant cats. *Americal Journal of Anatomy*, **181**, 419–24.

Vollmer, G., Siegal, G. P., Chiquet-Ehrismann, R., Lightner, V. A., Arnholdt, H. & Knuppen, R. (1990). Tenascin expression in the human endometrium and in endometrial adenocarcinomas. *Laboratory Investigations*, **62**, 725–30.

Waites, G. T., Wood, P. L., Walker, R. A. & Bell, S. C. (1988*a*). Immunohistological localization of human endometrial secretory protein, 'pregnancy-associated endometrial α_2-globulin' (α_2-PEG), during the menstrual cycle. *Journal of Reproductive Fertility*, **82**, 665–72.

Waites, G. T., James, R. F. L. & Bell, S. C. (1988*b*). Immunohistological localization of the human endometrial secretory protein pregnancy-associated endometrial α_1-globulin, an insulin-like growth factor-binding protein, during the menstrual cycle. *Journal of Clinical Endocrinology Metabolism*, **67**, 1100–4.

Waites, G. T., James, R. F. L. & Bell, S. C. (1989). Human 'pregnancy-associated endometrial α_1-globulin', an insulin-like growth factor-binding protein: immunohistological localization in the decidua and placenta during pregnancy emloying monoclonal antibodies. *Journal of Endocrinology*, **120**, 351–7.

West, D. C., Hampson, I. N., Arnold, F. & Kumar, S. (1985). Angiogenesis induced by degradation products of hyaluronic acid. *Science*, **228**, 1324–5.

7

Electrophysiology of the human myometrium

T. KAWARABAYASHI

Introduction

Every smooth muscle organ carries out its physiological roles through contractile activities: tonic and/or phasic contractions which vary according to the function of each organ. The three characteristics of contractive activity are amplitude, duration, and frequency. When combined, these elements determine the type of motility, and the contractile properties are generally correlated with the electrical activity of the plasma membrane. However, the influence of electrical activity varies from organ to organ. Some muscles do not generate action potentials, while others produce active responses. Differences in electrical properties might be expected to correlate with the different mechanisms by which bioactive substances and drugs affect the activity of smooth muscle. For this reason, the various types of smooth muscle have been classified according to their excitability. Bülbring and Tomita (1987) have placed myometrium in the group of spontaneously active and readily excitable muscles based on membrane excitability. The contractility of this muscle group is greatly influenced by changes in electrical activity.

However, one of the most important roles of the uterus is to retain a fetus by suppressing contractility until such time as adequate fetal growth can be achieved, and then to expel the fetus by rhythmic contraction. Long-term and short-term control mechanisms are essential to achieve this dual role. The activity of the myometrium is highly influenced by hormonal conditions to keep the fetus *in utero*, and by a variety of stimulants (oxytocin, prostaglandins, catecholamines, etc.) which promote expulsion of the fetus. The course of pregnancy and parturition vary between different species and myometrial functions would be expected to show similar variation. In the human, a periodicity consisting of one-minute of contraction and a few minutes of relaxation is essential for both mother and fetus. The mother can perform pushing efforts during the contraction phase, and the fetus can recover from the hypoxic state during the relaxation phase. This periodicity probably determines the fundamental characteristics of human uterine contractility.

This chapter focuses on the electrical activity and contraction of human myometrium.

Electrical activity in the human myometrium

Few studies have recorded the intracellular electrical activity of the human myometrium, though there have been many studies on the electrophysiological properties of animal myometrium. In 1971, Nakajima reported intracellular action potentials of human isthmic myometrium using a microelectrode. His description was limited to the mean resting potential (-46.4 mV), and the configuration of the action potentials (plateau-type). In 1982 therefore, we initiated electro-physiological experiments in human myometrium using the single sucrose-gap method.

The specimens consisted of small strips of pregnant human isthmic myometrium dissected from the lower uterine segment at the time of term Caesarean section with patients under epidural anaesthesia, prior to the administration of oxytocics. This material can be easily and consistently obtained from the human uterus without complications. We used the single sucrose-gap method to make a simultaneous record of spontaneous electrical and mechanical activity; this is the most stable method for recording long-term activities.

Methodology

Single sucrose-gap method

Human myometrium is composed of a complex lace-like arrangement of small muscle bundles, which are difficult to separate into discrete bundles. However, strips of myometrium, 1–1.5 mm in diameter and 6–7 mm in length, can be dissected along the longitudinal axis of the complex small muscle bundles under a binocular microscope and mounted onto a single sucrose-gap apparatus. This has four compartments, each separated by thin rubber with a small hole through which the muscle strip is passed. One end of the muscle strip is fixed and the other end is tied with silk thread and connected to a mechano-transducer in order to record an isometric contraction. One side of the compartments is filled with isotonic KCl and the other with calcium-free Krebs solution to suppress spontaneous activity. The two central chambers are perfused with sucrose and the test solution (Fig. 1). Electrical activities are recorded between the test solution

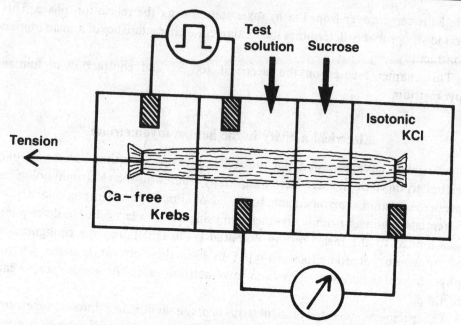

Fig. 1. Diagram of the single sucrose-gap apparatus.

and the isotonic KCl by Ag–AgCl electrodes, and current pulse can be applied
between Ca-free Krebs solution and the test solution through the hole in the
rubber using Ag–AgCl electrodes (Kawarabayashi, Kishikawa & Sugimori, 1988).
It is not possible to measure the parameters of individual spikes since these are
distorted, but distortion in the recording of slow changes of the membrane
potential is minimal (Coburn, Ohba & Tomita, 1975). Osa *et al.* showed that
spike, plateau and slow potentials in rat myometrium were distinguishable as the
basic potentials composing the membrane activities (Osa & Fujino, 1978);
furthermore, these potentials should be sufficient to allow recognition of the
relationship between the contraction and the electrical activities.

Microelectrode method

The procedure described by Inoue *et al.* in 1990 is fundamentally the same as
the one we used on pregnant rat myometrium (Kawarabayashi & Osa, 1976).
Small strips (5 × 20 mm; 1–1.5 mm thick) are prepared under a binocular
microscope, and connective tissue is carefully removed with fine scissors. The
muscle strip is lightly stretched across a small chamber, divided into two
compartments for electrical stimulation and recording. A microelectrode filled
with 3 mol/l potassium chloride (40 to 60 MΩ) is inserted into the cell to record

the intracellular membrane activity, and stimulating pulses are applied via a partition electrode as described by Abe and Tomita (1968).

Patch clamp method

The tight-seal technique has made it possible to study the properties of a single channel in a patch of living membrane, whether and how they open and close, the influence of membrane voltage, ionic composition, drugs, neurotransmitters, and other features. Ionic currents in whole cells, which underlie action potentials, are the sum of the current in many individual channels. Clean isolated single cells are essential for this technique. Small segments of myometrium are incubated in Ca-free physiological salt solution containing 0.3% collagenase for 80 min. After completion of the digestion, single cells are dispersed by gentle agitation with a blunt-tipped glass pipette. The cell suspension is filtered through a fine nylon mesh, and the cell sediment is resuspended in fresh physiological salt solution and stored at 10 °C (Okabe *et al.*, 1987). For whole-cell voltage clamp experiments, a patch glass-electrode is filled with a high potassium solution (142 mmol/l potassium) or a caesium-tetraethylammonium solution (120 mmol/l caesium and 20 mmol/l tetraethylammonium). The electrode resistance is 3 to 5 MΩ. An electrode with an internal tip diameter of approximately 1 μm is pushed against the cell membrane, and suction is applied. If the cell membrane is sufficiently clean, a very tight seal can be obtained. This preparation is known as the cell-attached patch with gigaΩ (10^9 Ω) seal. With seal resistance in the GΩ range, the patch of membrane inside the electrode is, electrically and chemically, isolated from the surrounding environment. After GΩ seal is achieved, the patch membrane is ruptured by negative pressure, and electrical responses are recorded with a patch clamp amplifier. For single-channel current recording, the pipette solution contains 100 mmol/l barium. After GΩ seal is obtained, a high potassium solution is superfused in the bath, and electrical responses are recorded through a patch clamp amplifier with a high-resistance feedback resistor. A few drops of the cell suspension are placed in a chamber on the stage of an inverted difference-interference microscope. The patch electrode is controlled by means of an electronically driven three-dimensional micromanipulator (Inoue *et al.*, 1990). *et al.*, 1990).

Passive electrical properties

Resting membrane potential

The resting membrane potential of a spontaneously active smooth muscle, such as intestine and myometrium, is lower than a non-spontaneously active smooth muscle. In these muscles, the resting potential is defined as the maximum polarization between action potentials recorded by the microelectrode method. If the tissue shows bursts of spontaneous activity, the value obtained during the quiescent period is taken as the membrane potential. In pregnant human myometrium, it is easier to measure the resting membrane potential because of the long-lasting quiescent period, since the frequency of the action potential is very low in comparison with that of the rat. However, it is obvious that many factors, such as faulty impalement, deficiencies in the microelectrodes, tip-potentials of the microelectrodes, stretching of the tissue, bathing temperature and so on, all affect the membrane potential. Therefore, it is difficult to compare data reported by different investigators even for the same tissue. The actual value of the resting membrane potential in term-pregnant human myometrium is about -46 to -50 mV (Nakajima, 1971; Inoue et al., 1990), and this is compatible with the values in term-pregnant rat myometrium (Kuriyama & Suzuki, 1976; Anderson, Kawarabayashi & Marshall, 1981). Even in isolated pregnant human myometrial cells dissected from the incisional edge of the lower uterine segment at the time of Ceasarean delivery, the mean resting membrane potential is -49.4 mV, the same as in intact tissue (Pressman et al., 1988).

The resting membrane potential of the myometrium is highly influenced by external potassium and sodium in animals. In the rat, when potassium is increased from the normal concentration (5.9 mM in Krebs solution), the membrane gradually depolarizes (Kanda & Kuriyama, 1980). On the other hand, when sodium is decreased, the membrane depolarizes and contracture develops in pregnant mouse (Osa, 1971) and rat (Kanda & Kuriyama, 1980) myometrium. It is considered that the contracture produced by Na removal is largely Ca dependent, and that an increase in Ca conductance, secondary to membrane depolarization and Na–Ca exchange, is involved in the Ca-dependent contracture (Masahashi & Tomita, 1983). In pregnant human myometrium, the resting membrane potential is primarily influenced by permeability for potassium ion, but sodium permeability also has an important role (Inoue et al., 1990).

Length constant

Fig. 2 shows the electrical responses of pregnant human myometrium evoked by various intensities of stimulation recorded at three different distances from the stimulating partition (Inoue et al., 1990). The amplitudes of the electrotonic potentials show outward rectification. Linear relations between the applied inward current intensities and the amplitudes of the electrotonic potential were seen at more than three places. There was a log-linear relationship between spatial decay of the electrotonic potential produced by a given current intensity and the distances

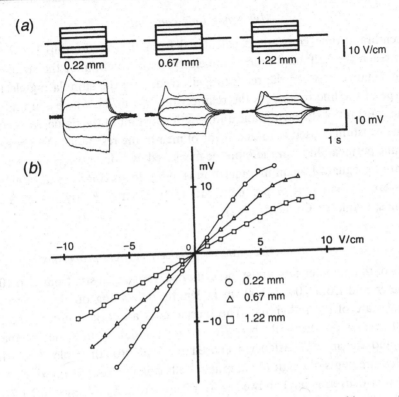

Fig. 2. The electrotonic potentials and the current–voltage relationships recorded at three different distances in pregnant human myometrium recorded by the microelectrode method. (*a*) Six traces of electrotonic potentials evoked by three different intensities of outward and inward current pulses are superimposed. Recordings were made at distances of 0.22, 0.67, and 1.22 mm from the partition stimulating electrode. In this preparation a large outward current evoked only an abortive action potential. (*b*) The current–voltage relationships obtained at three different distances from the partition electrode. (*a*) and (*b*) were obtained from the same preparation. (Modified from Inoue *et al.*, 1990, with permission.)

from the partition. This indicates an exponential decay of the electrotonic potential along the tissue. The length constant describes the efficiency with which a current will spread through the tissue. This content is significant in determining the propagation of action potentials through the tissue. The mean value of the length constant was 1.0 ± 0.1 mm, which was the distance at which the electronic potential decayed to $1/e$. This value is shorter than that measured in the longitudinal muscle of term-pregnant rat myometrium (2.9 mm) (Kuriyama & Suzuki, 1976), but is similar to that observed in the circular muscle of mid-pregnant rat myometrium (1.02 mm) (Kawarabayashi, 1978).

Membrane time constant

The membrane time constant is calculated from the relationship between the time to reach the half amplitude of the electrotonic potential at the steady state and the distance between the recording electrode and the stimulating electrode. The slope of the line represents the relationship of $\tau m/2\lambda$, where τm and λ are the time constant of the membrane and length constant of the tissue, respectively. The time constant is used as an indicator of membrane resistance. An increase in membrane permeability can therefore be measured as a decrease in τm. The time constant of pregnant human myometrium is 396 ± 46 ms (Inoue *et al.*, 1990); this value is larger than that of pregnant rats (180–228 ms) (Kuriyama & Suzuki, 1976; Sims, Daniel & Garfield, 1982).

Effect of reproductive state on passive electrical properties

The cells of the myometrium are spindle-shaped, ranging in size from 2 to 10 μm in diameter and from 200 to 600 μm in length, depending on the species and hormonal state of the individual. The muscle cells are largest during the later stages of pregnancy, primarily because of the stimulatory influence of the sex steroids and the muscle distention caused by fetal growth (Cole & Garfield, 1989). Measurements of longitudinal muscle cells isolated from the uteri of 21-day pregnant rats (delivering day), showed an average size of $232 \pm 74 \mu$m $\times 16.2 \pm 7.0 \mu$m (Tsukamoto *et al.*, 1991). Hormones, especially estrogen, and muscle distention also affect the electrical properties of the myometrium (Kawarabayashi & Marshall, 1981). In rat, the resting membrane potential gradually depolarizes (from -43 to -36 mV in circular, -45 to -41 mV in longitudinal muscle), and there is a progressive increase in the length constant (from 2.5 to 2.9 mm in longitudinal muscle) and the time constant (from 180 to 228 msec in longitudinal muscle) throughout pregnancy and delivery (Kuriyama & Suzuki, 1976; Anderson *et al.*, 1981). Thus a spontaneous action potential is more easily generated and propagated through the myometrium as pregnancy progresses. The overall excitability of the myometrium in late pregnancy culminates in the initiation and progress of labour. The same may occur in human myometrium, though this has not been verified because of the difficulty in obtaining early and mid-pregnancy myometrium.

Active electrical properties

Action potentials

In a small animal with a bicornuate uterus, such as the rat or mouse, the myometrium consists of a well-defined outer longitudinal layer and an inner

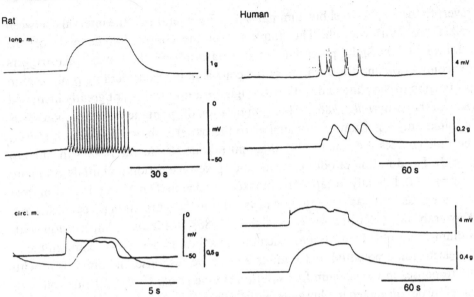

Fig. 3. Spontaneous electrical activities and contractions in longitudinal and circular muscle of pregnant rat (left column), and in pregnant human isthmic myometrium (right column). Activities in the rat were recorded by the microelectrode method, and human records were obtained by the single sucrose-gap method. Upper traces exhibit spike-type action potentials and lower the plateau-type. Each contraction is well synchronized with the action potential.

circular layer separated by an extensive vascular plexus; the electrophysiological characteristics of each muscle are different. The predominant types of action potentials in rat uteri at mid-pregnancy are spike in the longitudinal muscle and plateau in the circular muscle (Kawarabayashi & Osa, 1976). In human myometrium it is difficult to dissect the longitudinal and circular muscle and therefore difficult to distinguish the action potentials characteristic of these two layers. However, spike and plateau action potentials, can be distinguished from the pattern of traces using the microelectrode method (Inoue *et al.*, 1990) and single sucrose-gap method (Kawarabayashi *et al.*, 1986*a*). Plateau potentials are more frequently observed, but these do not allow prediction of whether the pattern of action potentials will be spike or plateau type before the onset of spontaneous activity. Fig. 3 shows the spontaneous electrical and mechanical activities in longitudinal and circular muscle of the pregnant rat (left column, recorded by a microelectrode method), and in pregnant human isthmic myometrium (right column, recorded by a single sucrose-gap method). The upper traces exhibit spike-type action potentials and contractions, and the lower traces, the plateau-type. All contractions are well synchronized with the action potentials. In the spike-type action potential, even a single spike effectively triggers a small contraction; the tension does not revert to the resting level but summates to a fused tetanus if the intervals between spikes are short enough. The amplitude of the contraction depends on the frequency of the spike potentials. In the plateau-type, the initial spike triggers the contraction and the duration of the contraction is considerably prolonged in proportion to the plateau duration, though the amplitude is not greatly increased (Kawarabayashi *et al.*, 1986*a*). The configuration of spontaneous action potentials in human myometrium is very similar to the pattern observed in rats; however, the time courses are remarkably different (about 10 s in rat vs 60 s in human) (Fig. 3). The duration of both plateau- and spike-type action potentials gradually decreases and finally disappears in excess calcium (7 mM) and calcium-free solutions, as well as with application of the calcium antagonist, diltiazem (Kawarabayashi, Kishikawa & Sugimori, 1986*b*). Moreover, superfusion with sodium-deficient (15.5 mM) and calcium-free solution increases the amplitude of the electrotonic potential and inhibits any active response, in comparison with the responses in the calcium-free solution (Inoue *et al.*, 1990). Calcium ions can therefore be considered to play an essential role in constituting the action potential, and sodium ions influence the generation of the action potential.

Pacemaker potentials

Myometrium is a spontaneously active and highly excitable muscle. Most of the uterine muscles show spontaneous rhythmic action potentials which arise in pacemaker cells, and are transmitted over the organ as a whole. As in other visceral smooth muscles, and the heart, uterine pacemaker activity is characterized by a slow depolarization of the muscle cell membrane culminating in generation of the action potential. As the pacemaker cells are not localized to a specific area of the myometrium, these cells can only be recognized by the pattern of electrical activity. It is said that all uterine muscle cells are capable of becoming pacemakers (Marshall, 1973). The frequency of pacemaker activity determines the rate of contraction. In pregnant rat myometrium, the slow depolarization is associated with a gradual increase in membrane resistance, presumably due to a reduction in potassium conductance, as judged from the increase in amplitude of the electrotonic potential recorded from a single cell (Kuriyama & Suzuki, 1976). It is also possible that the slow depolarization results from an increase in sodium permeability, since the pacemaker potential is dependent upon the presence of sodium in the external environment and is unaffected by the removal of calcium (Reiner & Marshall, 1976). The pacemaker potential is also observed in pregnant human myometrium, as shown in Fig. 4. The membrane potential gradually depolarizes and the action potential is ultimately evoked. Though steady current pulses are applied, evoked potentials are not regular and the pattern gradually

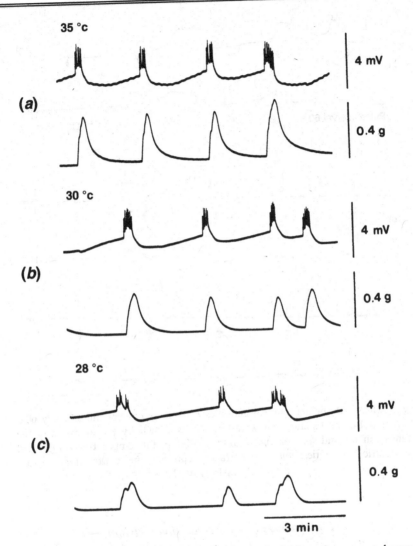

Fig. 4. Spontaneous electrical and mechanical activities of pregnant human myometrium recorded by the single sucrose-gap method at various temperatures (35 °C, 30 °C, and 28 °C). In this specimen, a pacemaker potential was observed. When the temperature was lowered, the gradient of the pacemaker potential, and the subsequent frequency of the activities decreased. Amplitude of contractions also decreased at lower temperature.

changes in accordance with the periodicity of the membrane (Fig. 5). The pacemaker potential is greatly influenced by temperature (Fig. 4); external magnesium ion suppresses the gradient of the pacemaker potential and the duration of each action potential (Kawarabayashi *et al.*, 1984; Kawarabayashi, Kishikawa & Sugimori, 1989).

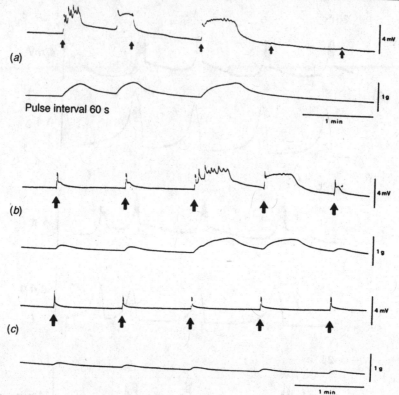

Fig. 5. Electrical and mechanical activities evoked by current pulses every 60 s. Current pulses of 1 s duration were applied as shown by the arrows and the intensity in (b) and (c) was the double of that in (a). Upper traces represent the electrical activities; the lower traces represent the contractions. (From Kawarabayashi *et al.*, 1988.)

Ion channels in the human myometrium

Calcium channels It is well known that contractions of the myometrium are related to an increase in the concentration of intracellular free calcium ion, and it is also known that a large difference in calcium concentrations exists between the extracellular fluid ($\sim 10^{-3}$ M) and intracellular cytosol ($\sim 10^{-7}$ M). Therefore, calcium influx from the extracellular space into the cytosol is very important in regulating myometrial contractility. Two types of channels for calcium influx have been suggested (Bolton, 1979). One is a potential-sensitive calcium channel that opens when the membrane depolarizes and is normally responsible for the action potential. The other type is a receptor-operated channel which is controlled or operated by a receptor for a stimulant substance. In pregnant human myometrium, two different types of voltage-dependent calcium channels have

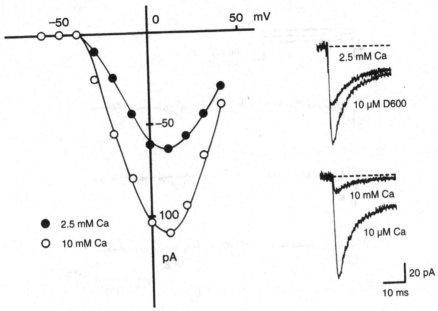

Fig. 6. The current–voltage relationships recorded from single smooth muscle cells dispersed from pregnant human myometrium. The amplitude of inward current was increased in proportion to concentrations of calcium, and the inward current was blocked by application of D600 or nicardipine or by superfusion of the calcium-free solution. (Effects of the latter two are not shown in the Figure.) (From Inoue *et al.*, 1990, with permission.)

been observed at the single-channel level using the patch clamp technique (Inoue *et al.*, 1990), and the inward calcium current was characterized by activation and inactivation properties (Young, Herndon-Smith & Anderson, 1991*b*). Fig. 6 shows the current–voltage relationships recorded from single smooth muscle cells dispersed from pregnant human myometrium. The amplitude of inward current was increased in proportion to concentrations of calcium, and the inward current was blocked by application of nicardipine or D600 (Fig. 6) or by superfusion of the calcium-free solution. Furthermore, the current–voltage relationships at different holding potentials indicated two types of inward currents. The maximum amplitude of inward current was evoked by a depolarizing pulse to 0 mV when the holding potential was − 60 mV, but the maximum amplitude of the depolarizing pulse was shifted to − 20 mV when the holding potential was − 100 mV (Inoue *et al.*, 1990). To confirm these results, single calcium channel currents were recorded by the patch clamp technique with the cell-attached configuration (Fig. 7). Two types of calcium channels distributed in pregnant human myometrium were identified. One of these had a single-channel conductance of 12 pS, and was

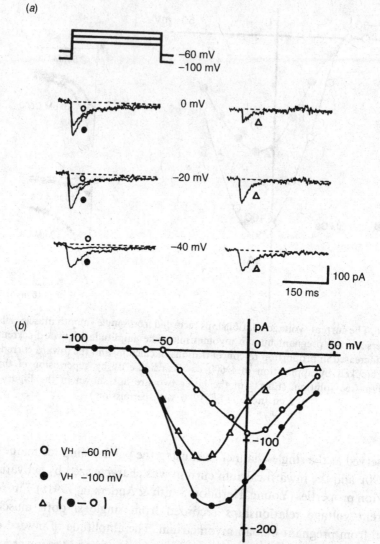

Fig. 7. The inward calcium current recorded from single smooth muscle cells isolated from pregnant human myometrium. The high-caesium solution in the pipette isolated the calcium current. Physiological salt solution (2.5 mM calcium) with 1 μM tetrodotoxin was superfused in the bath. (a) Traces in the left column were recorded by application of depolarizing pulses (300 ms in duration) to −40, −20, and 0 mV from holding potentials at −60 mV (open circles) and −100 mV (solid circles). Traces in the right column were obtained by subtracting inward currents recorded at the holding potential of −60 mV from those obtained at the holding potential of −100 mV. (b) The current–voltage relationships obtained at the holding potentials of −60 mV (open circles) and −100 mV (solid circles). The current–voltage relationship of the subtracted current (open triangles) was also plotted. The amplitudes of the inward currents were measured at the peak. (From Inoue et al., 1990, with permission.)

only activated by depolarizing pulses from a holding potential of -100 mV; this channel was inactivated at a holding potential of -60 mV. The second type had a single-channel conductance of 29 pS activated by depolarizing pulses from a holding potential of of -60 mV. Summated currents also showed different time courses for current relaxation; i.e. the 12 pS calcium channel (transient type: T-type) was rapidly inactivated, whereas the 29 pS calcium channel (long-lasting type: L-type) was slowly inactivated. The majority of the 12 pS calcium channels are likely to be inactivated at a normal resting potential of about -50 mV, as indicated by experiments that used the whole-cell voltage clamp technique (Inoue *et al.*, 1990). The physiological importance of the L-type current must be related to the formation of plateau potential, judging from its higher threshold potential and slower inactivation. Activation of the T-type calcium channel may be responsible for the spike component, and it may trigger activation of the long-lasting-type calcium channel.

Sodium channels Sodium ions may play an important role in generating the pacemaker potential and the action potential in uterine muscle. In the longitudinal muscle layer of pregnant rat myometrium, a fast sodium channel current (tetrodotoxin sensitive) was recorded from freshly isolated single cells using the whole cell voltage-clamp technique, and it was suggested that the fast sodium channel current might play a role in cell-to-cell conduction and possibly in regulation of spontaneous electrical activity (Ohya & Sperelakis, 1989). In cultured cells obtained from pregnant human myometrium, a large voltage-activated inward current was identified as sodium channel conductance by the following criteria: (1) removal of sodium from the bath eliminated the current; (2) the current was blocked by the sodium-channel-blocking agent, tetrodotoxin; (3) the current was observed in the absence of calcium (Young & Herndon-Smith, 1991a). The sodium current was large (maximal inward current 7.2 μ A/cm^2) and of short duration (decayed within 10 ms); the onset of activation was -40 mV, with a peak inward current at -10 mV. Steady-state voltage inactivation of this channel showed half-maximal inactivation at -67 mV, indicating that this channel is largely inactivated at normal resting potentials. The sodium currents do not appear to contribute to the rising phase of the action potential in human myocytes (Young & Herndon-Smith, 1991a). Further study is required to clarify the physiological role of sodium channels.

Potassium channels The potassium channels are involved in terminating action potentials and in returning the membrane potential to its resting level. Furthermore, the resting potential is primarily set by the permeability to potassium ion, and changes in the membrane potential can affect the initiation of the action potential and hence contraction. In pregnant human myometrium, it is believed that the changes in potassium permeability primarily affect the resting potential (Inoue *et al.*, 1990), and that this might be involved in the action of catecholamine β_2-agonist and the effect of high calcium on the duration of action potentials (Kawarabayashi *et al.*, 1984; Kawarabayashi *et al.*, 1986b). Though a single channel potassium current has not yet been recorded from the human myometrium, several studies of potassium current obtained from the myometrial cells of experimental animals by the patch-clamp technique have been reported (Coleman & Parkington, 1987; Kihira *et al.*, 1990; Toro, Stefani & Erulkar, 1990a). It has been suggested that calcium-activated potassium channels, which are controlled by intracellular calcium, are not activated by calmodulin but rather that calcium binds directly to the gating site for channel activation (Kihira *et al.*, 1990). Furthermore, three potassium currents (fast, intermediate and slow) are found in rat myometrium; the fast current is predominant in cells from estrus rats, whereas intermediate current is more frequent in cells from diestrus rats. In addition, norepinephrine potentiates the fast current and reduces the intermediate current (Toro *et al.*, 1990a). Using rat or pig myometrial potassium channels incorporated into lipid bilayers, it has been shown that myometrial β-adrenergic receptors may be coupled to a GTP-dependent protein that can directly gate calcium-activated potassium channels (Toro, Ramos-Franco & Stefani, 1990b).

Effect of reproductive state on active electrical properties

Near the end of pregnancy the circular muscle activities of the rat uterus exhibit characteristic changes that are a prerequisite for normal delivery. These changes consist of a progressive alteration in the configuration of action potentials from a single, plateau-type in early and mid-pregnancy to a repetitive train discharge at term (Osa & Fujino, 1978; Anderson *et al.*, 1981). The action potentials cause brief, irregular contractions during early and mid-pregnancy and regular contractions of longer duration at term. Furthermore, uterine volume (muscle stretching) and circulating estrogens may be more important than the fetoplacental unit in the evolution of circular muscle activity in the pregnant rat (Kawarabayashi & Marshall, 1981). The protein synthesis inhibitor, cycloheximide, can suppress the evolution of activity and delay parturition (Maruta & Osa, 1986). The action potential of longitudinal muscle exhibits a burst discharge of spikes and the pattern does not change throughout pregnancy. However, oestradiol hyperpolarizes the membrane and a burst of spikes is generated from a sustained depolarization. Progesterone, by contrast, slightly hyperpolarizes the membrane and typical burst discharges occur without sustained depolarization. Simultaneous treatment with progesterone and oestradiol produces a plateau potential (Kuriyama

& Suzuki, 1976). Although sex steroids affect membrane properties, the changes which occur during pregnancy cannot be explained by the action of such hormones. There is only one report which describes the electrical activity of human myometrium in early pregnancy (Kawarabayashi *et al.*, 1986a). The action potential is composed of a long plateau potential or abortive spikes superimposed on the long plateau. The duration tends to be longer than in term pregnancy.

Relationship between electrical activity and contraction

Contraction of the myometrium is related to the concentration of intracellular free calcium ion; the increase in intracellular calcium might arise from an influx of calcium from the extracellular space, the translocation of calcium ions in or near the cell membrane and/or the release of calcium from internal stores. Pregnant human myometrium usually generates spontaneous action potentials and extracellular calcium might enter the cell through the calcium channels during these action potentials. In our sucrose-gap experiments, contractions were always synchronized with the corresponding action potentials. Therefore, the amount of calcium which enters during the action potential is sufficient to activate the contractile mechanism and to release additional calcium from internal stores, thereby amplifying the transmembrane signals (Parkington & Coleman, 1990). On the other hand, the periodicity of one-minute contraction and a few minutes of relaxation is essential for mother and fetus during the stress of parturition. A long and hypertonic contraction decreases uteroplacental blood flow, causes fetal hypoxia, and small contractions cannot expel the fetus further. The myometrium has a spontaneous periodicity and thereby generates action potentials and contractions of appropriate duration. Under physiological conditions, the contractility of the uterus is regulated by changing the electrical activity.

Propagation of excitation

In human uterus, the resting tonus maintains uterine shape and fetal position. Resting tonus is maintained by random activation of the myometrium by action potentials. However, well-coordinated contraction is essential for successful expulsion of the fetus after the onset of labour. In order to achieve this coordination, many myometrial cells have to contract at the same time, and local contractions obtained by the coordination of the cells have to synchronize over the whole of the uterus as parturition progresses. Since small muscle strips of pregnant human myometrium exhibit spontaneous periodicity with one-minute contraction and a few minutes relaxation, this periodicity may facilitate coordinated contraction. In our clinical study, the qualitative characteristics of uterine contractions in labour were evaluated by a double guard-ring tocodynamometer attached to the fundus and the caudal part of the uterus. The percentages of both concurrent and synchronous contractions were higher than those of Braxton Hicks contractions, and both values increased significantly between 5 and 6 cm of cervical dilatation (Shinmoto *et al.*, 1991). Thus synchronization of local contractions results in the effective contractions of human parturition. However, the uterus does not have any specific conduction pathways for excitation. Instead, the action potential spreads into the surrounding cells in three-dimensions in accordance with their cable-like properties. The length constant of the membrane gradually increases throughout pregnancy in the rat, as described earlier (see p. 162), and the conduction velocity of the action potential in longitudinal preparations of pregnant rat myometrium increases from 9.2 cm/s at late pregnancy to 10.5 cm/s during delivery (Miller, Garfield & Daniel, 1989). Gap junctions, which are assumed to be the structure involved in electrical and chemical communication between cells, increase during parturition and disappear after delivery in experimental animals (Garfield, 1984). This structure is observed in human myometrium from women in pre-term labour (Garfield & Hayashi, 1981). These changes may contribute to the propagation of excitation during parturition.

Effects of ions and drugs on electrical activity and contraction

Calcium

Extracellular calcium has been shown to play an important role in the activation of smooth muscle, and the amplitude of the tension can be related to the external calcium concentration and consequently to the calcium influx in pregnant rat myometrium (Mironneau, 1973; Bengtsson, Chow & Marshall, 1984). Moreover, the inward calcium current may affect potassium conductance during the plateau potential in the circular muscle of pregnant rat myometrium, and the potassium conductance provides the plateau duration, and consequently the duration of the contraction (Osa & Kawarabayashi, 1977). In pregnant human myometrium, spontaneous contraction is strongly affected by external calcium; 2.5 mM calcium in Krebs solution is the most efficient concentration in terms of frequency, amplitude, and duration of whole contractions. Both excess calcium and low calcium suppress the generation of spontaneous contraction; however, the mechanism of these two types of suppression may differ. Calcium ions may play dual roles in the electrical activity of the myometrium: an excitatory role in action potential and an inhibitory role accomplished by membrane stabilization and calcium-mediated potassium activation. Therefore, the effects of excess calcium on spontaneous contractions may depend on the balance of excitatory and inhibitory effects. If the increase of calcium influx during the action potential is predominant, the amplitude of the contraction will increase; however, the contraction will be diminished if the generation of action potentials is suppressed by membrane stabilization and activation of the outward potassium current. By contrast, low calcium may decrease the influx of calcium and consequently suppress the contraction, since both the amplitude and duration of contraction are generally decreased in low calcium solution (Kawarabayashi *et al.*, 1986*b*, 1989).

Magnesium

Magnesium sulphate has been used as a tocolytic agent to prevent pre-term labour. The effect of magnesium on the spontaneous electrical and mechanical activities of the circular muscle of term pregnant rat uterus suggests that the effect is largely due to suppression of the plateau potential (Osa & Ogasawara, 1983). According to the whole-cell voltage clamp method on freshly isolated single pregnant rat myometrial cells, magnesium inhibits the calcium current, affecting mainly the transient component (Ohya & Sperelakis, 1990). In pregnant human myometrium, frequency, amplitude, and duration of spontaneous contractions all decrease with increases in external magnesium; the frequency change is the most significant (Kawarabayashi *et al.*, 1989*a*). Magnesium ion suppresses the gradient of pacemaker potential, and consequently the frequency of contraction (Kawarabayashi *et al.*, 1984).

Oxytocin

The effect of oxytocin on spontaneous electrical and mechanical activities in pregnant human myometrium has been investigated using the single sucrose-gap method (Kawarabayashi, Kishikawa & Sugimori, 1986*c*). Oxytocin potentiates spontaneous contractions by enhancing the plateau part of action potentials; the spike-type configuration becomes plateau (Fig. 8). This potentiation depends on the external calcium concentration, and the effects on frequency and amplitude of contractions may vary. Oxytocin evokes action potentials and contractions in high frequency; the duration of the action potential is short and the contraction is small in the presence of diltiazem (calcium antagonist) (Fig. 9). The results of the potassium contracture experiment also suggest that oxytocin evokes a contracture in the absence of an action potential by releasing calcium from intracellular storage sites. This possibility is supported by our recent study measuring intracellular calcium using Fura-2 in isolated cells of pregnant rat myometrium (Tsukamoto *et al.*, 1991).

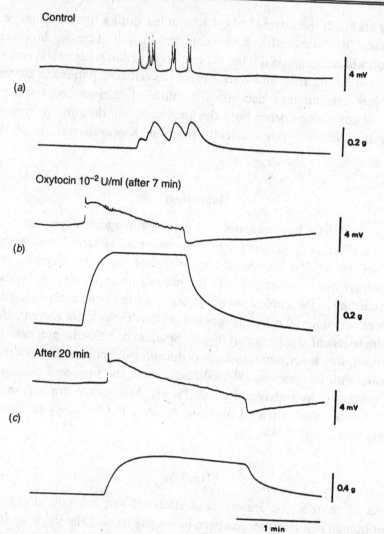

Fig. 8. Effect of 10^{-2} U/ml of oxytocin on spontaneous spike-type action potentials and contractions of pregnant myometrium recorded by the single sucrose-gap method. Trace (*a*) shows control and (*b*) represents responses 7 minutes after the introduction of oxytocin. Contraction trace was saturated in (*b*). Trace (*c*) shows the response after 20 minutes. The upper traces show the electrical activities, and the lower traces, the contractions. (From Kawarabayashi *et al.*, 1986c, with permission.)

The excitatory effect of oxytocin is modified by external magnesium ion in pregnant human myometrium. Relatively high magnesium (2.4 mM) suppresses the spontaneous activities; however, oxytocin enhances the contractions and the plateau part of action potentials to a greater extent than does the magnesium-free solution. In the potassium contracture experiment, the oxytocin-induced contracture

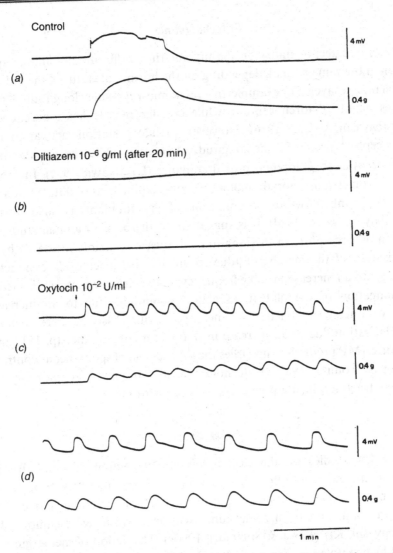

Fig. 9. Effect of 10^{-2} U/ml of oxytocin on spontaneous activities in the presence of 10^{-6} g/ml of diltiazem. Trace (*a*) is a control (plateau-type action potential), and (*b*) shows the responses to application of 10^{-6} g/ml of diltiazem. (*c*) and (*d*) are continuous records showing the effect of oxytocin in the presence of diltiazem. The upper traces show electrical activities, and the lower ones, the contractions. (Kawarabayashi *et al.*, 1986*c*, with permission.)

during the tonic phase is potentiated by magnesium. Magnesium may potentiate the excitatory effect of oxytocin at superficial sites of the plasma membrane, allowing the possibility of intracellular action (Kawarabayashi *et al.*, 1990*a*). The interaction between calcium and magnesium is probably very significant in the regulation of the action of oxytocin on uterine contractility.

Catecholamines

The effects of catecholamines on the myometrium differ among animal species, and even in the same animal, depending on the hormonal status of the individual and each muscle layer. For example, in a rat at mid-pregnancy longitudinal muscle possesses mainly β-adrenoceptors, while circular muscle has α-adrenoceptors (Kawarabayashi & Osa, 1976). However, in late gestation, activation of the α-adrenoceptors occurs in the longitudinal muscle, while the circular muscle switches from α- to β-adrenoceptor dominance (Kishikawa, 1981). In pregnant human myometrium, noradrenaline always exhibits α-excitatory action at $10^{-12}–10^{-6}$ g/ml; however β-inhibition of β_2-stimulant is also observed (Kawarabayashi et al., 1984). It is suggested on the basis of animal studies that activation of α-receptors in the longitudinal muscle is mainly mediated by slow depolarization of the membrane (due to an increase in chloride conductance) which leads to an increase in spike frequency; in the circular muscle it is mediated by prolongation of the plateau of action potentials (due to an increase in calcium conductance). β-action of the myometrium also includes membrane hyperpolarization due to an increase in potassium conductance (p. 161) and an increase in cAMP production underlies the suppression of spontaneous contraction (Bülbring & Tomita, 1987). Catecholamine action may fundamentally affect uterine contractility during pregnancy and parturition.

Other drugs

There are few studies on the electrophysiological action of other drugs on the human myometrium. Prostaglandin $F_{2\alpha}$ and methylergometrine maleate (methergin) potentiate the plateau part of the action potential and contraction of pregnant human myometrium (Kawarabayashi & Sugimori, 1985; Kawarabayashi, Kishikawa & Sugimori, 1990b). The action of methergin is not inhibited by phentolamine (an α-blocker). Plateau enhancement may be the main effects.

Conclusion

The myometrium has a spontaneously active and highly excitable membrane with many voltage dependent ion channels. Contractility of the myometrium is regulated by the electrical activity of this membrane. The main external controlling factors are sex steroid hormones. The balance of oestrogen and progesterone, and the changes during the course of the menstrual cycle, pregnancy and parturition, changes the pattern of action potentials and the effects of drugs such as catecholamines and oxytocin. Hormones also affect the conduction of excitation and produce morphological changes of cell size. All of these changes lead to synchronized contractions which are effective in expulsion of the fetus. It is particularly important for the fetus that the periodicity of the phasic contractions is strictly maintained.

Acknowledgements

The author is grateful to Professor T. Osa and Professor H. Nakano for their consistent encouragements in this work and to Dr K. Kitamura for his advice, and also to Mrs Lisa Tsukamoto for correcting the manuscript. This work was supported by a grant-in-aid for general scientific research (No. 03670793) from the Ministry of Education, Science and Culture, Japan.

References

Abe, Y. & Tomita, T. (1968). Cable properties of smooth muscle. *Journal of Physiology*, **196**, 87–100.

Anderson, G. F., Kawarabayashi, T. & Marshall, J. M. (1981). Effect of indomethacin and aspirin on uterine activity in pregnant rats: comparison of circular and longitudinal muscle. *Biology of Reproduction*, **24**, 359–72.

Bengtsson, B., Chow, E. H. M. & Marshall, J. M. (1984). Calcium dependency of pregnant rat myometrium: Comparison of circular and longitudinal muscle. *Biology of Reproduction*, **30**, 869–78.

Bolton, T. B. (1979). Mechanisms of action of transmitters and other substances on smooth muscle. *Physiology Reviews*, **59**, 606–718.

Bülbring, E. & Tomita, T. (1987). Catecholamine action on smooth muscle. *Pharmacology Reviews*, **39**, 49–96.

Coburn, R. F., Ohba, M. & Tomita, T. (1975). Recording of intracellular electrical activity with the sucrose-gap method. In *Methods in Pharmacology*, vol. 3, *Smooth Muscle*. Ed. E. E. Daniel and D. M. Paton, pp. 231–45, Plenum Press, New York.

Cole, W. C. & Garfield, R. E. (1989). Ultrastructure of the myometrium. In *Biology of the Uterus*. Ed. R. M. Wynn and W. P. Jollie, pp. 455–504, Plenum Press, New York.

Coleman, H. A. & Parkington, H. C. (1987). Single channel Cl- and K-currents from cells of uterus not treated with enzymes. *Pflügers Archives*, **410**, 560–2.

Garfield, R. E. & Hayashi, R. H. (1981). Appearance of gap junctions in the myometrium of women during labor. *American Journal of Obstetrics and Gynecology*, **140**, 254–60.

Garfield, R. E. (1984). Control of myometrial function in preterm versus term labor. *Clinical Obstetrics and Gynecology*, **27**, 572–91.

Inoue, Y., Nakao, K., Okabe, K. *et al.* (1990). Some electrical properties of human pregnant myometrium. *American Journal of Obstetrics and Gynecology*, **162**, 1090–8.

Kanda, S. & Kuriyama, H. (1980). Specific features of smooth muscle cells recorded from the placental region of the myometrium of pregnant rats. *Journal of Physiology*, **299**, 127–44.

Kawarabayashi, T. & Osa, T. (1976). Comparative investigations of alpha- and beta-effects on the longitudinal and circular muscles of the pregnant rat myometrium. *Japan Journal of Physiology*, **26**, 403–16.

Kawarabayashi, T. (1978). The effects of phenylephrine in various ionic environments on the circular muscle of mid-pregnant rat myometrium. *Japan Journal of Physiology*, **28**, 627–45.

Kawarabayashi, T. & Marshall, J. M. (1981). Factors influencing circular muscle activity in the pregnant rat uterus. *Biology of Reproduction*, **24**, 373–9.

Kawarabayashi, T., Ikeda, M., Sugimori, H. & Nakano, H. (1984). Effects of magnesium and catecholamines on spontaneous contraction of pregnant human isthmic myometrium. *Asia-Oceania Journal of Obstetrics and Gynaecology*, **10**, 375–84.

Kawarabayashi, T. & Sugimori, H. (1985). Effects of oxytocin and prostaglandin $F_{2\alpha}$ on pregnant human myometrium recorded by the single sucrose-gap method. Comparison of an *in vitro* experiment and an *in vivo* trial. *Asia-Oceania Journal of Obstetrics and Gynaecology*, **11**, 247–53.

Kawarabayashi, T., Ikeda, M., Sugimori, H. & Nakano, H. (1986a). Sponteneous electrical activity and effects of noradrenaline on pregnant human myometrium recorded by the single sucrose-gap method. *Acta Physiologia Hungaria*, **67**, 71–82.

Kawarabayashi, T., Kishikawa, T. & Sugimori, H. (1986b). Effects of external calcium and calcium antagonist, diltiazem, on isolated segments of pregnant human myometrium. *Asia-Oceania Journal of Obstetrics and Gynaecology*, **12**, 409–17.

Kawarabayashi, T., Kishikawa, T. & Sugimori, H. (1986c). Effect of oxytocin on spontaneous electrical and mechanical activities in pregnant human myometrium. *American Journal of Obstetrics and Gynecology*, **55**, 671–6.

Kawarabayashi, T., Kishikawa, T. & Sugimori, H. (1988). Characteristics of action potentials and contractions evoked by electrical-field stimulation of pregnant human myometrium. *Gynecological and Obstetric Investigations*, **25**, 73–9.

Kawarabayashi, T., Kishikawa, T. & Sugimori, H. (1989). Effects of external calcium, magnesium, and temperature on spontaneous contractions of pregnant human myometrium. *Biology of Reproduction*, **40**, 942–8.

Kawarabayashi, T., Izumi, H., Ikeda, M., Ichihara, J., Sugimori, H. & Shirakawa, K. (1990a). Modification by magnesium of the excitatory effect of oxytocin in electrical and mechanical activities of pregnant human myometrium. *Obstetrics and Gynecology*, **76**, 183–8.

Kawarabayashi, T., Kishikawa, T. & Sugimori, H. (1990b). Effect of methylergometrine maleate (methergin) on electrical and mechanical activities of pregnant human myometrium. *Gynecological and Obstetric Investigations*, **29**, 246–9.

Kihira, M., Matsuzawa, K., Tokuno, H. & Tomita, T. (1990). Effects of calmodulin antagonists on calcium-activated potassium channels in pregnant rat myometrium. *British Journal of Pharmacology*, **100**, 353–9.

Kishikawa, T. (1981). Alterations in the properties of the rat myometrium during gestation and post partum. *Japan Journal of Physiology*, **31**, 515–36.

Kuriyama, H. & Suzuki, H. (1976). Changes in electrical properties of rat myometrium during gestation and following hormonal treatments. *Journal of Physiology*, **260**, 315–33.

Marshall, J. M. (1973). The physiology of the myometrium. In *The Uterus*, pp. 89–109, Williams & Wilkins, Baltimore.

Maruta, K. & Osa, T. (1986). Blockage by cycloheximide of the prepartum changes in membrane activity and adrenergic response of the circular muscle of rat uterus. *Japan Journal of Physiology*, **36**, 971–83.

Masahashi, T. & Tomita, T. (1983). The contracture produced by sodium removal in the non-pregnant rat myometrium. *Journal of Physiology*, **334**, 351–63.

Miller, S. M., Garfield, R. E. & Daniel, E. E. (1989). Improved propagation in myometrium associated with gap junctions during parturition. *American Journal of Physiology*, **256**, C130–41.

Mironneau, J. (1973). Excitation–contraction coupling in voltage clamped uterine smooth muscle. *Journal of Physiology*, **233**, 127–41.

Nakajima, A. (1971). Action potention of human myometrial fibers. *American Journal of Obstetrics and Gynecology*, **111**, 266–9.

Ohya, Y. & Sperelakis, N. (1989). Fast Na^+ and slow Ca^{2+} channels in single uterine muscle cells from pregnant rats. *Americal Journal of Physiology*, **257**, C408–12.

Ohya, Y. & Sperelakis, N. (1990). Tocolytic agents act on calcium channel current in single smooth muscle cells of pregnant rat uterus. *Journal of Pharmacology Experimental Therapy*, **253**, 580–5.

Okabe, K., Terada, K., Kitamura, K. & Kuriyama, H. (1987). Features of 4-aminopyridine sensitive outward current observed in single smooth muscle cells from the rabbit pulmonary artery. *Pflügers Archives*, **409**, 561–8.

Osa, T. (1971). Effect of removing the external sodium on the electrical and mechanical activities of the pregnant mouse myometrium. *Japan Journal of Physiology*, **21**, 607–25.

Osa, T. & Kawarabayashi, T. (1977). Effects of ions and drugs on the plateau potential in the circular muscle of pregnant rat myometrium. *Japan Journal of Physiology*, **27**, 111–21.

Osa, T. & Fujino, T. (1978). Electrophysiological comparison between the longitudinal and circular muscles of the rat uterus during the estrous cycle and pregnancy. *Japan Journal of Physiology*, **28**, 197–209.

Osa, T. & Ogasawara, T. (1983). Effects of magnesium on the membrane activity and contraction of the circular muscle of rat myometrium during late pregnancy. *Japan Journal of Physiology*, **33**, 485–95.

Parkington, H. C. & Coleman, H. A. (1990). The role of membrane potential in the control of uterine motility. In *Uterine Function: Molecular and Cellular Aspects*. Ed. M. E. Carsten and J. D. Miller, pp. 195–248, Plenum Press, New York.

Pressman, E. K., Tucker, Jr. J. A., Anderson, Jr. N. C. & Young, R. C. (1988). Morphologic and electrophysiologic characterization of isolated pregnant human myometrial cells. *American Journal of Obstetrics and Gynecology*, **59**, 1273–9.

Reiner, O. & Marshall, J. M. (1976). Action of prostaglandin, $PGF_{2\alpha}$, on the uterus of the pregnant rat. *Naunyn-Schmiedeberg's Archives in Pharmacology*, **292**, 243–50.

Shinmoto, M., Kawarabayashi, T., Ikeda, M. & Sugimori, H. (1991). Qualitative evaluation of uterine contractions recorded by a double guard-ring tocodynamometer. *American Journal of Obstetrics and Gynecology*, (in press).

Sims, S. M., Daniel, E. E. & Garfield, R. E. (1982). Improved electrical coupling in uterine smooth muscle is associated with increased numbers of gap junctions at parturition. *Journal of General Physiology*, **80**, 353–75.

Toro, L., Stefani, E. & Erulkar, S. (1990a). Hormonal regulation of potassium currents in single myometrial cells. *Proceedings of the National Academy of Sciences, USA*, **87**, 2892–5.

Toro, L., Ramos-Franco, J. & Stefani, E. (1990*b*). GTP-dependent regulation of myometrial K–Ca channels incorporated into lipid bilayers. *Journal of General Physiology*, **96**, 373–94.

Tsukamoto, T., Kawarabayashi, T., Kaneko, Y., Kumamoto, T. & Sugimori, H. (1991). Intracellular calcium of longitudinal muscles isolated from pregnant rat myometrium. *Cell Biology International Report*, **15**, 637–44.

Young, R. C. & Herndon-Smith, L. (1991*a*). Characterization of sodium channels in cultured human uterine smooth muscle cells. *American Journal of Obstetrics and Gynecology*, **64**, 175–81.

Young, R. C., Herndon-Smith, L. & Anderson, Jr. N. C. (1991*b*). Passive membrane properties and inward calcium current of human uterine smooth muscle cells. *American Journal of Obstetrics and Gynecology*, **164**, 1132–9.

8

Hormonal control of myometrial function

S. BATRA

Introduction

Compared with other smooth muscles, the myometrium is unique by virtue of being a major target for ovarian steroids. The smooth muscle of the uterine vasculature may also be a target for oestrogen and progesterone. *In vivo*, both the myometrium and smooth muscle of the uterine vessels are subject to changes in the environment, be it physiological such as cyclic hormonal changes or pharmacological such as those observed after the administration of drugs or hormones. Consequently, the results of *in vivo* observations discussed in later sections may be very different from those seen *in vitro* with uterine strips. Another confounding aspect of myometrial studies is the diversity in the pattern of hormonal regulation of myometrial activity among different species.

Myometrial function

The ultrastructure and mechanisms of excitation and contraction of uterine smooth muscle are not very different from those of other smooth muscle cells. The cytoplasm is largely filled with myofilaments. Most ultrastructural studies of mammalian smooth muscle, including uterine muscle, have described myofilaments of only one diameter. Uterine smooth muscle contains both actin and myosin in proportions similar to those found in skeletal muscle; in the latter, actin and myosin exhibit a highly ordered management. The studies by Devine and co-workers (Devine, Somlyo & Somlyo, 1972) showed that the intracellular organization of contractile proteins in smooth muscle is different from that in skeletal muscle. The thick myosin and thin actin filaments occur in long random bundles throughout the smooth muscle cells; unlike skeletal muscle, the continuity of these filaments is not interrupted by Z-lines. There is also a third type of filament, the 100 Å intermediate filaments. The intermediate filaments are attached randomly at sites on the inner surface of the smooth muscle cells known as dense bodies. These sites provide a structural network and as well as points of attachment for filaments.

The major calcium sequestering organelle, the sarcoplasmic reticulum, in smooth muscles is less well developed than in skeletal muscle (Gabella, 1971; Devine et al., 1972). Consequently, these cells are more dependent on extracellular calcium than are skeletal and even cardiac muscle cells. Similar mechanisms are involved in the transport of calcium across the cell membrane of myometrial and other smooth muscle cells. They include voltage-dependent calcium channels, ATP-dependent calcium pumps, sodium–calcium exchange mechanisms and receptor-controlled calcium channels (Batra, 1987).

The mechanism of activation of the contractile machinery of smooth muscle has only recently been fully elucidated. The interactions between calcium and contractile proteins in smooth muscle are different from those in skeletal muscle. In particular, Ca^{2+} does not appear to react with troponin C as in the case of skeletal muscle, but with another Ca-binding protein, calmodulin (Kamm & Stull, 1985). The calcium–calmodulin complex activates a protein kinase known as myosin light chain kinase, with specific phosphorylation of the 20 kD light chain of smooth muscle myosin. Once phosphorylated, the myosin can react with actin to form contractile linkages. This interaction occurs in a cyclic fashion involving attachment, which acts as a power stroke, followed by detachment of cross-bridges and the splitting of one mole of ATP in each cycle. The cross-bridge activity results in either force generation and/or shortening of the muscle fibres. In contracted smooth muscle, myosin is more phosphorylated than in relaxed smooth muscle. The degree of phosphorylation and hence of contraction depends on the balance of the activities of kinase on the one hand, and of myosin phosphatase on the other.

Recent developments contribute to the belief that smooth muscle contractile mechanisms differ in several respects from that of skeletal muscle. In particular, the actomyosin interaction noted above was different from that in skeletal muscle. Furthermore, in smooth muscle extracellular calcium plays a dominant role in the activation of the contractile process (Daniel & Janis, 1975; Loutzenhiser et al., 1985; Batra, 1987). The earlier failure to recognize these differences was responsible for the slow progress in understanding the cellular mechanisms of excitation–contraction coupling and interaction of contractile proteins in smooth muscle.

Ovarian steroids

In 1896 Sokoloff reported that castration had a dramatic effect on the evolution of myometrial activity. By the turn of the century it was suggested that the ovaries

Table 1. *Plasma, oestradiol and progesterone concentration in guinea-pig, man and rabbit*

	Oestradiol pg/ml			Progesterone ng/ml		
	Non-pregnant	Mid-term	Full term	Non-pregnant	Mid-term	Full term
Guinea-pig	29.8	20.5	59.3	3.6	203	162
Man	106	5100	19 700	6.7	38.8	172
Rabbit	31.8	27.5	34.5	0.3	18	7

produce substances that influence the uterus. These observations were made many years before the chemical structure of oestrogen was elucidated. Despite this early start, knowledge in this area is still insufficient to allow a definitive statement on the influence of ovarian hormones on myometrial function. Even today it is not uncommon to find contradictory statements in the literature about the influence of ovarian steroids on uterine activity. Much confusion results from the fact that little attention has been paid to the inherent differences in hormonal regulation of myometrial activity among different species (Finn & Porter, 1975; Batra & Dahlander, 1984). This is well illustrated by the data shown in Table 1, compiled from a number of studies on the dynamics of ovarian steroids in three species during pregnancy (see Batra *et al.*, 1976, 1979; Batra, Sjöberg & Thorbert, 1980). In the guinea pig and rabbit, relatively small changes in plasma oestradiol occur during pregnancy; in others, plasma oestradiol levels increase by tenfold around mid-term and by a further fourfold at full term. The pattern of changes in plasma progesterone in all three species is strikingly different (Table 1). All show an increase. In the rabbit, however, the levels decline towards the end of pregnancy, consistent with the progesterone block theory (Csapo, 1956). In man, the levels continue to increase throughout pregnancy (Batra *et al.*, 1976; Andersson, Hancock & Oakey, 1985); plasma progesterone concentrations at full term are approximately fourfold higher than those at mid-term. In the guinea pig there is little difference between the levels at mid- and full term, although progesterone levels are 50–60 times higher than those in non-pregnant animals. Whereas in the non-pregnant guinea-pig, approximately 80% of the total plasma progesterone is protein-bound, at term nearly 100% of plasma progesterone exists in the bound form and is therefore probably devoid of biological activity. This is due to production of large amounts of a progesterone binding protein which is unique to this species; the biological function is not known. The consequence of elevated progesterone binding is that there is no change in the concentration of free progesterone despite a nearly 50-fold increase in total progesterone (Batra *et al.*, 1980).

In spite of these differences in plasma steroid levels and even myometrial concentrations of ovarian steroids in different species, the ability to develop forceful myometrial contractions during labour is a universal property of uterine smooth muscle in all species. Species differences must always be remembered in studies of the effects of ovarian steroids, particularly at the cellular level. Lack of attention to these differences has given rise to controversies on the role of progesterone in the initiation of parturition. This is illustrated by the argument that raged between the supporters and opponents of the progesterone block hypothesis. This provocative hypothesis has been a useful stimulus to research, but is not consistent with experimental observations in man (see Fuchs & Fuchs, 1984; Batra, 1985a). It originated with observations in the rabbit and remained a dominant theory for nearly two decades. Many conclusions in support of the hypothesis were extrapolated with impunity from the one species to many others.

It is not possible to cover in a single chapter all aspects of the influence of oestrogen and progesterone on myometrial function in all species. The effects of ovarian steroids on myometrial activity have been studied in considerable detail in the rabbit, a species in which the progesterone block theory finds strongest support. In the present discussion, much attention will focus on the rabbit, but comparisons and contrasts with the human myometrium will be emphasized.

Oestrogens

The involvement of oestrogens in RNA and protein synthesis is well established. Major biochemical and morphological changes follow administration of oestrogen. The effects on uterine blood flow and fluid accumulation occur within a few hours following oestrogen administration whereas mitosis in the glands and epithelium, hypertrophy of myometrial cells and uterine enlargement are late effects observed after 18–24 hours. Most if not all of these actions of oestrogens are mediated by interaction of oestrogen with specific nuclear receptors and are considered as truly genomic actions (Fig. 1). These effects of oestrogens are observed in all species that have been studied. In addition to these well-known effects, oestrogens can exert actions that are unrelated or not directly related to transcription by receptor bound oestrogen (see Fig. 1).

Effects on plasma membrane

A number of studies suggest that the plasma membrane may be the initial cellular site of steroid hormone interaction, prior to steroid entry into cytoplasm and interaction with the nuclear receptors. An example of direct effects of oestrogen on a plasma membrane was provided by Bergamini et al. (1985) who showed

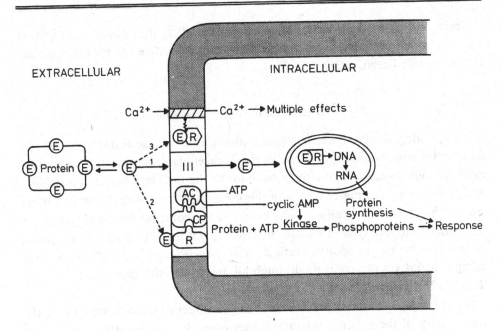

Fig. 1. Cellular mechanism(s) of oestrogen (E) action on the myometrium. Only the free (not protein bound) hormone is able to penetrate the cell membrane, and as shown in (1) combines in the nucleus with a specific receptor (R). The receptor complex subsequently binds to nuclear acceptor sites on the chromatin which results in the alteration of gene transcription, DNA-dependent RNA and protein synthesis and finally the synthesis of proteins (see Rories & Spelsberg, 1989, for different models of ovarian steroid action). The E molecule (2) may combine with a receptor in the plasma membrane, the existence of which is still not unequivocally acknowledged, and activate adenylate cyclase (AC) via a coupling protein (CP) to generate cyclic AMP which is the second messenger of hormonal action (for details see Michell, 1987). Thirdly (3) E after combining with a receptor (hypothetical) may directly influence the entry of calcium into the cell through membrane calcium channels. An increase in cytoplasmic Ca^{2+}, another key messenger for eliciting cellular responses, leads to multiple effects.

specific stimulation of adenylate cyclase activity within minutes following exposure to oestradiol of membrane prepared from secretory human endometrium.

High affinity binding of oestrogen to membrane fractions prepared from isolated uterine cells of ovariectomized rats was originally shown by Pietras & Szego (1975). Direct oestrogen-induced changes in membrane permeability were also observed with rapid changes (10–30 min) in calcium influx after addition of small amounts of oestradiol (10^{-9} M). The rapid elevation of uterine nuclear RNA labelling that follows administration of oestradiol to rats injected with ^{3}H-uridine (Means & Hamilton, 1966), could reflect a direct effect on membrane permeability causing a rapid increase in the activity of the intracellular nucleosides.

Szego and co-workers have presented evidence that the primary recognition site for steroid hormones, as for peptide hormones, is localized on the outer surface of the cell (see Szego, 1978).

Effects on excitation–contraction coupling

It is now widely accepted that, in smooth muscle as in cardiac and striated muscle, an effective stimulus leads to a rise in the intracellular concentration of ionized calcium. This so-called activator calcium forms the final link between excitation and contraction. The major source of this calcium in the myometrium and other smooth muscles is extracellular. The extent of the contribution from within the cell varies from one type of smooth muscle to another. The extent to which the plasma membrane, endoplasmic reticulum or mitochondria provide the activator calcium is not yet determined, although all are potentially capable of doing so (Batra, 1977; Grover, 1985).

Studies from our laboratory have also shown direct effects of oestrogen on the contractility of the isolated rat uterus. Oestrogen has an important inhibitory effect on calcium entry into uterine cells (Batra & Bengtsson, 1978). Oestrogens reduced the influx of calcium in both normal and depolarized uterine tissue but did not affect ^{45}Ca efflux. In the same study, it was shown that oestrogen had an inhibitory effect on the mechanical responses of the uterus: the amplitude of contractions induced by acetylcholine was considerably reduced. Furthermore, oestrogens blocked the second and relatively slow phase of the contraction without influencing the first rapid response. From this it was concluded that the major action of oestrogen was to prevent the influx of extracellular calcium and thereby to inhibit responses dependent on extracellular calcium. In another study it was shown that the non-steroidal oestrogen, diethylstilbestrol, caused significant inhibition of both ^{45}Ca influx and ^{3}H-nitrendipine binding in the oestrogenized rat myometrium (Batra, 1985b).

The inhibitory effect of oestrogens on myometrial activity *in vitro* has been confirmed in strips prepared from the non-pregnant human myometrium. The human myometrium *in vitro* was more sensitive to the effects of oestrogen than the rat myometrium (Fig. 2). The IC_{50} values for both spontaneous myometrial activity and vasopressin-induced contractions were less than 10 μM for oestradiol 17-β (Kostrzewska, Laudanski & Batra, 1992). In contrast to the rat myometrium, the inhibitory action of oestrogen (and progesterone) did not depend on retardation of the entry of extracellular calcium through voltage-dependent channels. Instead, there was inhibition of receptor-operated calcium channels and possibly also release of intracellular calcium. This conclusion was supported by the fact that there was greater inhibition by steroids of vasopressin-induced

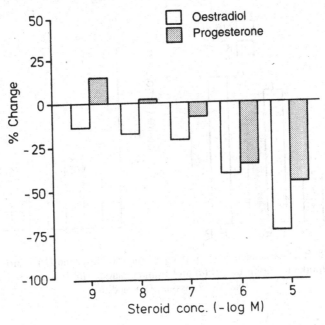

Fig. 2. Change in *in vitro* spontaneous response of the human myometrium to different concentrations of oestradiol and progesterone in the medium.

responses than of those induced by potassium depolarization (Kostrzewska *et al.*, 1992).

In vivo *effects*

The results obtained with myometria from rats and rabbits that had been oestrogenized for various lengths of time present a different picture. Oestrogen treatment usually led to an increase in contractility and ^{45}Ca influx in the isolated uteri (see Batra, 1987). In a recent study it was shown that both calcium uptake by the myometrium and the density of calcium channels and muscarinic cholinergic receptors was substantially higher in oestrogenized rabbits (Batra, 1990). The uptake of ^{45}Ca in the strips of urinary bladder from the same animals was not influenced by oestrogens (Fig. 3). The concentration of oestrogen receptors decreases substantially after short-term (1–5 days) or long-term (1–8 weeks) exposure to oestrogen (Batra *et al.*, 1987, and Fig. 4). Furthermore, the concentration of both cytosolic and nuclear receptors was decreased although uterine wet-weight increased more than 10-fold throughout the 8-week period of oestrogenization (Fig. 4). Uterine peroxidase-activity, which is highly dependent on oestrogen and which was undetectable in untreated animals, increased

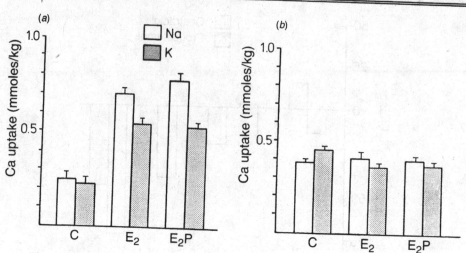

Fig. 3. Effect of oestrogen (E_2), oestrogen and progesterone (P) treatment on calcium uptake in rabbit uterus (*a*) and urinary bladder (*b*) incubated in sodium (Na) or potassium (K) medium.

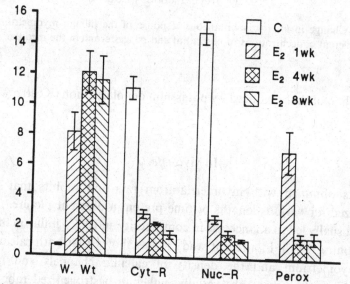

Fig. 4. Uterine wet weight (W.Wt, expressed in g) and cytosolic oestrogen receptors (Cyt-R, expressed as fmol × 100/mg protein), nuclear oestrogen receptors (Nuc-R, expressed as fmol × 100/mg protein) peroxidase (Perox) units in control (C) after 1 week (E_2-1 wk), 4 weeks (E_2 4 wk) and 8 weeks (E_2 8 wk) of oestrogen treatment in rabbits.

dramatically during the first week and then decreased by five-fold. Whether the effects of oestrogen treatment on membrane receptors are exclusively a result of interaction with intracellular receptors is still unknown since the time courses of changes in uterine weight, peroxidase activity and membrane receptors are not in concordance. It may be speculated that the responses mediated by the genomic action of oestrogen stem from the initial receptor interaction which translates into different individual responses with different time courses and durations. The duration depends probably on the length of the oestrogen treatment and may not have any direct relation to the number of oestrogen receptors (Fig. 4). The reduction of oestrogen receptors observed soon after oestrogen treatment (Batra *et al.*, 1987), and that is maintained with continuing treatment, may be an important part of an 'on' and 'off' mechanism.

The concept that, following initial stimulation, continued oestrogen treatment leads to desensitization and inhibition is supported by the data of Stormshak *et al.* (1976) who demonstrated that long-term administration of oestrogen to female rats induced a decrease in thymidine incorporation into DNA; thus continuation of oestrogen treatment leads to a refractory uterus. Mukku *et al.* (1981) reached a similar conclusion from their studies on thymidine incorporation in the uterus. Recently Haras, Samperez & Jouan (1989) have confirmed these studies and suggested that a specific protein inhibitor, the 105 kD protein, was synthesized with continuous exposure to oestrogen and was responsible for the reduction in the synthetic activity in the target organ.

Our recent data on peroxidase activity and oestrogen and other membrane receptors (Fig. 4) suggest an increase in synthesis of inhibitor protein by oestrogens. There may be a feedback control mechanism for this negative and positive effect of oestrogen. Tissues exhibiting a rapid and dramatic initial response to oestrogen, such as the uterus, rapidly become refractory to oestrogen, whereas other targets such as the tissues of the lower urinary tract show much slower desensitization (Batra & Iosif, 1992).

In addition to the above effects, the presence of oestrogen in the circulation would exert direct effects on the cell membrane and thereby myometrial activity (see also Batra, 1980). Together the genomic and non-genomic actions can lead to a complex situation. Unless great care is taken to analyse the separate parameters, erroneous conclusions are likely. The complexity of these mechanisms is illustrated in Fig. 5.

Progesterone

While the importance of progesterone in the maintenance of pregancy is widely acknowledged, the mechanism of action is poorly understood. Although the onset of labour in a variety of species is preceded by a fall in plasma progesterone, this is not seen in humans, monkeys and guinea-pigs (Finn & Porter, 1975; Batra, 1985a).

In the rabbit, the species in which evidence for the progesterone block hyopthesis

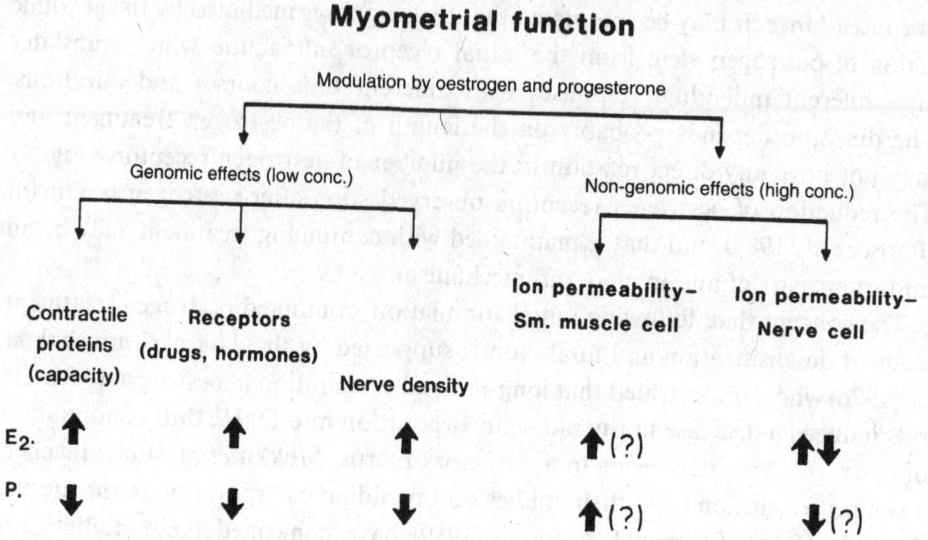

Myometrial function

Modulation by oestrogen and progesterone

Genomic effects (low conc.)   Non-genomic effects (high conc.)

			Ion permeability–	Ion permeability–
Contractile	Receptors		Sm. muscle cell	Nerve cell
proteins	(drugs, hormones)			
(capacity)		Nerve density		
E_2. ↑	↑	↑	↑(?)	↑↓
P. ↓	↓	↓	↑(?)	↓(?)

Fig. 5. Modulation by oestrogen (E_2) and progesterone (P) of myometrial function
and the possible mechanisms involved. Genomic mode of action which usually is
activated by very low concentration of E_2 leads to increased protein synthesis
resulting in specific effects as shown. Progesterone in this instant suppresses the
effect of E_2. Non-genomic action primarily resides in the cell membrane and is
not well understood.

was initially obtained, progesterone administration in physiological doses led to
a clear and rapid inhibition of myometrial activity (see Laudanski & Batra, 1984).
Withdrawal of progesterone by prostaglandin-induced luteolysis or by stopping
a progesterone infusion clearly resulted in augmented uterine contractions similar
to those observed during parturition.

The pseudopregnant rabbit is an excellent model for studying the influence of
progesterone on myometrial function since there are changes in progesterone
concentration almost identical to those in the pregnant rabbit except on a
contracted time scale (21 days rather than 31 days) (Fig. 6). Additionally, there
are relatively small changes in oestradiol levels, and in the pseudopregnant uterus
there is no fetal influence.

The effect of plasma progesterone elevation (day 6–12) and subsequent
withdrawal (day 18) can be observed in these studies on pseudopregnant animals
(Fig. 7). The weight of the uterus increased several fold, whereas oestrogen
receptors decreased, increasing toward the end of pseudopregnancy when the
progesterone level fell (Fig. 6 and Fig. 7). However, no significant change occurred
in uterine ^{45}Ca uptake or in the density of calcium channels or muscarinic
cholinergic receptors (Fig. 7). Thus the effect of progesterone on uterine activity
is probably not explained by alterations in uterine calcium uptake, calcium channel

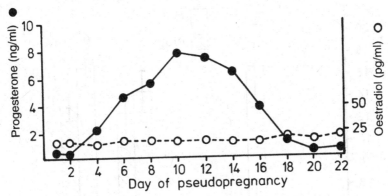

Fig. 6. Plasma oestradiol and progesterone concentration during pseudopregnancy
in the rabbit.

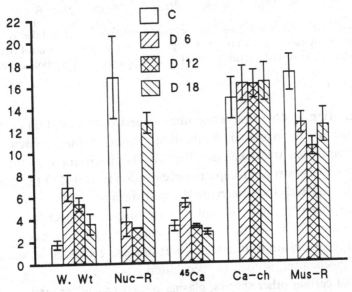

Fig. 7. Uterine wet weight (W.Wt, expressed in g), nuclear oestrogen receptor
(Nuc-R, expressed as fmol × 100/mg protein), ^{45}Ca uptake (^{45}Ca, expressed as
mmoles/kg), calcium channel density (Ca-ch, expressed as fmol × 10/mg protein)
and muscarinic cholinergic receptor density (Mus-R, expressed as fmol × 10/mg
protein) in control (C) and on day 6 (D 6), day 12 (D 12) and day 18 (D 18) of
pseudopregnancy in rabbits.

density or other cell surface receptors. To determine whether the changes observed
during pseudopregnancy were a result of changes in plasma progesterone levels,
similar studies were done in rabbits treated with progesterone to achieve
comparable levels. The data in Fig. 8 clearly confirmed this.

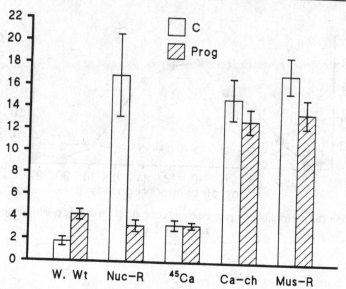

Fig. 8. Uterine wet weight, nuclear oestrogen receptor, ^{45}Ca uptake, calcium channel density and muscarinic cholinergic receptor density in control (C) and progesterone-treated (Prog) rabbits. See Fig. 7 for description of symbols and units.

It is interesting to note that while nuclear oestrogen receptors declined, the weight of the uterus increased, a situation similar to that encountered with continuous oestrogen treatment (see Fig. 4). This is contrary to the generally accepted view that oestrogen receptor concentration is related to the proliferative response. The very early increase in nuclear oestrogen receptors, within 1–6 hours, following oestrogen treatment is probably an adequate trigger for the series of events that follow. Whether the decline in receptor with continuous oestrogen or progesterone exposure is an integral part of these events, or serves as a type of feedback mechanism, is open to speculation.

In man and certain other species, plasma oestrogen and progesterone remain at high levels at the onset of labour. If the genomic response depends on the concentration of nuclear receptors, this response would probably be non-existent at term since the concentration of both oestrogen and progesterone receptors is very low (Giannopoulas & Tulchinsky, 1979). Furthermore, there is no significant change in the concentration of the steroids in plasma or their receptors in the myometrium before parturition (see Batra, 1985a).

Direct effects of progesterone

Little information is available on the direct (non-genomic) effects of progesterone in the human myometrium. In the rat, progesterone up to 20 μM has a negligible effect on spontaneous myometrial activity. However, in a recent study on the human myometrium, progesterone was found to be as potent as oestradiol in inhibiting spontaneous myometrial activity (Fig. 2), indicating species differences (Kostrzewska, Laudanski & Batra, 1992).

While the role of progesterone in parturition has been the subject of many studies, little attention has been paid to the active metabolites of progesterone. Progesterone is metabolized by the uterus to a number of 5α and 5β compounds. Many of these metabolites of progesterone, particularly those of the 5β reduced series, are more potent than progesterone in inhibiting uterine contractility. This raises the interesting possibility that the effect of progesterone on uterine contractility may actually be exerted through its metabolites. This is consistent with the observation that metabolites which are effective in inhibiting uterine contractility are also those which have anaesthetic effects *in vivo*. Because the kinetics of uterine and neuronal responses are extremely rapid, steroids may act at the membrane level to exert their effects upon these systems. The mechanism by which progesterone metabolites exert an anaesthetic effect appears to be related to their interaction with the receptors for gamma-aminobutyric acid$_A$ (GABA$_A$). Erdö (1984) has shown that a relatively high density of GABA$_A$ receptors is present in the rat uterus, and that these receptors can be activated by the progesterone metabolites, 3α, 5α-D-tetrahydroprogesterone (THP). Putnam *et al.* (1991) have presented convincing evidence that the inhibition of uterine contractions by progesterone and its metabolites is mediated by their interaction with the GABA$_A$ receptor in the uterus. The inhibitory responses were counteracted by the specific GABA$_A$ receptor inhibitor, pictrotoxin and not by the progesterone receptor antagonist, RU 486. The authors found that the progesterone metabolites were more potent than native progesterone in inhibiting myometrial contractions. These studies emphasize the importance of membrane effects and non-genomic actions of progesterone on myometrial activity.

Further insight into the steroid control of uterine contractility via GABA-ergic mechanisms arises from the work of Majewska & Vaupel (1991). They demonstrated that the GABA$_A$ agonist steroid THP relaxed uterine muscle while the GABA$_B$ antagonistic steroid pregnenolone sulphate potentiated contractions. Because of the rapidity of these effects they suggested a membrane rather than a nuclear mechanism of action. The multiple paths by which ovarian steroids can influence myometrial activity illustrated in Fig. 5 do not include the metabolites of ovarian steroids, though these may be of great importance.

Steroids and uterine vasculature

The first evidence for an effect of oestrogen on uterine blood flow was provided by Markee, Wells & Hinsey (1936) who showed that acute oestrogen administration in the rabbit caused vasodilatation of the uterine blood vessels. This effect has been repeatedly confirmed in various mammals and seems to occur in both the myometrium and endometrium. It is independent of cholinergic, histaminergic and adrenergic mediation. Furthermore, oestrogens do not alter blood flow in the renal or mesenteric vasculature (Altura & Altura, 1977).

The mechanism by which oestrogens modify uterine blood flow, blood pressure and vascular tone may involve either a direct action on the smooth muscle or a selective modification of the constrictor and dilator actions of other neurohumoral substances. Either would result in biochemical alterations in the smooth muscle cell and/or changes in cell membrane permeability to ions (see Fig. 5).

In addition to the rapid effects of oestrogen on uterine blood flow (the so-called early response) other cellular changes occur including hypertrophy and hyperplasia of vascular smooth muscle and alterations in collagen and elastin content. This anabolic response is thought to be mediated by an initial interaction between oestrogen and its intracellular receptor. However, a recent study showed that oestradiol 17-β was able to increase uterine blood flow in the absence of demonstrable RNA synthesis, indicating the non-genomic character of the response (Penny, Fredrick & Parker, 1981). The swiftness of the oestrogen response would seem to suggest a direct (non-genomic) action (Fig. 9). The direct effects could relate to both the inhibition of calcium entry or/and calmodulin inhibition within the cell (Kostrzewska et al., 1988). It should also be noted that nuclear oestrogen receptors have been demonstrated in the human uterine artery (Batra & Iosif, 1987), and direct inhibition of noradrenaline and depolarization-induced contractions of human uterine arteries by diethylstilboestrol have been reported (Kostrzewska et al., 1988). Thus nuclear-mediated (genomic) responses are responsible for the biosynthetic activity, hypertrophy and hyperplasia of vascular smooth muscle, while a rapid response such as the increase in blood flow is probably the result of a non-nuclear and more direct mode of action.

Data on the effect of progesterone on the uterine vasculature are limited. Treatment with progesterone following oestrogenization of rabbits reduced the elevation of blood flow (Batra et al., 1985a,b). This agrees with previous reports on uterine blood flow (Resnik, 1977). In vitro studies on isolated human uterine arteries have shown that whereas high concentrations of progesterone (μM range) inhibit contractile activity, very low concentrations (1–10 nM) increase the response of the uterine arteries to vasopressin (Fig. 10). The significance of this finding awaits further elucidation (Kostrzewska et al., 1992). It is interesting to note that cell surface binding sites for progesterone have been found in human sperm (Blackmore et al., 1991). These receptors differed from intracellular receptors as judged by the lack of antagonism by the progesterone antagonist

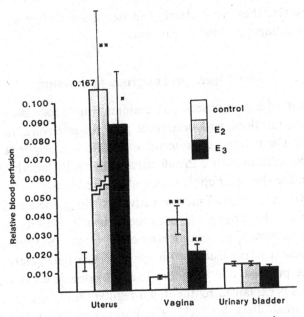

Fig. 9. Effect on blood flow of 0.5 μg/kg oestradiol-17β (E_2) and oestriol (E_3) in rabbit genitourinary tissues measured after one hour of administration. Statistical significance of differences from controls is represented by *$p < 0.05$, **$p < 0.01$, ***$p < 0.001$ (for details see Batra *et al.*, 1986).

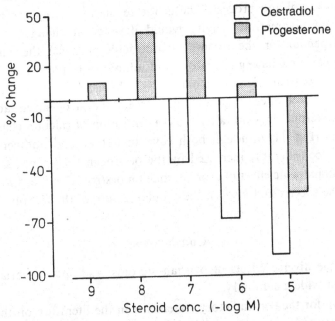

Fig. 10. Change in *in vitro* vasopressin-induced contractions of the human uterine artery exposed to different concentrations of oestradiol and progesterone.

RU 486. However, they were clearly functional since they elicited, following progesterone binding, an influx of calcium.

Oestrogen–progesterone interaction

The development of a mature secretory endometrium depends on the sequential action of oestradiol alone and oestradiol plus progesterone. In women cyclic treatment with a sequential contraceptive produces endometrial cycles which closely resemble normal cycles. Proliferative activity, including DNA synthesis, is prominent in the glandular epithelium and stroma during oestrogen treatment. Secretory activity, cessation of mitotic activity in the glands, and persistence of DNA synthesis in the stroma are prominent during combined oestrogen and progesterone treatment. The requirement of oestrogen priming for subsequent progesterone action is consistent with the evidence that oestrogen stimulates synthesis of the progesterone receptor. The antagonistic effect of progesterone on this synthesis is explained by the down-regulation of oestrogen receptors by progesterone (Hsueh, Peck & Clark, 1976; Batra et al., 1987). The synergism and antagonism between oestrogen and progesterone is dependent on the sequence and duration of exposure to these hormones, and can be satisfactorily explained by regulation of their intracellular receptors. However, species and organ differences make it difficult to make global statements about the interaction between oestradiol and progesterone in the regulation of myometrial function. The effect on myometrial activity would depend on changes in contractile capacity (dependent on the amount of contractile proteins), the number of cell surface receptors mediating excitatory and inhibitory responses, and membrane permeability, particularly to calcium. No change in ^{45}Ca uptake in the myometrium is seen after progesterone treatment of oestrogenized rabbits (Batra, 1986). Progesterone does not alter the concentration of calcium channels in the myometrium (Fig. 11) although both calcium uptake and number of calcium channels are considerably increased by the oestrogen treatment (Batra, 1985b). Thus, the antagonistic effect of progesterone on oestrogen-induced responses can vary with the species and also on the cellular nature of the response.

Conclusions

In view of the diverse effects of ovarian steroids, and species variability, it is difficult to provide a summary.

The reason for the contradictory statements in the literature on the influence of ovarian steroids on myometrial activity stems not only from the species variability but also from the lack of distinction between data obtained *in vitro*

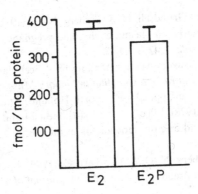

Fig. 11. Lack of effect of progesterone (E_2P) on oestrogen-induced (E_2) increase on calcium channel density in the myometrium (see also Batra, 1987).

and *in vivo*. The latter is well summarized by Finn & Porter (1975). Very few investigators use multiple techniques, yet these are crucial to the study of myometrial physiology. It is rare to find reports which correlate physiological or morphological response of the myometrium or uterine vasculature with steroid levels in blood and/or tissue. Furthermore, the uterus is composed of several specialized cells (epithelium, stroma, glands) and each cell type may respond differently.

In species such as man and other primates, in which there are cyclic changes, oestrogen–progesterone synergism and antagonism are an important component of the regulation of reproductive function. In species such as the rabbit which does not show oestrus, a study of oestrogen–progesterone interaction could not be extrapolated to other species.

The effects of steroids on the uterine vasculature are clearly of critical importance in the cyclic changes in the non-pregnant myometrium, in the quiescence of the myometrium during pregnancy and in the evolution of myometrial activity during parturition. The uterotropic effects of steroids during pregnancy and their inhibitory action on myometrial activity, and the increased blood supply to the uterus all work towards providing an ideal environment for the growing fetus.

References

Altura, B. M. & Altura, B. T. (1977). Influence of sex hormones, oral contraceptives and pregnancy on vascular muscle and its reactivity. In *Factors Influencing Vascular Reactivity*. Ed. O. Carrier and S. Shibata, pp. 221–54, Igaku-Shoin Ltd, Tokyo.

Andersson, P. J. B., Hancock, K. W. & Oakey, R. E. (1985). Non-protein-bound oestradiol and progesterone in human peripheral plasma before labour and delivery. *Journal of Endocrinology*, **104**, 7–15.

Batra, S., Bengtsson, L. Ph., Grundsell, H. & Sjöberg, N.-O. (1976). Levels of free and protein-bound progesterone in plasma during late pregnancy. *Journal of Clinical Endocrinological Metabolism*, **42**, 1041–7.

Batra, S. (1977). The importance of calcium binding by subcellular components of smooth muscle. In *Excitation Contraction Coupling in Smooth Muscle*. Ed. R. Casteels, T. Godfraind and J. C. Ruegg, pp. 225–32, North-Holland, Amsterdam.

Batra, S. & Bengtsson, B. (1978). Effects of diethylstilboestrol and ovarian steroids on the contractile responses and calcium movements in rat uterine smooth muscle. *Journal of Physilogy*, **276**, 329.

Batra, S., Owman, Ch., Sjöberg, N.-O. & Thorbert, G. (1979). Relationship between plasma and uterine estradiol in pseudopregnant rabbits. *Journal of Reproduction and Fertility*, **56**, 1–7.

Batra, S. (1980). Estrogen and smooth muscle function. *Trends in Pharmacological Sciences*, **1**, 268.

Batra, S., Sjöberg, N.-O. & Thorbert, G. (1980). Sex steroids in plasma and reproductive organs of the female guinea-pig. *Biology of Reproduction*, **22**, 430–7.

Batra, S. & Dahlander, K. (1984). Steroids and uterine contractility. In *Uterine Contractility*. Ed. S. Bottari, J. P. Thomas, A. Vokaer and R. Vokaer, pp. 251–60, Masson Publishing, New York.

Batra, S. (1985a). On the role of estradiol and progesterone in parturition: an updated proposal. *Acta Obstetrica Gynecologica*, **64**, 671–2.

Batra, S. (1985b). Characterization of [³H]-nitrendipine binding to uterine smooth muscle plasma membrane and its relevance to inhibition of calcium entry. *British Journal of Pharmacology*, **85**, 767–74.

Batra, S., Bjellin, L., Sjögren, C., Iosif, S. & Widmark, E. (1986). Increases in blood flow of the female rabbit urethra following low dose estrogens. *Journal of Urology*, **104**, 1360–2.

Batra, S. (1986). Effect of estrogen and progesterone treatment on calcium uptake by the myometrium and smooth muscle of the lower urinary tract. *European Journal of Pharmacology*, **127**, 37–42.

Batra, S. (1987). Calcium and uterine contractility. In *Control and Management of Parturition*. Ed. C. Sureau and G. Germain, pp. 208–16, John Libbey Eurotext Ltd, London.

Batra, S. & Iosif, S. (1987). Nuclear estrogen receptors in human uterine arteries. *Gynecological and Obstetric Investigations*, **24**, 250–5.

Batra, S. & Owman, C., Rydhström, H. & Sjöberg, N.-O. (1987). Modulation by continuous oestrogen treatment and by progesterone of oestrogen receptors in the rabbit uterus. *Journal of Endocrinology*, **115**, 199–203.

Batra, S. (1990). Influence of chronic oestrogen treatment on the density of muscarinic cholinergic receptors and calcium channels in the rabbit uterus. *Journal of Endocrinology*, **125**, 185–9.

Batra, S. & Iosif, S. (1992). Effect of estrogen treatment on the peroxidase activity and estrogen receptors in the female rabbit urogenital tissues. *Journal of Urology* (in press).

Bergamini, C. M., Pansini, F., Bettochi, S. Jr et al. (1985). Hormonal sensitivity of adenylate cyclase from human endometrium: modulation by estradiol. *Journal of Steroid Biochemistry*, **22**, 299–303.

Blackmore, P. F., Neulen, J., Lattanzio, F. & Beebe, S. J. (1991). Cell surface-binding sites for progesterone mediate calcium uptake in human sperm. *Journal of Biological Chemistry*, **266**, 18655–9.

Csapo, A. I. (1956). Progesterone 'block'. *American Journal of Anatomy*, **88**, 273–92.

Daniel, E. E. & Janis, R. A. (1975). Calcium regulation in the uterus. *Pharmacology Therapy B*, **1**, 695–729.

Devine, C. E., Somylo, A. V. & Somylo, A. P. (1972). Sarcoplasmic reticulum and excitation-contraction coupling in mammalian smooth muscles. *Journal of Cell Biology*, **52**, 690.

Erdö, S. L. (1984). Identification of GABA receptor binding sites in rat and rabbit uterus. *Biochemical and Biophysical Research Communications*, **125**, 18–24.

Finn, C. A. & Porter, D. G. (1975). *The Uterus*, p. 178, Elek Science, London.

Fuchs, A.-R. & Fuchs, F. (1984). Endocrinology of human parturition: a review. *British Journal of Obstetrics and Gynecology*, 91, 948–67.

Gabella, G. (1971). Caveolae intracellulares and sarcoplasmic reticulum in smooth muscle. *Journal of Cell Science*, **8**, 601.

Giannopoulas, G. & Tulchinsky, D. (1979). Cytoplasmic and nuclear progestin receptors in human myometrium during menstrual cycle and in pregnancy at term. *Journal of Clinical Endocrinology Metabolism*, **49**, 100–6.

Grover, A. K. (1985). Calcium-handling studies using isolated smooth muscle membranes. In *Calcium and Contractility*. Ed. A. K. Grover and E. E. Daniel, pp. 245–69, The Humana Press, New York.

Haras, D., Samperez, S. & Jouan, P. P. (1989). Positive and negative effects of estradiol-17β in the rat uterus. *Journal of Steroid Biochemistry*, **33**, 1073.

Hsueh, A. J. W., Peck, E. J. Jr. & Clark, J. H. (1976). Control of uterine estrogen receptor levels by progesterone. *Endocrinology*, **98**, 438.

Kamm, K. E. & Stull, J. T. (1985). The function of myosin and myosin light chain kinase phosphorylation in smooth muscle. *Annual Review in Pharmacological Toxicology*, **25**, 593–620.

Kostrzewska, A., Laudański, T. & Batra, S. (1988). Effect of calcium and calmodulin antagonists on contractile responses of the human uterine artery. *British Journal of Pharmacology*, **94**, 1037–42.

Kostrzewska, A., Laudański, T. & Batra, S. (1992). Effect of ovarian steroids and diethylstilboestrol on the contractile responses of the human myometrium and intramyometrial arteries. *European Journal of Pharmacology* (in press).

Laudański, T. & Batra, S. (1984). Hormonal factors in the regulation of myometrial activity. In *Uterine Contractility*. Ed. S. Bottari, H. J. P. Thomas, A. Vokaer and S. Vokaer, pp. 241–50, Masson Publishing USA Inc, New York.

Loutzenhiser, R., Leyten, P., Saida, K. & van Breemen, C. (1985). Calcium compartments and mobilization during contraction of smooth muscle. In *Calcium and Contractility*. Ed. A. K. Grover and E. E. Daniel, pp. 61–92, The Humana Press, New York.

Majewska, M. D. & Vaupel, D. B. (1991). Steroid control of uterine motility via γ-aminobutyric acid$_A$ receptors in the rabbit: a novel mechanism? *Journal of Endocrinology*, **131**, 427–34.

Markee, J. W., Wells, W. M. & Hinsey, J. C. (1936). Studies on uterine growth. III. A local factor in the rabbit uterus. *Anatomical Records*, **64**, 221–30.

Means, A. R. & Hamilton, T. H. (1966). Early estrogen action: concomitant stimulations within two minutes of nuclear synthesis and uptake of RNA precursor by the uterus. *Proceedings of the National Academy of Sciences, USA,* **56**, 1594–8.

Michell, R. H. (1987). How do receptors at the cell surface send signals to the cell interior? *British Medical Journal,* **295**, 1320–3.

Mukku, V., Kirkland, J., Hardy, M. & Stancer (1981). Stimulatory and inhibitory effects of estrogen and antiestrogen on uterine cell division. *Endocrinology,* **109**, 1005.

Penny, L. L., Frederick, R. J. & Parker, G. W. (1981). 17-β-estradiol stimulation of uterine blood flow in oophorectomized rabbits with complete inhibition of uterine ribonucleic acid synthesis. *Endocrinology,* **109**, 1672–6.

Pietras, R. J. & Szego, C. M. (1975). Endometrial cell calcium and oestradiol action. *Nature,* **253**, 357–9.

Putnam, C. D., Brann, D. W., Kolbeck, R. C. & Mahesh, V. B. (1991). Inhibition of uterine contractility by progesterone and progesterone metabolites: Mediation by progesterone and gamma amino butyric acid$_A$ receptor systems. *Biology of Reproduction,* **45**, 266–72.

Resnik, R. (1977). The effect of progesterone on estrogen-induced uterine blood flow. *American Journal of Obstetrics and Gynecology,* **128**, 251–4.

Rories, C. & Spelsberg, T. C. (1989). Ovarian steroid action on gene expression: mechanisms and models. *Annual Review in Physiology,* **51**, 653–81.

Sokoloff, A. (1896). Über den Einfluß der Ovarien-Extirpation auf Strukturveränderungen des Uterus. *Archive für Gynäkologie,* **51**, 286–9.

Stormshak, F., Leake, R., Wertz, N. & Gorski, J. (1976). Stimulatory and inhibitory effects of estrogen on uterine DNA synthesis. *Endocrinology,* **99**, 1501.

Szego, C. M. (1978). Parallels in the modes of action of peptide and steroid hormones: membrane effects and cellular entry. In *Structure and Function of the Gonadotrophins.* Ed. K. W. McKerns, pp. 431–72, Plenum Press, New York.

9

Neurotransmitters in the myometrium

MARTIN STJERNQUIST AND NILS-OTTO SJÖBERG

Autonomic uterine innervation

For more than a century it has been known that the uterus receives an extensive nerve supply. During the last decade of the 19th century Langley and Anderson described the autonomic innervation of the uterus (Langley & Anderson, 1895). They found the sympathetic nerves to originate in the 3rd–5th lumbar segments of the spinal cord, and then enter the 4th–6th lumbar ganglia of the sympathetic chain to continue, via the inferior mesenteric ganglia, in the two hypogastric nerves. The parasympathetic or pelvic nerves have their origin in the first 3 to 4 sacral roots and, after forming the two pelvic nerves, meet the sympathetic nerves in the paracervical tissue, giving the impression of a ganglion formation, which has been given the name of Frankenhäuser's plexus or ganglion. The active ganglia are found very close to the utero-vaginal junction, and are also located within the vaginal wall (Sjöberg, 1967). These peripheral ganglia are a relay not only for the parasympathetic nerves but also for a considerable proportion of the sympathetic nerves, as shown in denervation experiments (Sjöberg, 1967). These findings conflict with the classic concept of the organization of the autonomic nervous system, in which the sympathetic post-ganglionic nerve fibres are supposed to derive from cell bodies located at a considerable distance from the effector organ. The post-ganglionic nerve fibres originating in cell bodies at the utero-vaginal junction have been termed 'short adrenergic neurons' and seem to be a feature unique to the genital organs (Sjöstrand, 1965; Sjöberg, 1967).

The division of the autonomic nervous system into two parts, the sympathetic (adrenergic) and parasympathetic (cholinergic), is incomplete from a functional and morphological point of view. Thus, the presence of so-called 'non-adrenergic, non-cholinergic' (NANC) neuronal mechanisms has been demonstrated in miscellaneous organ preparations. The development of immunocytochemical techniques has made it possible to demonstrate several peptides in nervous tissue.

These have been termed 'neuropeptides', and 'peptidergic' nerves have been encountered in various organs including the uterus. Both *in vivo* and *in vitro* several of these neuropeptides exert biological effects and thus seem to possess regulatory properties.

Hence, when discussing the innervation of the myometrium we have to consider not only the adrenergic and cholinergic, but also the peptidergic nerves.

Adrenergic nerves

The concept of a peripheral relay in the uterine sympathetic innervation (Langley & Anderson, 1985), was unrecognized for many years. However, histofluorescence techniques and fluorometric determinations of tissue concentrations of the noradrenaline (NA) transmitter showed that the uterus is supplied by fibres originating in adrenergic ganglion formations in the upper part of the vaginal wall or in the parametrial tissue outside the utero-vaginal junction (Owman & Sjöberg, 1966). Adrenergic ganglia are also encountered at these sites in humans (Owman, Rosengren & Sjöberg, 1967), and their location corresponds to that of Frankenhäuser's ganglion. The sympathetic innervation of the female reproductive tract is complex. Hence, the ovarian nerve supply originates from a source entirely different from that of the rest of the internal female reproductive organs, i.e. the intermesenteric and renal plexuses as well as the superior hypogastric plexus and the hypogastric (presacral) nerve. By contrast, the adrenergic innervation of the oviduct, uterus and vagina originates not only from the paracervical ganglia (forming short adrenergic neurons) but also from the prevertebral, inferior mesenteric ganglia. In the male, the short adrenergic neurons seem to be the exclusive source of sympathetic nerves directed to the reproductive organs (Sjöstrand, 1965).

The adrenergic innervation of the uterus has been studied by means of formaldehyde histochemistry in many species, including man. The paracervical ganglia are usually scattered as smaller or larger clusters of ganglion cells in the adipose connective tissue immediately outside the utero-vaginal region, often in relation to blood vessels. Groups of nerve cells are also present in the periphery of the upper part of the vaginal wall, as well as in the adjacent adventitia. Groups of smooth nerve fibres emitting a formaldehyde-induced fluorescence of low intensity are often seen to issue from the ganglion formations.

Bundles of smooth nerve fibres are also seen in the connective tissue outside the uterus proper, following the uterine arteries. In animals possessing a bicornuate uterus, the muscle coat of the uterine horns consists of an outer longitudinal coat and an inner layer separated by a well-developed vascular plexus. Several bundles of nerves course along the vessels in this plexus, providing

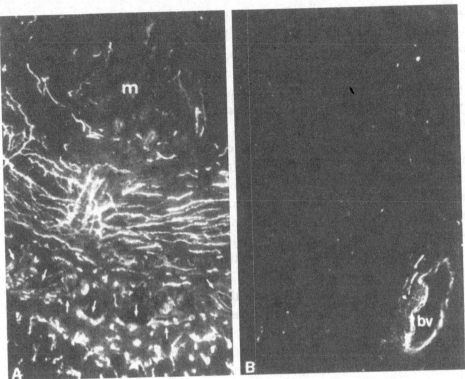

Fig. 1. Fluorescence photomicrographs of adrenergic nerves in transversely sectioned uterine horns from cat. × 121. A Non-pregnant animal showing dense innervation of circular and longitudinal smooth muscle layers of the myometrium (lower half of Figure), as well as fibres extending into the mucosa (m). Several blood vessels are supplied, particularly well seen between the muscle layers (arrows). B Late pregnancy, preparation oriented in the same manner as in A. The uterine wall is entirely devoid of fluorescent, noradenaline-containing axons, except for a few, isolated fibres in association with blood vessels (bv), large calibred at this stage of pregnancy. (Reproduced from Alm *et al.*, 1986, by courtesy of the Editors of *Neuroscience*.)

a well-developed nerve supply to both vascular and non-vascular smooth musculature (Fig. 1A). Within the muscle layers, the nerve fibres usually follow the general direction of the smooth muscle cells. A particularly dense supply of adrenergic nerve fibres is found in the smooth muscle coats of the tubal end of the uterine horn and in the cervix, whereas innervation in the main parts of the horns is less dense. In addition, adrenergic nerve terminals often run in the stroma of the endometrium, sometimes close to vessels and occasionally very close to the glandular epithelium.

The tubal end of the uterine horns (in species with a bicornuate uterus, e.g. the guinea-pig) are usually attached by a fibrous ligament to the medial third of the lower two ribs. It has been shown by electron microscopy that the ligament also contains smooth muscle elements. Cutting of this ligament leads to considerable shortening of the uterine horns. The ligament contains a large number of nerves with high fluorescence intensity running longitudinally (Thorbert, 1978). Some of these fibres have a beaded appearance, typical of the terminal part of the nerve; others are smooth in outline. The adjacent connective tissue also contains moderately fluorescent nerves, running parallel to the suspensory ligament.

The adrenergic nerve supply shows considerable regional variation in the human uterus (Owman et al., 1967). In the uterine fundus, scattered nerve terminals are scarce except where the intramural portion of the oviduct penetrates the uterine wall. The innervation pattern, with nerve terminals running close to smooth muscle fibres and following their direction, is also seen in the corpus which receives more numerous adrenergic terminals than the fundus. There are more adrenergic nerve fibres in the cervix than in the rest of the uterus. Fluorescent fibres have not been detected in the endometrium. Adrenergic ganglion formations are located in the periphery of the smooth-muscle wall in that part of the cervix adjacent to the vagina. Numerous bundles of post-ganglionic axons project from the clusters of ganglion cells.

The guinea-pig has spontaneous ovulations with cyclic, progesterone-secreting corpora lutea of about 14 days' duration. Uterine motility is not influenced by progesterone, and the placenta is steroid-secreting. This laboratory animal has therefore often been chosen as a suitable model for human reproductive endocrinology.

The guinea-pig uterus is innervated by adrenergic nerve terminals, originating from several sources (Thorbert, 1978). Approximately half of the total innervation in the cervix originates from post-ganglionic fibres running in the hypogastric nerves; the remainder is supplied by fibres from the short adrenergic neurons arising in the paracervical ganglia. The hypogastric nerves also carry fibres which contribute about one third of the adrenergic innervation in the uterine horns, another third deriving from the paracervical ganglia, and the remaining third entering the uterus via the suspensory ligaments which attach the tubal end of the uterine horn to the lower ribs. It is notable that this latter innervation, representing a considerable fraction of the total NA content of the uterine horn, is restricted to a very small part of the horn adjacent to the oviduct. However, the adrenergic innervation here is not interrelated with that supplying the rest of the horns. Although the nerves arrive via the suspensory ligament, their exact origin is not yet established.

Cholinergic nerves

It has not been possible to define exactly the cholinergic innervation of the uterus; there are technical problems and considerable species variation. It is doubtful if histochemistry or electron microscopy can distinguish truly cholinergic nerve fibres. Inhibitors of pseudocholinesterase may not be specific in tissues from certain species. Acetylcholinesterase may be present in tissues in other than cholinergic nerve fibres. Non-adrenergic nerves may store regulator peptides (see below) and are therefore not simple cholinergic nerves.

Choline acetyltransferase activity has been detected in the human myometrium (Thorbert, 1978), showing that acetylcholine (ACh) is synthesized in this tissue. The paracervical ganglia contain numerous acetylcholinesterase-positive cells (Kanerva, 1972). Neural storage of the enzyme has been demonstrated in the uterus of man, cat (Fig. 2, Fig. 3), and rat, but is absent in rabbits and guinea-pigs (Owman & Sjöberg, 1966; Thorbert, 1978). In the latter species the uterine artery and its primary ramifications to the uterus have dense plexuses of cholinesterase-containing nerves (Thorbert, 1978). The distribution corresponds to the perivascular adrenergic plexus, suggesting that the two systems might run close together. Close to the uterus, and at the point of vascular entry into the organ, there is no acetylcholinesterase activity; the adrenergic plexus, by contrast, can be followed into the uterine wall.

The histochemical properties of specific acetylcholinesterase and of butyryl-cholinesterase and the conditions for selective inhibition of pseudocholinesterase, were originally studied in cat tissue (Holmstedt, 1957). Cholinergic neurons are selectively revealed when the cholinesterase staining is performed after inhibition of pseudocholinesterase (Alm *et al.*, 1986). Some of the cholinesterase activity might also be associated with non-adrenergic nerves. For example, sensory neurons containing substance P have been shown to contain acetylcholinesterase (Papka *et al.*, 1985). However, the paucity of substance P-immunoreactive nerve fibres in cat uterus is not consistent with the distribution of acetylcholinesterase activity. Cholinesterase activity might also be located within adrenergic nerves.

Immunohistochemical studies show that the cat uterus is also rich in VIP-containing nerve fibres which originate in the same paracervical ganglia as the adrenergic nerves. These peptidergic fibres would seem to constitute a system apart from the adrenergic innervation of the uterus, but in both number and localization they are very similar to the acetylcholinesterase-positive fibres (Alm *et al.*, 1986). VIP may therefore co-exist with ACh.

Peptidergic nerves

Vasoactive intestinal polypeptide (VIP)

Vasoactive intestinal polypeptide (VIP) is a 28-amino acid peptide originally isolated from porcine small intestine (Said & Mutt, 1970). The peptide shares part of its amino acid sequence with secretin and glucagon, and was first thought to be a gut hormone. Immunocytochemical investigations have shown VIP to

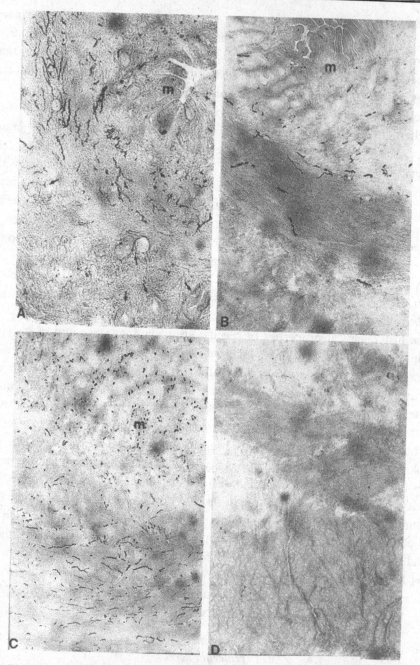

Fig. 2. Acetylcholinesterase (AChE) activity in cross-sectional feline uterine horns.
×125. A Non-pregnant animal showing positively stained nerve fibres in the
myometrium, particularly well recognizable in the circular layer. Also myometrial
blood vessels are supplied (arrows). Axons extend into the mucosal layer (m).
B Mid-pregnancy. In the tissue surrounding the fetus (perifetal uterus) there is a
marked reduction in the number of AChE-containing nerve fibres, both in the

be located exclusively in nerves in mammals, the most extensive VIP-innervation being found in the gut (Fahrenkrug, 1979). VIP-containing nerves are often confined to sphincter regions (Helm *et al.*, 1981). The peptide has a broad range of biological effects, including relaxation of vascular and non-vascular smooth muscle and stimulation of exocrine gland secretion (Said, 1982). Evidence is accumulating that VIP constitutes a true neurotransmitter, though no specific pharmacological blocking agent has been found to substantiate this hypothesis. Like many other regulatory peptides, VIP is derived from a precursor peptide, consisting of a longer amino acid chain, and called prepro-VIP (Itoh *et al.*, 1983). This precursor peptide splits into shorter peptide chains: the 28-amino acid peptide VIP, and the 27-amino acid PHI (peptide with NH_2-terminal histidine and COOH-terminal isoleucine).

The female genital tract receives an extensive innervation by VIP-containing nerves (Alm *et al.*, 1977; Huang *et al.*, 1984). In addition to their perivascular localization, the nerve fibres run in the submucosa and in the myometrium, where they are closely associated with non-vascular smooth muscle cells (Fig. 4). The VIP-innervation is particularly concentrated in the cervical region and in the isthmus of the Fallopian tube. The nerves have the same origin as most adrenergic nerves, the paracervical ganglia. There are considerable species differences in the extent of VIP-nerve supply to the myometrium. They are particularly dense in the cat (Ottesen *et al.*, 1981; Alm *et al.*, 1986). Relatively few fibres are found in the human myometrium (Helm *et al.*, 1981).

VIP inhibits spontaneous motor activity in myometrial strips from various species (Ottesen *et al.*, 1981, 1982), and also inhibits uterine activity *in vivo* (Ottesen, Söndergaard & Fahrenkrug, 1983). Myometrial strips obtained at the end of pregnancy seem to be unresponsive to VIP (Ottesen *et al.*, 1982).

A high concentration of VIP is found in the human endometrium without change during the menstrual cycle (Goodnough *et al.*, 1979). Measurements by xenon clearance shows that VIP enhances blood flow in the goat myometrium (Ottensen *et al.*, 1980).

Caption for fig. 2 (*cont.*).
smooth musculature and in the mucosa (m). C Mid-pregnancy. In the tissue located between the fetuses (parafetal uterus) from the same horn as in B, the nerve supply is better preserved than perifetally, and the fibres are particularly visible in the circular smooth musculature. AChE-positive axons are also found scattered in the mucosa (m). D Late pregnancy, fetus-containing horn. AChE activity is no longer visible in any part of the uterine wall. (Reproduced from Alm *et al.*, 1986, by courtesy of the Editors of *Neuroscience*.)

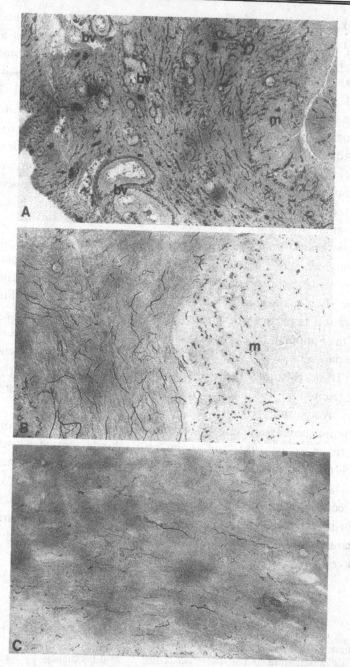

Fig. 3. AChE-activity in the feline uterine cervix. × 100. A Non-pregnant animal. The nerve supply is well developed in the smooth musculature, the circular layer being particularly prominent. Fibres extend into the mucosal layer (m). Numerous blood vessels (bv) are surrounded by nerve plexuses and transversely cut bundles are seen to run mainly in the outer parts of the cervix (arrows). B The total number of AChE-positive axons in the upper cervix seemed essentially unaltered

Neuropeptide Y (NPY)

Neuropeptide Y (NPY) (Y is the terminal amino acid tyrosine) is a 36-amino acid peptide belonging to the pancreatic family of neuropeptides, and originally isolated from porcine brain (Tatemoto, 1982). The presence of NPY has been shown immunocytochemically in nerves both of the central and peripheral nervous systems (Sundler *et al.*, 1989). The NPY-containing nerves are predominantly located around blood vessels, and seem to co-exist with NA in an extensive population of sympathetic nerves (Lundberg *et al.*, 1982; Stjernquist *et al.*, 1987, 1991). NPY induces vasoconstriction both through direct effects and via a potentiation of the contractile effect of NA (Lundberg & Tatemoto, 1982), though the peptide has also been shown to suppress the release both of NA and ACh from pre-synaptic nerve terminals (Stjernquist & Owman, 1987). The existence of different subpopulations of post-synaptic receptors for NPY has been postulated – the so-called Y_1 and Y_2 receptors (Schwartz *et al.*, 1989).

Stjernquist and co-workers (1983) described a considerable number of immunoreactive fibres in the uterine horns of the rat, particularly in the cervix. These were in the smooth muscle coat, around large- and medium-sized arteries, and sometimes in the subepithelial layer (Fig. 5). The pattern of NPY-immunoreactive nerve fibres in the guinea-pig myometrium closely resembles that of fibres exhibiting tyrosine hydroxylase staining. Accordingly, NPY-immunoreactive cells are present in the paracervical ganglia. Thus NPY and NA may co-exist in the adrenergic nerves, although they may not be as complete in the reproductive tract as in other peripheral tissues (Owman *et al.*, 1986), NPY fibres are also found among smooth muscle cells in the human uterus, particularly in association with blood vessels (Owman *et al.*, 1986).

Experiments on smooth muscle preparations from rats suggest that NPY is without postjunctional effect either on resting tension or on spontaneous smooth muscle activity (Stjernquist *et al.*, 1983), whereas it markedly inhibits neurally induced contraction (Figs. 6, 7).

Substance P (SP) and calcitonin gene-related peptide (CGRP)

Substance P (SP, P=powder) was discovered by von Euler and Gaddum in extracts from gut and brain; it could induce atropine-resistant contraction of gut

Caption for fig. 3 (*cont.*).
during mid-pregnancy. However, due to increase in the organ volume, the nerve plexus tends to appear less dense, as illustrated here, both in the smooth musculature (left half of picture) and in the mucosa (m). C A substantial amount of AChE-positive nerve fibres remain in the cervix at late pregnancy. (Reproduced from Alm *et al.*, 1986, by courtesy of the Editors of *Neuroscience*.)

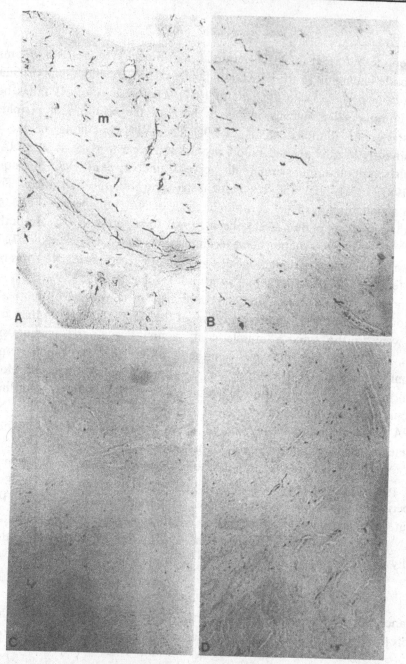

Fig. 4. VIP-immunoreactive nerve fibres in feline uterine horn. × 125. A Transversely sectioned organ from non-pregnant animal. Positively stained fibres are seen in the circular smooth muscle layer as well as in the mucosa (m). Also some perivascular fibres are visible (arrows). B Mid-pregnancy. Sterile (empty) horn from animal with fetuses only in one of the horns. Several VIP-positive axons are seen in the myometrium. The density of the nerve plexuses appear less

smooth musculature *in vitro* (Von Euler & Gaddum, 1931). The sequence of 11 amino-acids was determined in 1971 (Chang, Leeman & Niall, 1971); SP is widely distributed in nerves of the gut (Sundler, Håkanson & Leander, 1980), and is also present in primary afferent sensory neurons; it seems to be the mediator of antidromic vasodilatation in inflammatory reactions of various organs (Lundberg *et al.*, 1984).

CGRP is a 37-amino acid peptide obtained by alternative processing of the mRNA transcript (Amara *et al.*, 1982). The peptide has been detected in a number of peripheral organs. CGRP seems to be mainly confined to sensory neurons, but is also known to be a potent vasorelaxant and to induce contraction of intestinal smooth muscle (Sundler *et al.*, 1985).

Alm and colleagues (1978) have described SP-immunoreactive nerves beneath the uterine serosal epithelium, sometimes extending between the cells, and also in fibres related to non-vascular smooth muscle cells in the myometrium. SP was also found in isolated nerve fibres, but not in cell bodies, within the pelvic ganglia. In the rat, the number, but not the distribution, of uterine SP fibres is similar to that of VIP fibres (Papka, Cotton & Taurig, 1985). SP co-exists with CGRP in capsaicin-sensitive nerves within the uterus, further suggesting that they are sensory in nature (Gibbins *et al.*, 1985). The two peptides correlate in nerve fibres in the human uterus (Samuelson *et al.*, 1985). Although SP and CGRP seem to co-exist in some uterine nerve fibres, the effects of exogenously applied peptides on isolated myometrium strips are different. In humans, SP increases the smooth muscle tension (in which VIP induces relaxation) while CGRP diminishes spontaneous contractions (Samuelson *et al.*, 1985).

Galanin

Some nerve fibres in the paracervical ganglia contain galanin (Stjernquist *et al.*, 1988, Fig. 8). This is a 29-amino acid peptide isolated from porcine small intestine, deriving its name from the presence of N-terminal glycine and C-terminal alanine (Tatemoto *et al.*, 1983). Galanin nerve fibres have been traced both in the central and peripheral nervous systems (Rökaeus *et al.*, 1984). Nerve fibres containing galanin have been traced in the uterine cervix and horn, particularly in the outer

Caption for fig. 4 (*cont.*).
prominent due to enlargement of the organ. C In the perifetal tissue (from the same animal as in B, mid-pregnancy) very few weakly immunoreactive nerves are found. D In the parafetal regions of the same fetus-containing horn as in C VIP nerves are preserved almost to the same extent as in the empty horn illustrated in B. (Reproduced from Alm *et al.*, 1986, by courtesy of the Editors of *Neuroscience*.)

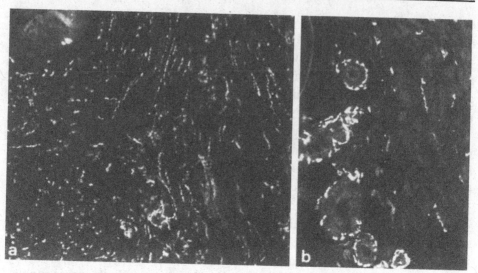

Fig. 5. Rat uterine cervix. (*a*) NPY immunofluorescent fibres form a dense network in the smooth musculature. × 150. (*b*) Intensely immunoreactive fibres innervate paracervical blood vessels. × 170. (Reproduced from Stjernquist *et al.*, 1983, by courtesy of the Editors of *Neuroscience Letters.*)

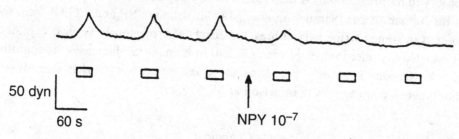

Fig. 6. Rat uterine cervix *in vitro*. Inhibitory effect of NPY (molar concentration) on the contractile response induced by transmural nerve stimulation (indicated by bars). (Reproduced from Stjernquist *et al.*, 1983, by courtesy of the Editors of *Neuroscience Letters.*)

part of the smooth musculature. Scattered fibres have also been found in the basal endometrium. Galanin exerts a contractile effect on isolated preparations of uterine horn from oestrogen-treated spayed rats; the effect on the uterine cervix is weaker (Stjernquist *et al.*, 1988, Fig. 9).

Gastrin-releasing peptide (GRP)

Gastrin-releasing peptide (GRP) was first isolated from the porcine non-antral gastric mucosa, and comprises 27 amino acids (McDonald *et al.*, 1978). Its seven

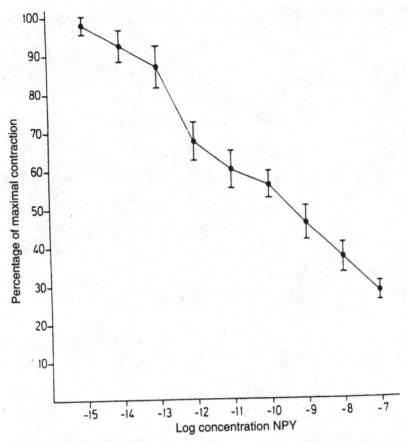

Fig. 7. Concentration–response curve showing inhibitory effect of NPY on the response to electrical nerve stimulation of the rat uterine cervix. *Ordinate*: Contraction amplitude, expressed as percentage of the response to electrical stimulation in Krebs–Ringer solution without NPY. *Abscissa*: logarithm of NPY concentration (M) in the organ chamber. Results are given as mean $+/-$SEM, $n = 5$–6 preparations. (Reproduced from Stjernquist *et al.*, 1983, by courtesy of the Editors of *Neuroscience Letters*.)

COOH-terminal amino acid sequence is identical with that of bombesin, a 14-àmino acid peptide originally isolated from amphibian skin. Since bombesin itself has not been isolated in mammals, GRP has been suggested as the mammalian counterpart. The biologically active site is the C-terminal region common to both peptides. Accordingly, GRP and bombesin have similar functional properties, i.e., contraction of smooth muscle and induction of secretion from both exocrine and endocrine glands (McDonald *et al.*, 1981). GRP-immunoreactivity has been found in nerve fibres from various organs (Moghimzadeh *et al.*, 1983).

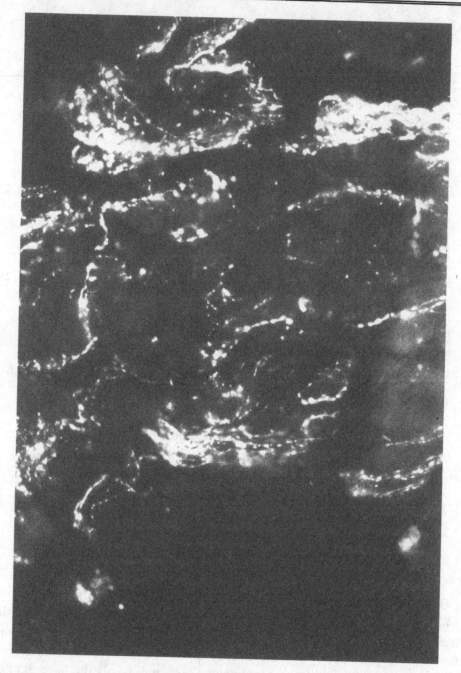

Fig. 8. Immunocytochemical demonstration of galanin in cryostat sections of paracervical tissue from rat. × 180. Numerous galanin-immunoreactive nerve fibres surround non-immunoreactive cell bodies. (Reproduced from Stjernquist *et al.*, 1988, by courtesy of the Editors of *Regulatory Peptides*.)

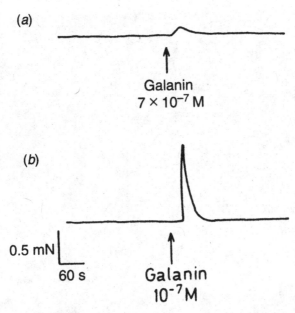

Fig. 9. Smooth muscle preparations from rat uterine cervix (*a*) and horn (*b*) *in vitro*, showing contractile effects of galanin. Note difference in effect between the two uterine preparations. *Abscissa*: time (s), *ordinate*: contractile force (mN). (Reproduced from Stjernquist *et al.*, 1988, by courtesy of the Editors of *Regulatory Peptides*.)

The distribution of GRP in the uterus is different from that of SP or galanin (Stjernquist *et al.*, 1986). The number of immunoreactive fibres in the myometrium is larger, with an even distribution throughout the smooth muscle layers. No GRP fibres are present in the mucosa or in association with blood vessels. The paracervical ganglia harbour several GRP-immunoreactive cell bodies, with GRP-positive fibres coursing among both stained and unstained cells (Fig. 10).

The contractile action of galanin is only short-lasting but GRP induces a more protracted response, including enhanced tone and frequent oscillations (Stjernquist *et al.*, 1986). As with galanin the effect is more pronounced in the horns, particularly in oestrogen-treated animals (Stjernquist *et al.*, 1988, Fig. 11).

Enkephalins

Enkephalins comprise two pentapeptides – met- and leu-enkephalin – differing only in their COOH-terminal residues (methionine and leucine respectively). They were originally isolated from brain tissue (Hughes *et al.*, 1975), and were the first recognized opiate receptor ligands of endogenous origin. Enkephalins have been demonstrated immunocytochemically both in the central and peripheral nervous

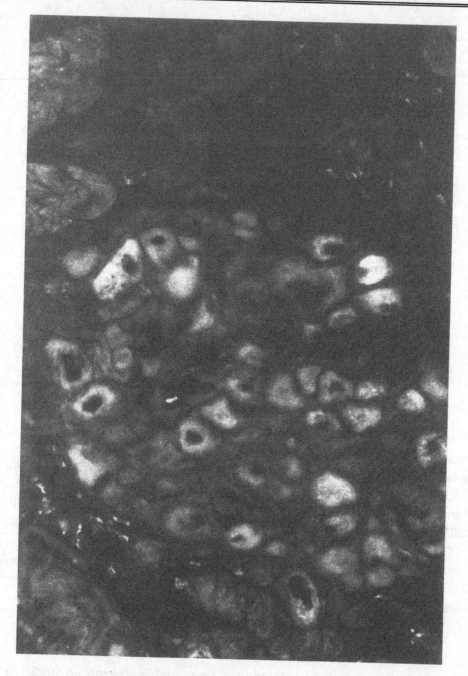

Fig. 10. Immunocytochemical demonstration of GRP in paracervical tissue from rat. × 200. GRP-immunofluorescent cell bodies and nerve fibres in the paracervical ganglia.

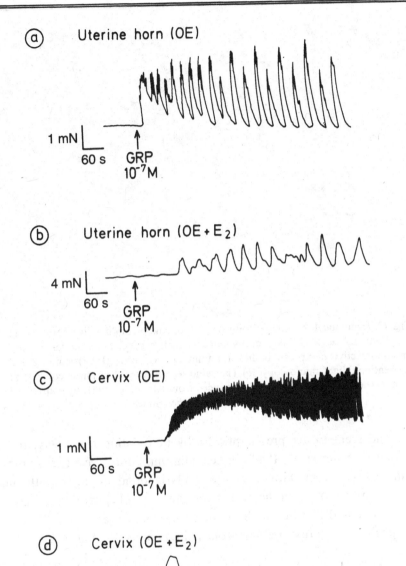

Fig. 11. Isolated smooth muscle preparations from rat uterine horn A, B and cervix C, D. Animals were oophorectomized (OE), and those illustrated in B and D in addition treated with oestradiol (E_2). The clonic contractions are more pronounced but have a lower frequency in tissues from oestrogen-treated animals. Note also the stronger effect in uterine horns as compared with cervix. (Reproduced from Stjernquist *et al.*, 1986, by courtesy of the Editors of *Regulatory Peptides*.)

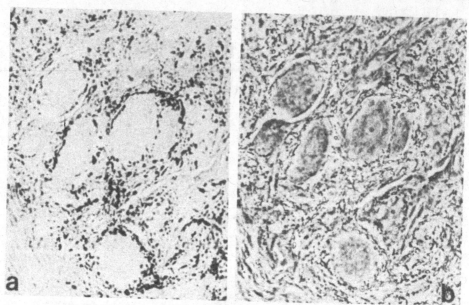

Fig. 12. Immunocytochemical demonstration of enkephalin in feline paracervical ganglionic tissue. × 370. Numerous immunoreactive nerve fibres surround non-immunoreactive nerve cell bodies. (*a*) Immunoperoxidase (PAP) staining and conventional light microscopy. (*b*) The same section viewed in phase contrast to demonstrate nerve cell bodies. (Reproduced from Alm *et al.*, 1981, by courtesy of the Editors of *Histochemistry*.)

systems, and seem to act presynaptically by modulating the release of other transmitters (Sundler *et al.*, 1980). Enkephalin-immunoreactive nerve fibres are sparse in the female genital tract, and are regularly found among smooth muscles cells only in the cervix. As in the case of substance P, enkephalin fibres have also been recognized in the pelvic ganglia among non-reactive ganglion cells, although the enkephalin fibres are more numerous (Alm *et al.*, 1981, Fig. 12).

Interaction between different uterine neurotransmitters

The neural regulation of the uterine smooth musculature is highly complex. This complexity is compounded by the finding of several systems of peptidergic nerves with smooth muscle activity in the uterus. The isolated cervix preparation from spayed rats, with and without treatment with oestrogen, has turned out to be a valuable tool in the elucidation of several of these mechanisms (Stjernquist & Owman, 1985).

Cervical smooth muscle from oophorectomized and oestrogen-treated rats exhibits spontaneous activity which completely disappears within an hour (Fig. 13). The preparations from oophorectomized but otherwise untreated rats,

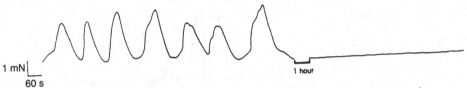

Fig. 13. Spontaneous smooth muscle activity in isolated uterine cervix preparation from oophorectomized rat treated with oestradiol. Note disappearance of spontaneous contractions after an equilibration period of one hour. (Reproduced from Sternquist & Owman, 1985, by courtesy of the Editors of *Acta Physiologica Scandinavica*.)

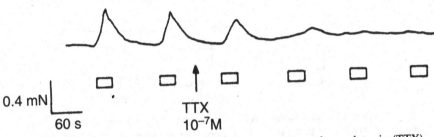

Fig. 14. Example of experiment showing inhibitory effect of tetrodotoxin (TTX) on contractile response of rat uterine cervix *in vitro* (spayed, oestrogen-treated animal) induced by electrical field stimulation (indicated by bars). (Reproduced from Stjernquist & Owman, 1985, by courtesy of the Editors of *Acta Physiologica Scandinavica*.)

however, manifest continuous smooth muscle activity with no tendency to exhaustion. Experiments with transmural electrical stimulation have been performed on cervix preparations from oestrogen-treated animals, while untreated animals have mainly been used for tests on spontaneous motor activity. Electrical field stimulation results in contractile responses, provided serial pulses are used to obtain regular and reproducible contractions. Thus, pulse series of 30 s duration were applied every two minutes with a frequency of 3 Hz (with 1 ms duration and 9 V over the electrodes). Addition of the nerve-blocking drug, tetrodotoxin, to the organ chamber characteristically abolishes about 85% of the contraction amplitude, indicating that this fraction of the smooth muscle response is due to stimulation of the nerves with the release of transmitter (Fig. 14). The remaining 15% is probably the result of direct electrical activation of the smooth muscle cells in the cervix preparation.

ACh and metacholine induce contractions in the isolated rat uterine cervix, and the smooth muscle activity achieved with transmural electrical stimulation is blocked by atropine (Fig. 15) or scopolamine, as well as by tetrodotoxin (Stjernquist & Owman, 1985). Hence, there is pharmacological evidence of a cholinergic motor innervation of the cervical smooth muscle tissue.

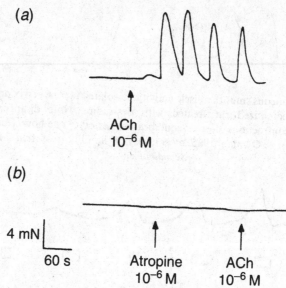

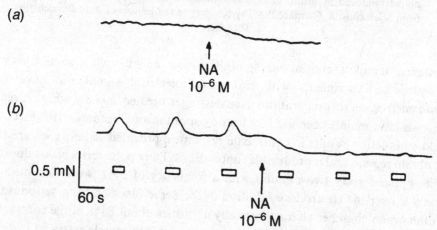

Fig. 15. Effect of acetylcholine (ACh) on isolated cervical smooth muscle from spayed, oestrogen-treated rat (a) ACh alone, and (b) after atropine. (Reproduced from Stjernquist & Owman, 1985, by courtesy of the Editors of *Acta Physiologica Scandinavica*.)

Fig. 16. Inhibitory effect of noradrenaline (NA) on (a) resting tension and (b) the response to electrical field stimulation (indicated by bars) of isolated cervix from spayed oestrogen-treated rats. (Reproduced from Stjernquist & Owman, 1985, by courtesy of the Editors of *Acta Physiologica Scandinavica*.)

NA reduces resting tension as well as spontaneous smooth muscle activity in the cervix, the effects being modified by adrenoceptor antagonists (Stjernquist & Owman, 1985, Figs. 16, 17, 18), suggesting the presence of post-junctional adrenergic receptors. However, the contractions induced by electrical field

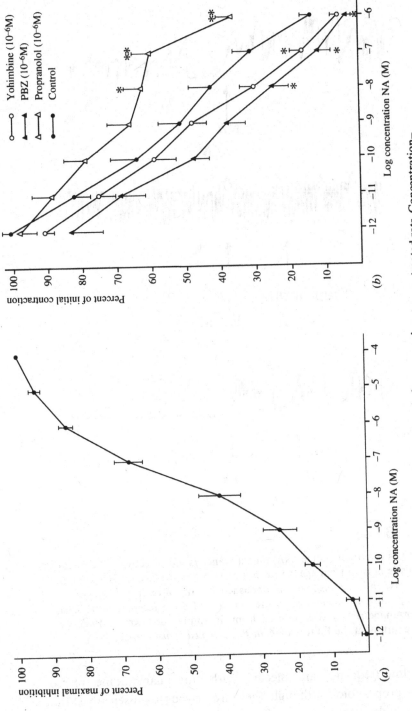

Fig. 17. Isolated uterine cervix from spayed oestrogen-treated rats. Concentration–response curves showing (a) inhibitory effect of noradrenaline (NA) on resting tension. (b) Mean effects and SEM of NA on response of uterine cervix to transmural nerve stimulation in controls and in the presence of the adrenergic blocking agents: yohimbine, phenoxybenzamine (PBZ), and propranolol. (Reproduced from Stjernquist & Owman, 1985, by courtesy of the Editors of *Acta Physiologica Scandinavica*.)

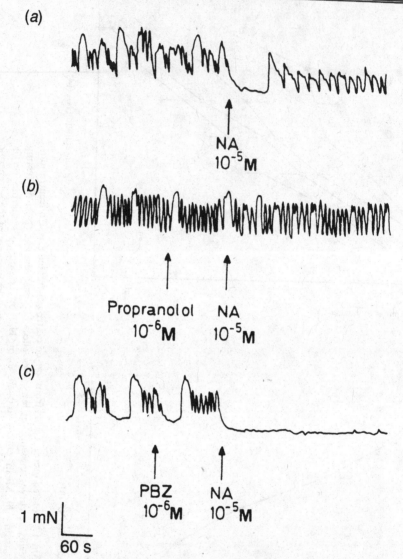

Fig, 18. Effects of noradrenaline (NA) on spontaneous motor activity of cervical smooth muscle *in vitro* from spayed rat not receiving oestrogen. (*a*) NA inhibits motor activity. (*b*) The response is abolished by the β-receptor antagonist, propranolol, and it is potentiated in the presence of the α-receptor antagonist phenoxybenzamine (PBZ). (Reproduced from Stjernquist & Owman, 1985, by courtesy of the Editors of *Acta Physiologica Scandinavica*.)

stimulation at low frequency are affected neither by guanethidine, phenoxy-benzamine nor propranolol, although they are tetrodotoxin-sensitive. In the absence of clear evidence of a neural release of NA directly affecting the smooth musculature of the rat cervix, the functional role of the adrenergic nerves remains

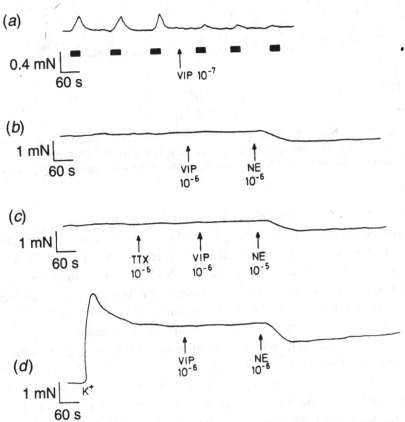

Fig. 19. Isolated cervix from oophorectomized, oestrogen-treated rat. (*a*) Inhibitory effect of VIP on contractions induced by electrical nerve stimulation (indicated by bars). (*b*) VIP is without effect on resting tension, which is reduced by noradrenaline (NA). (*c*) The responses to VIP and NA are not influenced by the nervous blocking agent, tetrodotoxin (TTX). (*d*) The same pattern of responses to VIP and NA is demonstrated on a preparation precontracted by exchanging sodium in the organ chamber against potassium. (Reproduced from Stjernquist & Owman, 1984, by courtesy of the Editors of *Regulatory Peptides*.)

an enigma. The observation that NA inhibits the electrically induced contractile response, which is antagonized by adrenergic blockers, would indicate a role for the adrenergic fibres as pre-junctional modulators of the cholinergic motor nerves, though the effect might also be the result of a direct action of NA on the smooth muscle cells.

Like NA, VIP inhibits spontaneous activity as well as neurally evoked contractions of the rat uterine cervix, but leaves the resting tension unaffected (Stjernquist & Owman, 1984, Figs. 19, 20). Thus, post-junctional VIP receptors would seem to be present, possibly together with pre-junctional receptors located on the cholinergic axons.

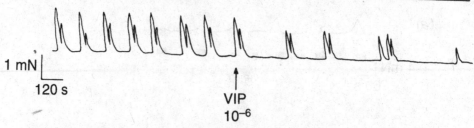

Fig. 20. Inhibitory effect of VIP on rhythmically contracting isolated cervix preparation from oophorectomized rat not treated by oestrogen. (Reproduced from Stjernquist & Owman, 1984, by courtesy of the Editors of *Regulatory Peptides*.)

NPY also blocks the response to transmural stimulation, but its effect differs from that of NA and VIP in leaving both the resting tension and spontaneous smooth muscle activity unaffected (Stjernquist *et al.*, 1983, Figs. 6, 7). There is so far no evidence of any post-junctional NPY receptors in the rat cervix; conceivably the inhibitory effect on the neurally evoked smooth muscle activity is mediated by pre-junctional receptors reducing the release of ACh.

The concentration–response curves to ACh and carbacholine are to a varying degree depressed and right-shifted in the presence of NA, but not in the presence of NPY or VIP (Stjernquist & Owman, 1987, Fig. 21). The electrically induced cholinergic contraction is potentiated in tissues from animals pre-treated with reserpine or 6-OHDA, but only at high stimulation frequencies (Fig. 22). Histochemically, both sympatholytics abolish NA from the cervical nerve fibres, whereas immunoreactive NPY is still found. Tyramine administered in the organ bath was found to reduce the contraction amplitude during electrical nerve stimulation by a β-adrenoceptor-sensitive mechanism (Fig. 23). In the presence of neostigmine, the amplitude could be reduced by NA but not by NPY or VIP; these had an inhibitory effect in the absence of neostigmine (Fig. 24). The results offer further support for the view that, although the cervical smooth muscle cells are equipped with adrenoceptors, the neurogenic motor response at low stimulation frequencies is mainly cholinergic. It appears that neurally released NA is able to exert an effect on these muscle cells primarily at high frequencies. There is no clear-cut evidence that the inhibitory effects of neural NPY or VIP on the cervix of spayed, oestrogen-treated rats are mediated by post-junctional receptors.

Pregnancy-induced changes in nerves of the myometrium

Knowledge of pregnancy-induced changes in the adrenergic innervation is most complete in the guinea-pig and discussion will mostly be confined to this animal.

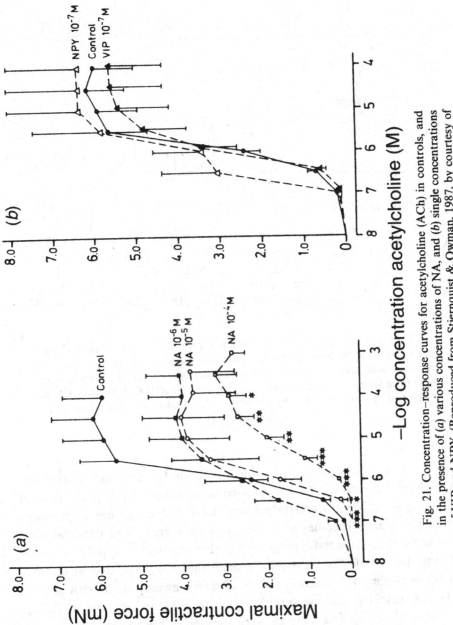

Fig. 21. Concentration–response curves for acetylcholine (ACh) in controls, and in the presence of (a) various concentrations of NA, and (b) single concentrations of VIP and NPY. (Reproduced from Sjernquist & Owman, 1987, by courtesy of the Editors of *Acta Physiologica Scandinavica*.)

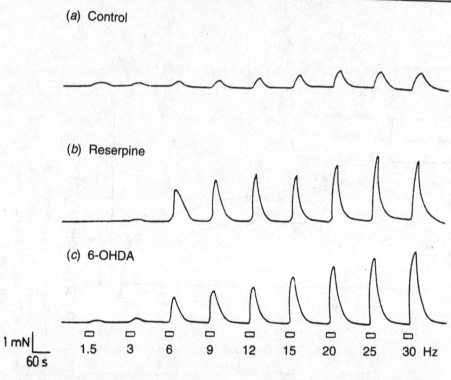

Fig. 22. Representative tracings from isolated rat cervix subjected to electrical field stimulation. With increasing stimulation frequencies, preparations from (a) control animals show a less prominent potential of the contractile response than those from animals treated with (b) reserpine or (c) 6-OHDA. (Reproduced from Stjernquist & Owman, 1987, by courtesy of the Editors of *Acta Physiologica Scandinavica*.)

Pregnancy in the guinea-pig lasts 63–65 days. The uterus is in five distinct parts: (1) the cervix; (2) the tubal end of the uterine horn; (3) the empty uterine horn in a unilateral pregnancy; (4) the fetus-containing horn with 'perifetal' tissue surrounding the conceptus; and (5) 'parafetal' tissue between fetuses. Demarcation between the fetuses becomes less evident as they grow, and parafetal tissue diminishes so that, at the end of pregnancy, the horn contains only perifetal tissue.

During the first 10 days of (bilateral) pregnancy the tissue content of NA in both horns is almost doubled; from 10–15 days onward, uterine NA shows a steady fall, reaching non-measurable concentrations at the time of delivery (Owman *et al.*, 1975). The same changes are seen in the fetus-containing horn during unilateral pregnancy. In the empty horn, however, the high concentration of NA in early pregnancy is maintained until 50 days; there is a rapid fall in the next two weeks to non-measurable levels. The changes in NA content of the cervix are very similar to those seen in the sterile horn (Owman *et al.*, 1975). The

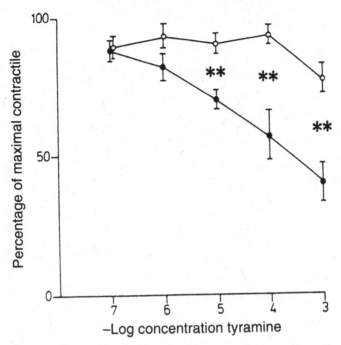

Fig. 23. Increasing concentrations of tyramine diminishes the amplitude of the contractions induced by transmural electrical stimulation of isolated rat cervix (●), the effect being counteracted by propanolol (○). (Reproduced from Stjernquist & Owman, 1987, by courtesy of the Editors of *Acta Physiologica Scandinavica*.)

tubal end of the uterine horn, whether or not it contains fetuses, is the only region in which the concentration of neuronal NA remains unchanged throughout pregnancy (Thorbert, 1978).

The adrenergic nerve plexus is a permanent structural component of sympathetically innervated organs. When the tissue mass changes, the sympathetic nerves adapt so that the neuro-effector relationship remains constant. But the situation for the uterus during pregnancy is the reverse: the massive enlargement is accompanied by a dramatic decay in the sympathetic innervation including degeneration of the adrenergic nerve endings. Since axonal uptake of NA is the major process for transmitter inactivation of the receptor, it is likely that alterations in neuronal uptake of NA will result in entirely different myometrial reactions to circulating catecholamines. Changes in adrenergic functions within the myometrium are not solely a reflection of altered reactivity of the post-junctional adrenoceptors, but represent profound alterations in the entire sympathetic innervation of the organ.

The decrease in the NA-synthesizing capacity with advancing pregnancy, in combination with the almost total loss of uterine NA transmitter (Thorbert, 1978),

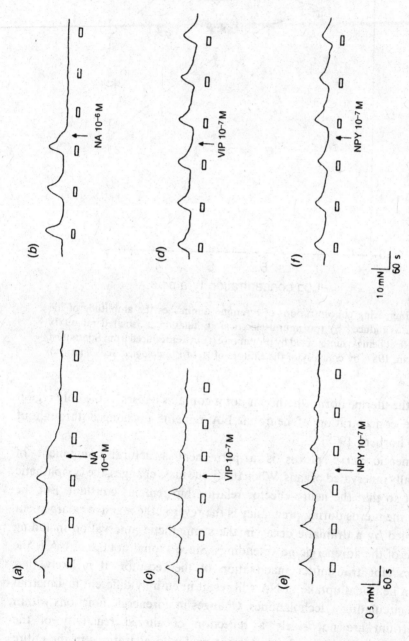

Fig. 24. Electrical field stimulation of isolated rat cervix before (left panel) and after (right panel) addition of 10^{-7} M neostigmine to the organ chamber. Note that NA, but not VIP or NPY, inhibits the contractions in the presence of neostigmine. (Reproduced from Stjernquist & Owman, 1987, by courtesy of the Editors of *Acta Physiologica Scandinavica*.)

seems to be the consequence of degeneration of the adrenergic nerve plexus in the fetus-containing horn; in the empty horn the nerves are structurally intact. Since the reduction in tyrosine hydroxylase activity and NA concentration in the uterine horns occurs whether or not fetuses are present, it is probably not the result of a local action of the conceptus on the uterine muscle. However, the magnitude of the changes in the fetus-containing uterine horn may be related to the location and size of the conceptus. Hormonal mechanisms are also involved; the short adrenergic neurons supplying the female reproductive tract are especially sensitive to the action of sex steroids. However, since the adrenergic nerves do not change uniformly throughout the uterus and cervix, it is unlikely that the nerve degeneration is solely due to systemic humoral factors. Instead, the neuronal changes may be caused by local hormonal effects. Interactions between neurons and target cells are also of fundamental importance in the establishment and maintenance of nerve connections.

The restoration of the uterine adrenergic innervation post-partum shows considerable regional differences (Thorbert, 1978). In the cervix, the NA concentration becomes normal shortly after delivery. The restoration is slower in the sterile uterine horn; it may be the result of 'refilling' of NA in functionally impaired but structurally intact nerves, combined with a regenerative process in the adrenergic nerve plexus. The restitution is, however, slower in the sterile uterine horn than in the cervix. Pre-pregnancy concentrations of NA in this horn are not reached until three months post-partum. Restitution in the fetus-containing uterine horn is incomplete even six months after pregnancy. A 'normal' neuromuscular relationship may never be re-established following a first pregnancy. The degree of normalization is much less than that following cytotoxic axon degeneration produced by administration of 6-ODHA or antiserum to nerve growth factor (NGF). Explanations for this include: (1) the pregnancy-induced degeneration is more complete and collateral sprouting from intact axons is limited; (2) the effect on the ganglion cells during pregnancy is different from that of the neurotoxic agents; or (3) the properties of the target organ have changed to such an extent that it no longer represents a natural template for the outgrowth of a dense adrenergic nerve plexus.

Nevertheless, the guinea-pig is highly fertile even immediately following a pregnancy. Thus the extensive adrenergic innervation present in the uterus of virgin animals is not required for pregnancy, and the small amount of innervation established post-partum is sufficient to fulfil the requirements of adrenergic smooth muscle control during pregnancy. In the human myometrium a degeneration/regeneration cycle takes place in the second and following pregnancies, but with a lower amplitude than the decay occurring during the first pregnancy. The adrenergic innervation supplying the uterus before the first pregnancy may not represent a final stage of development, and the 'normal' adrenergic innervation may be that established after the first pregnancy. The uterine adrenergic nerves in earlier phases may not have been involved in motor control, but rather have had functions such as trophic or metabolic regulation during the differentiation and growth of the myometrial smooth muscle cells.

The human myometrium is also extensively supplied with adrenergic nerve terminals (Owman *et al.*, 1967). In the second trimester of pregnancy the number and density of fibres with formaldehyde-induced fluorescence become reduced, and practically no fluorescent fibres are found at term (Thorbert, 1978). Incubation of myometrial tissue in the presence of α-methyl-NA does not increase the number of histochemically visible adrenergic nerves. These observations are consistent with the sharp reduction in NA concentration during the second trimester, so that the concentration of uterine NA at term is only 2% of that in non-pregnant subjects. A similar pattern of pregnancy-induced reduction occurs in tyrosine hydroxylase activity, as well as in the activity of the subsequent enzyme in the biosynthesis of NA, namely aromatic L-amino acid decarboxylase (Thorbert, 1978). During pregnancy, the human uterus increases its weight about 30-fold, the gain being predominant in the corpus. Hence, weight gain in the isthmus, from which the study materials were obtained, is probably relatively less. Thus, the reductions in the concentrations of NA, tyrosine hydroxylase, and the decarboxylating enzyme at term do not depend solely on an altered nerve-to-muscle ratio due to an increased muscle mass, but reflect real reductions in the total uterine content of the adrenergic transmitter and its synthesizing enzymes.

In the light of the regional distribution of the uterine adrenergic nerve supply, the sensitivity of the nerves to sex steroids, and the profound changes during pregnancy, it is tempting to suggest that the nerves play a functional part in pregnancy and labour. The suspensory ligament, which is homologous to the ligamentum ovarii proprium in humans, provides the entrance for that part of the uterine adrenergic innervation which is restricted to the tubal end of the uterine horn. Uterine contractions have a distinct propagation pattern, with the first increase in intramural, myometrial pressure occurring at one of the two tubo-uterine junctions. This site has been designated as the uterine pacemaker. After the initial increase in intramural pressure in the pacemaker area, the wave spreads in all directions to involve the whole organ. Because of the location of the pacemaker, the predominant direction of propagation is downwards. It is possible that the adrenergic innervation of this pacemaker area could be engaged in the initiation of labour. In addition, at the end of pregnancy the myometrium shows signs of denervation and supersensitivity to NA; this may increase the sensitivity of the smooth muscle to circulating myoactive substances near term and during labour. The degeneration and functional inactivation of the nerves which occurs before this supersensitivity develops may be one of the factors maintaining myometrial quiescence during the growth of the conceptus. The cervical adrenergic nerves are structurally unimpaired and are thus able to control sphincter functions in this region through pregnancy. The adrenergic innervation of the cervix, together with VIP, is hyperactive at term and may be part of an intricate regulatory control of the sphincter during passage of the conceptus.

The normal decay of the NA transmitter in the course of pregnancy may be disturbed in pathological conditions (Rydhström, Walles & Owman, 1988). In patients undergoing Caesarean section because of abruptio placentae, impending asphyxia, dystocia, or pre-eclampsia, the myometrial NA concentrations are 6–10 times higher than in normal pregnancy. By contrast, a Caesarean section for a premature breech, transverse position of the fetus, or prolapse of the umbilical cord, is associated with normal NA concentrations (Rydhström, Walles & Owman, 1988). Thus, the abnormal concentrations do not reflect the emergency situation as such. The increased concentration of myometrial NA in late pregnancy is probably part of the primary pathophysiological condition associated with sympathetic overactivity, resulting in disturbed myometrial circulation and/or motor activity.

There is a major reduction in the neural acetylcholinesterase activity of the feline myometrium; at term almost no positively stained fibres are present in the uterine horns (Alm *et al.*, 1986, Fig. 2). A small number of positive fibres remain in the wall of the sterile (empty) horn during unilateral pregnancy. The reduction is less prominent in the cervix, particularly in its lower part (Fig. 3). Distinct changes are found during early and mid-pregnancy in those parts of the uterine wall which are distended by the growing conceptus. The nerve supply is less affected in the non-distended portions between the fetuses, and especially in the empty horn of a unilateral pregnancy. No reduction in the number of nerve fibres can be found in the cervix at these stages of pregnancy.

In cats and rats there is a considerable reduction in the number of uterine VIP-immunoreactive nerve fibres at the end of pregnancy (Stjernquist *et al.*, 1985; Alm *et al.*, 1986), corresponding to a reduction in radioimmulogically determined VIP concentration (Fig. 25). In contrast, the concentration of VIP in the cervix is not altered (Fig. 25); there is a well-preserved nerve supply, especially in the lower part of the cervix. This is similar to the NA content of the uterus during pregnancy in guinea-pigs (Owman *et al.*, 1975), supporting the view that the autonomic nerves of the uterine horns and of the cervix react differently. In view of the rapid return to normal of rat uterine VIP levels following delivery (Stjernquist *et al.*, 1985), the VIP nerves may only be subject to functional changes rather than the more profound structural degeneration in the adrenergic nerve plexus. The acetylcholinesterase activity of the uterine nerves shows the same pregnancy-related fluctuations as VIP, which may indicate that the changes are associated with the same system of nerves.

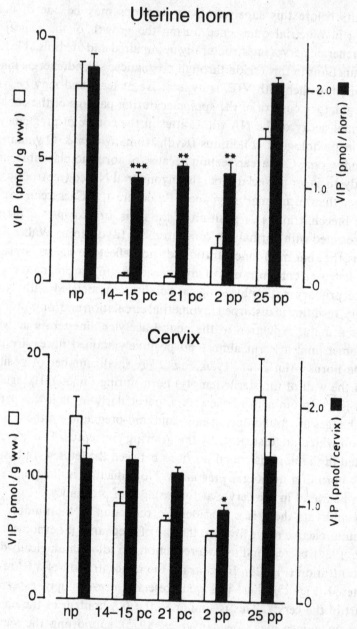

Fig. 25. Radioimmunoassay of VIP in uterine horn and cervix of non-pregnant animals (np), and at various stages before and after delivery: 14–15 and 21 days post-coitum (pc) and 2 and 25 days post-partum (pp). The VIP levels are expressed either on an organ wet weight (ww) basis or as peptide content in the entire horn or cervix. Values are means and SEM of tissue from five animals in each group. Comparison of total organ content of VIP in non-pregnant controls and in separate stages of pregnancy according to Student's *t*-test. (Reproduced from Stjernquist *et al.*, 1985, by courtesy of the Editors of *Biology of Reproduction*.)

Effects of sex steroids on myometrial innervation

The adrenergic nerves of the genital tract have functional properties that differ from those of the rest of the peripheral sympathetic system (Owman & Sjöberg, 1977; Thorbert, 1978). A notable difference is the remarkable sensitivity of the genital adrenergic nerves to sex steroids. Oestrogen, for example, increases NA content of individual adrenergic fibres, whereas progesterone causes a reduction (Falck *et al.*, 1975). Experiments involving ovariectomy and re-implantation of ovarian tissue (Falck *et al.*, 1974) have suggested that adrenergic transmitter concentrations are influenced by the ovaries. The steroid-mediated fluctuations in NA take place at a rate sufficiently high to be measurable in the course of a single oestrous cycle (Thorbert, 1978). It is unlikely that the changes in transmitter concentrations are the result of the hormone-induced alteration in volume of the target organ, since there is often a dissociation between the two variables. Moreover, studies on the uterus after early androgenization of female rats show that the local adrenergic neurons are a separate target system for the hormones which affect the early differentiation of the hypothalamus (Broberg *et al.*, 1974).

Conclusions

The female reproductive organs have extensive autonomic innervation. The sympathetic nerves to the smooth muscle coats of the Fallopian tube, uterus, and vagina comprise a mixture of short adrenergic nerves from utero-vaginal ganglion formations and fibres originating in the inferior mesenteric ganglion.

The adrenergic nerves of the uterus are uniquely sensitive to the action of ovarian sex steroids. Through these effects and additional mechanical effects exerted by the growing conceptus, the uterus undergoes a complete – and entirely physiological – adrenergic denervation in the course of pregnancy, with a slow and incomplete restitution post-partum. This reflects a particularly high degree of plasticity in the myometrial autonomic nerve plexus. The changes may be functionally associated with the maintenance of pregnancy, initiation of labour, and expulsion of the fetus during parturition. VIP in cholinergic nerves supplying the cervical sphincter may also be involved.

The major motor innervation of the uterine cervix appears to be cholinergic in nature, to be subject to axo-axonal cross-talk from adjacent adrenergic fibres, and to be modulated by both VIP and NPY. Substance P is present in primary sensory nerves, extending branches into vascular as well as non-vascular smooth musculature of the uterus, and distributing among the neurons forming the peripheral autonomic ganglia. In this way, both smooth muscle contractility and ganglionic transmission may be modulated by the nociceptive transmitter, substance P. Numerous other peptides have been identified in the uterine nerves: enkephalins, CGRP, PHI, GRP, and galanin. These peptides exert both direct and indirect effects on the smooth musculature in different parts of the reproductive tract.

In view of the specialized neurobiological and functional properties of the autonomic innervation of the female reproductive tract, and on the basis of the peculiar sensitivity of these adrenergic, cholinergic, and peptidergic nerves to the effect of humoral interactions, it would seem reasonable to view this part of the autonomic nervous system as a peripheral neuro-endocrine mechanism, regulating smooth muscle functions.

References

Alm, P., Alumets, J., Håkanson, R. & Sundler, F. (1977). Peptidergic (vasoactive intestinal peptide) nerves in the genito-urinary tract. *Neuroscience*, **2**, 751–4.

Alm, P., Alumets, J., Brodin, G., Håkanson, R., Sjöberg, N.-O. & Sundler, F. (1978). Peptidergic (substance P) nerves in the genito-urinary tract. *Neuroscience*, **3**, 419–25.

Alm, P., Alumets, J., Håkanson, R. *et al.* (1981). Enkephalin-immunoreactive nerve fibers in the feline genito-urinary tract. *Histochemistry*, **72**, 351–5.

Alm, P., Owman, Ch., Sjöberg, N.-O., Stjernquist, M. & Sundler, F. (1986). Histochemical demonstration of a concomitant reduction in neuronal vasoactive intestinal polypeptide (VIP), acetylcholinesterase and noradrenaline of cat uterus during pregnancy. *Neuroscience*, **18**, 713–26.

Amara, S. G., Jonas, V., Rosenfeld, M. G., Ong, E. S. & Evans, R. M. (1982). Alternative RNA processing in calcitonin gene expression generates mRNAs encoding different polypeptide products. *Nature*, **298**, 240–4.

Broberg, A., Nybell, G., Owman, Dh., Rosengren, E. & Sjöberg, N.-O. (1974). Consequence of neonatal androgenization and castration for future levels of norepinephrine transmitter in uterus and vas deferens of the rat. *Neuroendocrinology*, **15**, 308–12.

Chang, M. M., Leeman, S. E. & Niall, H. D. (1971). Amino-acid sequence of substance P. *Nature (New Biology)*, **232**, 86–7.

Fahrenkrug, J. (1979). Vasoactive intestinal polypeptide: measurement, distribution and putative neurotransmitter function. *Digestion*, **19**, 149–69.

Falck, B.,Gårdmark, S., Nybell, G., Owman, C., Rosengren, E. & Sjöberg, N.-O. (1974). Ovarian influence on the content of norepinephrine transmitter in guinea pig and rat uterus. *Endocrinology*, **19**, 1475.

Falck, B., Owman, Ch., Rosengren, E. & Sjöberg, N.-O. (1975). Reduction by progesterone of the estrogen-induced increase in transmitter level of the short adrenergic neurons innervating the uterus. *Endocrinology*, **84**, 958–9.

Gibbins, I. L., Furness, J. B., Costa, M., MacIntyre, I., Hilliyard, C. J. & Girgis, S. (1985). Co-localization of calcitonin gene-related peptide-like immunoreactivity with substance P in cutaneous, vascular and visceral sensory neurons of guinea pigs. *Neuroscience Letters*, **57**, 125–30.

Goodnough, J. E., O'Dorisio, R. T. M., Friedman, C. I. & Kim, K. H. (1979). Vasoactive intestinal polypeptide (VIP) in tissues of the human female reproductive tract. *American Journal of Obstetrics and Gynecology*, **134**, 579–89.

Helm, G., Ottesen, B., Fahrenkrug, J. *et al.* (1981). Vasoactive intestinal polypeptide (VIP) in the human female reproductive tract: distribution and motor effects. *Biology of Reproduction*, **25**, 227–34.

Holmstedt, B. (1957). A modification of the thiocholine method for the determination of cholinesterase. *Acta Physiologica Scandinavica*, **40**, 331–7.

Huang, W. M., Gu, J., Blank, M. A., Allen, J. M., Bloom, S. R. & Polak, J. M. (1984). Peptide-immunoreactive nerves in the mammalian female genital tract. *Histochemical Journal*, **16**, 1297–310.

Hughes, J., Smith, T. W., Kosterlitz, H. W., Fothergill, L. A., Morgan, B. A. & Morris, H. R. (1975). Identification of two related pentapeptides from the brain with potent opiate agonist activity. *Nature*, **258**, 577–9.

Itoh, N., Obata, K., Yanaihara, N. & Okamoto, H. (1983). Human preprovasoactive intestinal polypeptide contains novel PHI-like peptide, PHM-27. *Nature*, **304**, 547–9.

Kanerva, L. (1972). Development, histochemistry and connections of the paracervical (Frankenhäuser) ganglion of the rat uterus. *Acta Institute Anatomy University Helsinki*, Suppl. **2**, 1–31.

Langley, J. N. & Anderson, H. K. (1985). The innervation of the pelvic and adjoining viscera. Part 4. The internal generative organs. *Journal of Physiology* (*London*), **19**, 122–30.

Lundberg, J. M. & Tatemoto, K. (1982). Pancreatic polypeptide family (APP, BPP, NPY and PYY) in relation to sympathetic vasoconstriction resistant to alpha-adrenoceptor blockade. *Acta Physiologica Scandinavica*, **116**, 339–42.

Lundberg, J. M., Terenius, L., Hökfelt, T. *et al.* (1982). Neuropeptide Y (NPY)-like immunoreactivity in peripheral noradrenergic neurons and effects of NPY on sympathetic function. *Acta Physiologica Scandinavica*, **116**, 477–80.

Lundberg, J. M., Hökfelt, T., Martling, C.-R., Saria, A. & Cuello, C. (1984). Substance P-immunoreactive sensory nerves in the lower respiratory tract of various mammals including man. *Cell Tissue Research*, **235**, 251–61.

McDonald, T. J., Nilsson, G., Vagne, M., Ghatei, M., Bloom, S. R. & Mutt, V. (1978). A gastrin releasing peptide from non-antral gastric tissue. *Gut*, **19**, 767–74.

McDonald, T. J., Ghatei, M. A., Bloom, S. R. *et al.* (1981). A qualitative comparison of canine plasma gastroenteropancreatic hormone response to bombesin and the porcine gastrin-releasing peptide (GRP). *Regulatory Peptides*, **2**, 293–304.

Moghimzadeh, E., Ekman, R., Håkanson, R., Yanaihara, N. & Sundler, F. (1983). Neuronal gastrin-releasing peptide in the mammalian gut and pancreas. *Neuroscience*, **10**, 553–63.

Ottesen, B., Fahtenkrug, J., Wagner, G. *et al.* (1980). Effects of VIP in the female genital tract. *Endocrinology Japan*, **1**, 71–8.

Ottesen, B., Larsen, J.-J., Fahrenkrug, J., Stjernquist, M. & Sundler, F. (1981). Distribution and motor effect of VIP in female genital tract. *American Journal of Physiology*, **240**, E32–6.

Ottesen, B., Ulrichsen, H., Fahrenkrug, J. *et al.* (1982). Vasoactive intestinal polypeptide and the female genital tract: relationship to reproductive phase and delivery. *American Journal of Obstetrics and Gynecology*, **143**, 414–20.

Ottesen, B., Söndergaard, F. & Fahrenkrug, J. (1983). Neuropeptides in the regulation of female genital smooth muscle contractility. *Acta Obstetrica Gynecologica Scandinavica*, **62**, 591–2.

Owman, Ch. & Sjöberg, N.-O. (1966). Adrenergic nerves in the female genital tract of the rabbit. *Zeitschrift Zellforschung*, **74**, 182–97.

Owman, Ch., Rosengren, E. & Sjöberg, N.-O. (1967). Adrenergic innervation of the human female reproductive organs: a histochemical and chemical investigation. *Obstetrics and Gynecology*, **30**, 763–73.

Owman, Ch., Alm, P., Rosengren, E., Sjöberg, N.-O. & Thorbert, G. (1975). Variations in the level of uterine norepinephrine during pregnancy in guinea pig. *American Journal of Obstetrics and Gynecology*, **122**, 961–4.

Owman, Ch. & Sjöberg, N.-O. (1977). Influence of pregnancy and sex hormones on the system of short adrenergic neurons in the female reproductive tract. In *Endocrinology*. Ed. V. H. T. James, pp. 205–9, Excerpta Medica, Amsterdam.

Owman, Ch., Stjernquist, M., Helm, G., Kannisto, P., Sjöberg, N.-O. & Sundler, F. (1986). Comparative histochemical distribution of nerve fibers storing noradrenaline and neuropeptide Y (NPY) in human ovary, Fallopian tube, and uterus. *Medical Biology*, **64**, 57–65.

Papka, R. E., Cotton, J. P. & Taurig, H. N. (1985). Comparative distribution of neuropeptide tyrosine-, vasoactive intestinal polypeptide-, substance P-immunoreactive, acetylcholinesterase-positive and noradrenergic nerves in the reproductive tract of the female rat. *Cell Tissue Research*, **242**, 475–90.

Rökaeus, Å, (1987). Galanin: a newly isolated biologically active neuropeptide. *Trends in Neuroscience*, **10**, 158–64.

Rökaeus, Å., Melander, T., Hökeflt, T. *et al.* (1984). A galanin-like peptide in the central nervous system and intestine of the rat. *Neuroscience Letters*, **47**, 161–6.

Rydhström, H., Walles, B. & Owman, Ch. (1989). Myometrial norepinephrine in human pregnancy. Elevated levels in various disorders leading to cesarean section. *Journal of Reproductive Medicine*, **34**, 901–4.

Said, S. I. & Mutt, V. (1970). Polypeptide with broad biological activity: isolation from small intestine. *Science*, **169**, 1217–18.

Said, S. I., ed. (1982). *Vasoactive Intestinal Polypeptide*. Raven Press, New York.

Samuelson, U. E., Dalsgaard, C.-J., Lundberg, J. M. & Hökfelt, T. (1985). Calcitonin gene-related peptide inhibits spontaneous contractions in human uterus and fallopian tube. *Neuroscience Letters*, **62**, 225–30.

Schwartz, T. W., Funlendorff, J., Langeland, N., Tögersen, H., Jörgensen, J. C. & Sheikh, S. P. (1989). Y1 and Y2 receptors for NPY – the evolution of PP-fold peptides and their receptors. In *Neuropeptide Y*. Ed. V. Mutt, K., Fuxe, T. Hökfelt & J. M. Lundberg, pp. 143–51, Raven Press, New York.

Sjöberg, N.-O. (1967). The adrenergic transmitter of the female reproductive tract: distribution and functional changes. *Acta Physiologica Scandinavica*, Suppl. **305**, 1–32.

Sjöstrand, N. O. (1965). The adrenergic innervation of the vas deferens and the accessory male genital glands. *Acta Physiologica Scandinavica*, **65**, Suppl. **257**, 1–82.

Stjernquist, M., Emson, P., Owman, Ch., Sjöberg, N.-O., Sundler, F. & Takemoto, K. (1983). Neuropeptide Y in the female reproductive tract. Distribution of nerve fibers and motor effects. *Neuroscience Letters*, **39**, 279–84.

Stjernquist, M. & Owman, Ch. (1984). Vasoactive intestinal polypeptide (VIP) inhibits neurally evoked smooth muscle activity of rat uterine cervix *in vitro*. *Regulatory Peptides*, **8**, 161–7.

Stjernquist, M., Alm, P., Ekman, R., Owman, Ch., Sjöberg, N.-O. & Sundler, F. (1985).

Levels of neural vasoactive intestinal polypeptide (VIP) in rat uterus are markedly changed in association with pregnancy, as shown by immunocytochemistry and radioimmunoassay. *Biology of Reproduction*, **33**, 157–63.

Stjernquist, M. & Owman, Ch. (1985). Cholinergic and adrenergic neuronal control of smooth muscle function in the non-pregnant rat uterine cervix. *Acta Physiologica Scandinavica*, **124**, 429–36.

Stjernquist, M., Ekblad, E., Owman, Ch. & Sundler, F. (1986). Neuronal localization and motor effects of gastrin releasing peptide (GRP) in rat uterus. *Regulatory Peptides*, **13**, 197–205.

Stjernquist, M., Owman, Ch., Sjöberg, N.-O. & Sundler, F. (1987). Coexistence and cooperation between neuropeptide Y and norepinephrine in nerve fibers of guinea pig vas deferens and seminal vesicle. *Biology of Reproduction*, **36**, 149–55.

Stjernquist, M. & Owman, Ch. (1987). Interaction of noradrenaline, NPY and VIP with the neurogenic cholinergic response of the rat uterine cervix *in vitro*. *Acta Physiologica Scandinavica*, **131**, 553–62.

Stjernquist, M., Ekblad, E., Owman, Ch. & Sundler, F. (1988). Immunocytochemical localization of galanin in the rat male and female genital tracts and motor effects *in vitro*. *Regulatory Peptides*, **20**, 335–43.

Stjernquist, M., Ekblad, E., Nordstedt, E. & Radzuweit, C. (1991). Neuropeptide Y (NPY) co-exists with tyrosine hydroxylase and potentiates the adrenergic contractile response of vascular smooth muscle in the human uterine artery. *Human Reproduction*, **6**, 1034–8.

Sundler, F., Håkanson, R. & Leander, S. (1980). Peptidergic nervous system in the gut. *Clinical Gastroenterology*, **9**, 517–43.

Sundler, F., Brodin, E., Ekblad, E., Håkanson, R. & Uddman, R. (1985). Sensory nerve fibers: distribution of substance P, neurokinin A and calcitonin gene-related peptide. In *Tachykinin Antagonists*. Proceedings of the Fernström Symposium, Ed. R. Håkanson and F. Sundler, vol. 6, pp. 3–14, Elsevier, Amsterdam.

Sundler, F., Ekblad, E., Grunditz, T., Håkanson, R., Luts, A. & Uddman, R. (1989). NPY in peripheral non-adrenergic neurons. In *Neuropeptide Y*. Ed. V. Mutt, K. Fuxe, T. Hökfelt and J. M. Lundberg, pp. 93–102, Raven Press, New York.

Tatemoto, K. (1982). Neuropeptide Y: the complete amino acid sequence of the brain peptide. *Proceedings of the National Academy of Sciences, USA*, **79**, 5485–9.

Tatemoto, K., Rökaeus, Å., Jörnvall, H., McDonald, T. J. & Mutt, V. (1983). Galanin – a novel biologically active peptide from porcine intestine. *FEBS Letters*, **164**, 124–8.

Thorbert, G. (1978). Regional changes in structure and function of adrenergic nerves in guinea pig uterus during pregnancy. *Acta Obstetrica Gynecologica Scandinavica*, Suppl. **305**, 1–32.

Von Euler, U. S. & Gaddum, J. H. (1931). An unidentified depressor substance in certain tissue extracts. *Journal of Physiology*, **72**, 74–87.

10

Prostaglandins and uterine activity

J. J. MORRISON AND S. K. SMITH

Introduction

Prostaglandins were discovered in the 1930s by the Swedish scientist Ulf Von Euler in Stockholm. He observed that human semen and extracts of sheep vesicular glands lowered arterial blood pressure on intravenous injection and stimulated various isolated intestinal and uterine smooth muscle preparations (Von Euler, 1934). The active principle was a lipid-soluble acid different from all other known substances (Von Euler, 1936). It was many years later before their key role in human reproduction became fully evident and much is yet to be learnt about their synthesis, catabolism and mechanism of action.

Prostaglandins originate at or near their site of action as do the related products of archidonic acid metabolism, leukotrienes and thromboxanes, collectively termed the eicosanoids. The eicosanoids can influence the activity of numerous cell types including platelets, neutrophils, monocytes, endothelial cells, vascular and smooth muscle cells, and regulate physiological and pathological processes in all body systems including the reproductive tract. This influence has been largely attributed to an action at the cell membrane level but it is becoming apparent that prostaglandins may have a wider role to play within the cell. They can regulate gene expression (Acarregui et al., 1990) which adds a new dimension to prostaglandins and their effects on DNA replication, transcription and translation.

The importance of lipids in the initiation of uterine activity and parturition was first suggested by Luukkainen and Csapo in the early 1960s (Luukkainen & Csapo, 1963). Intravenous infusion of a lipid emulsion into pregnant rabbits resulted in an increased responsiveness of uteri to oxytocin. A component of the lipid emulsion was demonstrated to be phosphatidylcholine containing an essential fatty acid (Lanman, Herod & Thau, 1972, 1974; Ogawa, Herod & Thau, 1970). It was subsequently found that parturition could be induced in the rabbit by the maternal intravenous administration of arachidonic acid (Nathanielsz, Abel & Smith, 1973). Prostaglandins are of critical importance in the initiation and maintenance of human labour. They have been used in pregnancy since 1967, first for induction of labour (Karim *et al.*, 1968), and later for termination of pregnancy (Karim & Filshie, 1970), for preparing the cervix for induction (Calder & Embrey, 1973), and for the treatment of post-partum haemorrhage (Tagaki *et al.*, 1976; Keirse, 1989). Suppression of endogenous prostaglandin synthesis by inhibition of the cyclooxygenase pathway with indomethacin can arrest pre-term labour in some women (Zuckerman, Reis & Rubinstein, 1974).

Our knowledge about the role of prostaglandins in uterine activity has expanded rapidly but the overall picture of production and action is still rather fragmentary. This review examines the experimental evidence for the importance of prostaglandins in uterine activity at parturition.

Intra-uterine synthesis and metabolism of prostaglandins

All the intra-uterine tissues have the potential for prostaglandin synthesis but it is not yet clear which provides the most important contribution (Mitchell, 1986) or how the various synthetic pathways in the different tissues are coordinated to obtain the required level of prostaglandin production, in the appropriate place and at the appropriate time. *In vitro* experiments are complicated by the fact that *in vivo* compartments are lost, a factor which is particularly relevant to the cyclooxygenase system which is regulated in the cell by peroxides. Under *in vitro* conditions interactions between prostaglandins and other active endogenous compounds such as cAMP, cGMP, ATP, leukotrienes, kinins and catecholamines are lost. We will describe the control of uterine prostaglandin biosynthesis by examining the controlling factors in the myometrium, the endometrium, the fetal membranes and placenta.

Prostaglandin production in the myometrium

Immunohistochemical localization of cyclooxygenase and prostacyclin (PGI_2) synthetase shows that both of these enzymes are located in myometrium cells (Moonen, Klok & Kierse, 1985). Prostacyclin appears to be the main prostaglandin formed in myometrium in contrast to the endometrium, in which prostaglandins of the E and F series are predominant (Abel & Kelly, 1979; Christensen & Green, 1983).

It is not clear what controls prostaglandin synthesis in the myometrium but the concentrations of cyclooxygenase and prostacyclin synthetase enzymes in the non-pregnant and pregnant uterus have been reported (Moonen, Klok &

Kierse, 1984). Pregnant myometrium showed a three-fold increase in cyclooxygenase content per milligram microsomal protein, as measured using monoclonal antibodies against the enzyme and immunoradiometric assay, compared to the non-pregnant myometrium. There was also an increase in prostacyclin synthetase but it was much less than the cyclooxygenase increase and had a different subcellular distribution, i.e. in the non-microsomal fraction. An increase in myometrial vascularization, as occurs in pregnancy, might be contributed to by an increased production of prostacyclin but this is not compatible with the finding that PGI_2 synthetase is located predominantly in smooth muscle and not in myometrial blood vessels. The role of prostacyclin and the reason for the increase in pregnancy are speculative. The increase in cyclooxygenase content can be explained as an attempt to produce more contractile prostaglandins relative to prostacyclin but there is no increase over the last few weeks of pregnancy or with the onset of labour (Moonen et al., 1984).

Moonen et al. studied the influence of uterine anatomy in pregnancy on myometrial cyclooxygenase and PGI_2 synthetase concentrations and found major differences between the localization of both. Cyclooxygenase concentrations increased gradually, but markedly, from the uterine fundus towards the lower uterine segment. PGI_2 synthetase concentrations showed no such trend but were higher in myometrium underneath the placental bed than in the myometrium from the opposite side of the uterus (Moonen, Klok & Keirse, 1986).

Prostaglandin production in the endometrium

In 1965 Pickles and co-workers demonstrated high concentrations of prostaglandins in the endometrium and menstrual fluid (Pickles et al., 1965). Both epithelial and stromal components have the capacity to synthesize prostaglandins (Schartz, Markiewicz & Gurpide, 1987; Lumsden, Brown & Baird, 1984). Estradiol (Domnie, Poyser & Wunderlich, 1974), progesterone (Horton & Poyser, 1976) and the adrenal steroids (Markiewicz & Gurpide, 1988) are among the many factors implicated in the control of prostaglandin synthesis in the endometrium. Prostaglandin production in the endometrium has been linked with dysfunctional uterine bleeding and menorrhagia (Smith et al., 1981a,b). For the purposes of discussion of prostaglandins and uterine activity in pregnancy and labour, the endometrium has by this time become decidualized and we shall refer to the decidual production of prostaglandins below.

Prostaglandin synthesis in the amnion, chorion, decidua and placenta

Most of the arachidonic acid present in mammalian cells is esterified in the sn.-2 position of glycerophospholipids. In order to define the tissue origins of unesterified arachidonic acid found in amniotic fluid during early labour the fatty acid composition of intra-uterine tissues was examined and it was shown that esterified arachidonic acid accounts for between 9 and 20% of the total fatty acid content of fetal membranes, placenta, umbilical cord, decidua and myometrium (Keirse, 1978, 1990; Schwarz *et al.*, 1975). These tissues all contain phospholipases which can release free arachidonic acid needed for eicosanoid synthesis. The concentration of arachidonic acid in amniotic fluid increases several fold during labour (Keirse *et al.*, 1977*a*). This mobilization of arachidonic acid has been attributed to phospholipase A_2 (PLA_2), which exhibits substrate specificity for phosphatidylethanolamine (PE)-containing arachidonic acid (Okazaki *et al.*, 1978; Schultz *et al.*, 1975) and a phosphatidylinositol (PI)-specific phospholipase C (PLC), coupled with diacylglycerol and a monoacylglycerol lipase, in fetal membranes (Bleasdale & Johnston, 1984; Ohazaki *et al.*, 1981*a*; Keirse, 1990). The arachidonic acid content of PE and phosphatidylcholine (PC) in the fetal membranes is decreased during labour; this decrease is large enough to account for the arachidonic acid required for the prostaglandin production associated with parturition (Okita, MacDonald & Johnston, 1982*a*).

Karim reported an increase in prostaglandin levels in amniotic fluid associated with labour (Karim & Devlin, 1967). Subsequently it has been demonstrated that after the onset of labour and throughout active labour, the levels of PGE_2 and $PGF_{2\alpha}$ and/or other metabolites are elevated in amniotic fluid (Keirse, Mitchell & Turnbull, 1977*b*; Satoh *et al.*, 1979; Ghodgaonkar *et al.*, 1979), maternal plasma (Satoh *et al.*, 1979; Ghodgaonkar *et al.*, 1979; Green *et al.*, 1974) and urine (Satoh *et al.*, 1979; Hamberg, 1974) compared to the level of these substances prior to the onset of labour.

Relative importance of the amnion

The relative importance of each of the intra-uterine tissues as a source of prostaglandins involved in the initiation of uterine activity and parturition is not yet clear. Amnion may play an active role and it has a greater capacity to synthesize prostaglandins than other intra-uterine tissues (Okazaki *et al.*, 1981*b*). The specific activity of the PG synthetase complex is also higher in amnion compared to other fetal tissues. The activity of PG synthetase in human amnion increases dramatically during the later stages of gestation, being several times higher at term than in early pregnancy (Okazaki *et al.*, 1981*b*). There was no comparable change in enzymatic activity in chorion laeve and decidua vera. Okazaki *et al.* demonstrated that while amnion has a capacity for synthesis of prostaglandins, the ability to inactivate prostaglandins is limited with low activity of 15-hydroxyprostaglandin dehydrogenase (Okazaki *et al.*, 1981*b*). They also demonstrated that the specific activities of phospholipase A_2 and C increase in human amnion as gestation advances but remain unchanged in chorion laeve and decidua vera (Okazaki *et al.*, 1981*a*).

Transfer of prostaglandins across the fetal membrane

Prostaglandins are produced by the amnion and are associated with the onset of human labour.

The question arises as to how they are transferred across the fetal membranes. It has been shown that PGE_2 can transfer across the membranes without being metabolized before the onset of labour, and that the transfer of PGE_2 was greater after the onset of labour (Nakla *et al.*, 1986). Another report, however, contradicts this finding, suggesting that most of the endogenous PGE_2 produced by the amnion (or exogenous PGE_2) does not cross the amnion and chorion unmetabolized (Roseblade *et al.*, 1990). The problem with this type of research is that *in vitro* experiments may not accurately reflect the dynamic *in vivo* process making interpretation of results difficult.

Phospholipases and regulation of prostaglandin synthesis

The sources of arachidonic acid to support prostaglandin production in human fetal membranes during early labour are phosphatidylethanolamine and phosphatidylinositol (Okita *et al.*, 1982*a*) which are substrates for PLA_2 and PLC, respectively.

Okazaki *et al.* showed that PLA_2 activity in fetal membranes is calcium dependent and has an alkaline pH optimum (pH 8.0) (Okazaki *et al.*, 1978). The liberation of arachidonic acid from glycerophospholipids is the first step in prostaglandin biosynthesis and this may be a rate-limiting step. The periparturitional gene expression of PLA_2 has been studied in human placentae and fetal membranes (Aitken, Rice & Brennecke, 1990) using a cDNA clone for non-pancreatic PLA_2. Steady-state levels of messenger RNA (mRNA) for PLA_2 were increased in placentae obtained after spontaneous-onset labour and normal vaginal delivery as compared with placentae from elective Caesarean section. Interestingly, however, the steady-state levels of mRNA encoding PLA_2 in amnion and chorion were less than of placenta, and in the former tissues there was no significant change in association with the onset of labour at term. This led Aitken *et al.*, 1990, to suggest that the enzyme of central regulatory significance may be cyclooxygenase rather than PLA_2.

Mammalian cells contain at least five immunologically distinct PLC enzymes that appear to be separate gene products (Rhee *et al.*, 1989). Several PLC enzymes have been purified to homogeneity leading to many unsystematically named enzymes and therefore problems with nomenclature. The use of Greek letters (α, β, γ, δ, ε) to designate the PLC enzymes with different primary structures has helped in differentiation. The enzyme purified, characterized and DNA sequenced from guinea-pig uterus is PI-PLC (α) with a molecular mass of 62 kD (Bennett *et al.*, 1988).

Initial studies on PLC activity in fetal membranes and decidua found it to be primarily in the cytosolic fraction of amnion, having a pH optimum of 6.5 to 7.5, and requiring calcium for activity. PLC specific activity increases approximately five-fold between early second trimester and term (Okazaki *et al.*, 1981*a*). Bala *et al.* characterized the major phosphoinositide-specific PLC of human amnion and found it to be attributable to a single isoform (mol. wt. 85 000) (Bala, Thakur & Bleasdale, 1990). This isoform catalysed the calcium-dependent hydrolysis of both phosphatidylinositol and phosphatidylinositol-4,5-biphosphate. They found that the PLC activity of amnion cells isolated at 38–41 weeks gestation declined >80% during the initial 2–5 days of culture as did basal production of PGE_2. In contrast, both vasopressin and epidermal growth factor (EGF) stimulated prostaglandin production was equal on day 2 and day 5 and appeared to be independent of PLC activity. These findings indicate that regulation of prostaglandin biosynthesis can occur at the level of arachidonic acid mobilization or by modultion of the cyclooxygenase system.

Other factors which may alter the arachidonic acid cascade in intrauterine tissues are amines (Sagawa, Bleasdale & Di Renzo, 1983) and catecholamines (Di Renzo, Venincasa & Bleasdale, 1984*a*; Di Renzo, Anceschi & Bleasdale, 1984*b*).

Uterine contractility and prostaglandin function at the cellular level

Calcium mobilization

Calcium is necessary for smooth muscle contraction and is a common denominator in linking excitation at the cell membrane with the actin-myosin interaction. Prostaglandins are produced at or near their site of action and their contractile effect is based on their ability to mobilize calcium. PGE_2 and $PGF_{2\alpha}$ cause release of calcium from microsomal preparations of myometrium enriched in sarcoplasmic reticulum (Carsten, 1974*a*, Carsten & Miller, 1977). In bovine pregnant uterus, PGE_2 had a greater effect than $PGF_{2\alpha}$. The effects of PGE_2 on cellular calcium transport were also observed in term pregnant human uterus obtained at caesarian hysterectomy (Carsten, 1973). $PGF_{2\alpha}$ is more potent in stimulating myometrial activity in preparations of pregnant than non-pregnant bovine uterus (Carsten

1974*b*). *In vitro* experiments in calcium-free solution provide additional evidence for the requirement of calcium release from intracellular stores in PGE_2-induced uterine contractions (Villar, D'Ocon & Anselmi, 1985).

The prostaglandin receptor

Although receptors for prostaglandins in the myometrium of non-pregnant women have been identified, there is relatively little information on pregnant myometrium (Giannopoulos *et al.*, 1985). In contrast to oxytocin, the number of PGE and $PGF_{2\alpha}$ receptors changes little in the human myometrium during pregnancy and labour (Carsten & Miller, 1987). Some studies have shown PGE_2 and $PGF_{2\alpha}$ receptors to be homogenous (Giannopoulos *et al.*, 1985; Carsten & Miller, 1987) while others have reported high and lower affinities for each prostaglandin (Hoffman *et al.*, 1983). The affinity of the PGE receptor for PGE_2 is 10- to 20-fold higher than the affinity of the PGF receptor for $PGF_{2\alpha}$, a factor which may explain the greater potency of PGE_2 as a stimulant of uterine activity.

Carsten and Miller have demonstrated that in purified subcellular fractions from bovine and human pregnant myometrium, prostaglandin receptors are found in the cell membrane fraction and the sarcoplasmic reticulum (Carsten & Miller, 1981). The affinity of cell membrane and sarcoplasmic reticulum for PGE_2 was the same with the average kD for PGE_2 and PGE_1 being 2.50 and 3.05 nM, respectively; the same receptor was specific for both prostaglandins. Their studies indicated, however, that there were separate receptors for $PGF_{2\alpha}$ and a series of inactive prostaglandins which exhibited low competitive effects on PGE_2 binding.

Second messengers

It is clear that there are prostaglandin receptors on the cell surface and in the intracellular organelles and that receptor binding is for prostaglandin action. What is not clear is whether prostaglandin binding to some or all of its cellular receptors is required for action. In any case, this binding results ultimately in the alteration of intracellular events working largely through the pathway of second messengers.

Phosphoinositides

The phosphoinositides are components of cell membranes and account for approximately 3–5% of the phospholipid content (Abdel-Latif, 1986). Phosphatidylinositol exists in the cell membrane as a glycerol backbone with a fatty acid attached in position 1, arachidonic acid in position 2 and inositol attached in position 3 through a phosphate group. Approximately 10–20% of the phosphatidylinositol is further phosphorylated at positions 4 and 5 of inositol (Carsten & Miller, 1990).

Binding of agonist, such as a prostaglandin, to a receptor, activates PLC after stimulation of a G protein (Fuse & Tai, 1987). PLC enzymes are phosphodiesterases which can hydrolyse phosphatidylinositol-4,5-biphosphate to diacylglycerol (DAG) and inositol-1,4,5-triphosphate (IP$_3$) (Berridge, 1984). Mammalian cells contain at least five immunologically distinct PLC enzymes that appear to be separate gene products and which have limited amino acid sequence similarity to enzymes catalysing the same chemical reaction (Rhee *et al.*, 1989). One explanation is that each isozyme has a defined function in processing different physiological responses allowing for further diversity in regulation. While it is held that several isozymes exist there is controversy as to whether the active form is the membrane-bound or soluble form. The consensus is that only membrane-bound enzyme mediates second messenger production but it is possible that there is translocation of the two forms (Wilson, 1990). However, most of the phosphoinositide-specific PLC activity in human amnion at term was found to be attributable to a single isoform (mol.wt. 85 000) (Bala *et al.*, 1990).

The IP$_3$ released mobilizes intracellular calcium from the sarcoplasmic reticulum (Carsten & Miller, 1985). Specific binding of IP$_3$ to endoplasmic reticulum has been analysed by Scatchard plots (Guillemette *et al.*, 1987). This release of calcium from the sarcoplasmic reticulum is mediated by a channel rather than a carrier as it is not altered at lower temperature; it was assumed that an increase in the viscosity of the lipid bilayer would not affect a channel mechanism (Smith, Smith & Higgins, 1985). The site of action also appears to be solely at the endo(sarco)-plasmic reticulum to promote calcium release (Delfert *et al.*, 1986).

The IP$_3$ is broken down in the cytoplasm in a stepwise fashion to inositol biphosphate (IP$_2$), inositol monophosphate (IP$_1$) and inositol by specific phosphomonoesterases (Storey *et al.*, 1984). In the cell membrane inositol is used for the resynthesis of phosphatidylinositol.

Diacylglycerol (DAG) is the other compound formed when PLC acts upon phosphatidylinositol-4,5-biphosphate in the cell membrane. The actions appear to be three-fold:

1. It activates protein kinase C. This may stimulate the release of arachidonic acid and prostaglandins (Wijkander & Sundler, 1989; Zakar & Olson, 1989). It may also regulate the release of arachidonic acid through inhibition of acyl transferase thereby increasing free available arachidonate and stimulating prostaglandin synthesis (Fuse, Iwanga & Tai, 1989). Protein kinase C has been identified in fetal membranes (Okazaki, Ban & Johnston, 1984) and in

uterus (Baraban *et al.*, 1985) and in many systems that use IP_3 as a second messenger.

2. It is converted to phosphatidic acid (PA) (Takuwa, Takuwa & Rasmussen, 1986). The exact role of PA is not clear but it may in some way be involved in a late effect of the agonist and it has been suggested that it may enhance the calcium releasing effects (Brass & Laposata, 1987).

3. DAG usually contains arachidonic acid thereby directly providing for prostaglandin synthesis within the cell. This may explain why the effect of oxytocin is reduced in the presence of a prostaglandin synthesis inhibitor (Chan, 1983) and it has been shown that oxytocic agents can increase the synthesis of prostaglandins in human pregnant myometrium (Hensby *et al.*, 1986).

In summary, prostaglandins, like many other agonists, stimulate myometrial PLC to hydrolyse phosphoinositides (Ruzycky & Crankshaw, 1988; Scherey, Read & Steer, 1987; Breuiller-Fouche *et al.*, 1991; Shieman & Buxton, 1991) and the second messengers IP_3 and DAG account, at least in part, for the contractile response. This system of second messengers does not act alone but interacts in a complex fashion with other messengers and regulatory proteins as described below.

Cyclic AMP

Adenosine $3',5'$-cyclic monophosphate (cAMP) is a second messenger involved in the action of numerous drugs and hormones. In uterine tissue it was initially recognized for its role in myometrial relaxation. Beta adrenergic receptor stimulation results in myometrial relaxation (Mahon, Reid & Day, 1967). The mechanism of this action appears to be through the formation of cAMP and a stimulatory GTP-binding protein (Litime *et al.*, 1989). Other relaxing agents have been shown to work via cAMP (Yang *et al.*, 1973).

The role of cAMP is more complex than a simple involvement in myometrial relaxation. It was demonstrated that PGE_1 and PGE_2, which are uterine contractile agents, result in increased synthesis of cAMP in rat myometrium as did epinephrine which is a relaxant (Vesin & Harbon, 1974). It has been proposed that relaxation induced by stimulation of β-adrenergic receptors is the result of combined effects of both a cAMP dependent and a cAMP-independent process (Dokhac, Mokhtari & Harbon, 1986). The coupling of adrenergic and prostaglandin receptors to other components of the adenylate cyclase complex was studied in uteri obtained from pregnant rats at different stages of gestation. It appeared that guanine–nucleotide regulatory proteins may also play a role in controlling responses to receptor-mediated agonists under differing hormonal conditions (Tanfin & Harbon, 1987). It was suggested that the response to PGE_2 was converted from a G_s-mediated stimulation of adenylate cyclase in the oestrogen-dominated myometrium to a G_i-mediated inhibition of cAMP production in the final stages of gestation.

There are many unanswered questions in the area of prostaglandins, second messengers and the role of cAMP. Further studies are necessary to provide a better understanding of the nature of their interactions.

Cyclic GMP

It was originally held that contractile effects were mediated through cyclic guanosine monophosphate (cGMP) and relaxant effects through cAMP (Goldberg *et al.*, 1973). The exact role of cGMP is still unclear. In guinea-pig myometrium it was shown that cGMP was increased but the contractions preceded this increase (Diamond & Hartle, 1976). It was later shown that there was no correlation between elevation of cGMP and contraction or relaxation in the rat myometrium (Diamond, 1983).

G proteins

Guanine nucleotide binding proteins provide a regulatory link between action at a receptor site and intracellular activity. Receptor-stimulated PLC activity is mediated through a G protein (Cockcroft & Gomperts, 1985; Fuse & Tai, 1987). This may well be a mechanism of activation of PLA_2 (Clark *et al.*, 1988; Welsh, Dubyak & Douglas, 1988). GTP is necessary for the action of PLC in the presence of physiological cation concentrations (Fulle *et al.*, 1987) and also for the IP_3 induced calcium release from sarcoplasmic reticulum (Vesin & Harbon, 1974). Pregnancy suppresses G protein coupling to phosphoinositide hydrolysis in guinea-pig myometrium which may contribute to diminished contractile sensitivity during pregnancy or at least be a regulatory event in the processes maintaining uterine quiescence in pregnancy (Arkinstall & Jones, 1990).

In summary, the myometrium possesses extracellularly directed G-protein coupled receptors which can be occupied by prostaglandins producing many diverse physiological actions. By working via their effect on adenylate cyclase, cAMP, cGMP, protein kinases and PLC catalyzed hydrolysis of membrane phosphatidylinositol-4,5-biphosphate to IP_3 and DAG, prostaglandins can mobilize calcium leading to uterine muscle contraction.

The interaction of prostaglandins and oxytocin

The first clue to an interaction between prostaglandins and oxytocin was the demonstration that indomethacin and meclofenamate, both prostaglandin synthetase inhibitors, antagonized the contractile effects of oxytocin on isolated uterus from the pregnant rat (Vane & Williams, 1973). Similarly an increase in oxytocin sensitivity is prevented by administration of prostaglandin synthetase inhibitors (Chan, 1983). Prostaglandin synthetase inhibitors have been shown to antagonize the contractile effect of oxytocin but not of $PGF_{2\alpha}$ on the isolated uterus of the rat and human (Dubin, Ghodaonkar & King, 1979; Garrioch, 1978). Oxytocin at physiological concentration stimulates immediate release of free arachidonic acid from dispersed human decidual cells (Wilson, Liggins & Whittaker, 1988). The suggestion, therefore, is that oxytocin can enhance phospholipase activity.

The *in vitro* effect of oxytocin on phosphoinositide hydrolysis has been studied in gestational myometrium by measuring the production of inositol phosphates in tissue explants prelabelled with ^{3}H-inositol. A significant increase in all three inositol phosphates was elicited by oxytocin in myometrium and this was accompanied by increased arachidonic acid release and PGE_2 and $PGF_{2\alpha}$ production (Scherey *et al.*, 1988). The hydrolysis of phosphatidylinositol in their homogenates showed a precursor–product relationship for the production of diacylglycerol, monoacylglycerol, and arachidonic acid, indicative of a sequential action of PLC and diacylglycerol lipase. Thus oxytocin can use inositol lipid signalling to mobilize free arachidonic acid for prostaglandin production and to release intracellular calcium during excitation–contraction coupling.

The effect of prostaglandins on oxytocin and its receptors is less clear. There is a close relationship between enhanced oxytocin responsiveness of pregnant rat uteri and increased prostaglandin synthesis; suppression of PG synthesis attenuates the oxytocin responsiveness and markedly reduces oxytocin binding sites (Chan, 1987) with no change in binding affinity. The conclusion from another study was that the concerted effect of oxytocin and prostaglandins on myometrial contraction did not involve modulation of the oxytocin receptor by prostaglandins (Engstrom, Atke & Vilhardt, 1988). More recent reports have demonstrated that naproxen sodium can suppress both oxytocin receptor and gap junction formation, prolong gestation, double the duration of parturition by 24 hours or longer and increase fetal mortality in rats (Chan *et al.*, 1991; Chan & Chen, 1992). Treatment with an oxytocin antagonist did not have the same effect on myometrial oxytocin receptors and gap junction formation on days 21–23 of gestation, but does increase the duration of parturition and fetal mortality without prolonging gestation. Thus prostaglandins appear to be important in the regulation of oxytocin receptor and gap junction formation and play a critical role in the initiation of labour.

Prostaglandins and uterine activity – a possible role in modulation of potassium channels

Potassium (K^+) channels are the largest category of ion channels and are associated with dampening of cellular activity. Large conductance calcium-activated K$^+$-channels (BK$_{Ca}$) have been described in pregnant rat (Kihira *et al.*, 1990) and non-pregnant (Ashford, Khan & Smith, 1991) and pregnant (Khan *et al.*, 1992) human myometrium. They are similar to those of a variety of cell types including smooth muscle cells of gastrointestinal (Benham *et al.*, 1986; Singer & Walsh, 1987), tracheal (Green, Foster & Small, 1991) and vascular (Benham *et al.*, 1986; Williams *et al.*, 1988) origin.

Many functions have been assigned to smooth muscle BK$_{Ca}$ channels including membrane repolarization (Benham *et al.*, 1986; Singer & Walsh, 1987), contribution to slow wave activity (Singer & Walsh, 1987) and regulation of vascular tone through membrane potential (Brayden & Nelson, 1992). Several potassium channel openers have been shown to be uterine relaxants in the rat (Piper *et al.*, 1990). Potassium channel modulation is a widespread phenomenon in both nerve and muscle cells and produces marked changes in cellular electrical activity (Pfaffinger & Siegelbaum, 1990). G proteins (Van Dongen *et al.*, 1988) and cAMP (Levitan, 1988) may have some role in regulation of potassium channel function. IP$_3$, as described above, releases calcium from intracellular stores (Berridge & Irvine, 1984) and thus can lead to the opening of calcium-activated potassium channels (Trautmann & Marty, 1984). IP$_3$ has also been shown in neuronal tissue to influence potassium current through a Ca^{2+}-independent mechanism (Dutar & Nicoll, 1988). Protein kinases may exert some action on K$^+$-channel function (Ewald, Williams & Levitan, 1985). There is evidence suggesting that potassium channels may be a site of action for arachidonic acid and other fatty acids (Kim & Clapham, 1989; Ordway, Walsh & Singer, 1989). The lipoxygenase products of arachidonic acid may also be involved in modulation of potassium channel function (Belardetti *et al.*, 1988; Kurachi *et al.*, 1989).

An understanding of the electrophysiology of K$^+$-channels may provide some information concerning the onset of myometrial activity in labour. The conversion of the electrically silent pregnant uterus to being highly excitable at term represents a dramatic physiological event which is poorly understood. Whatever mechanisms regulate uterine muscle activity in labour, prostaglandins are intimately involved. Further experiments are necessary to clarify the complex network of interactions between prostaglandins, second messengers and potassium channels and their contribution to myometrial activity.

Prostaglandins and the initiation of labour

Three major theories have been considered by investigators concerning the initiation of labour. The first one is the so-called 'progesterone block hypothesis' of Csapo (Csapo, 1970). The second one, the oxytocin theory, was first introduced in 1906, when the uterotonic action was described by Sir Henry Dale (Dale, 1906). The third theory involves the concept that the fetus may regulate the initiation or course of parturition and was first mentioned over 100 years ago by Speigelberg (cited by Thorburn, 1979). Various combinations of these three theories have been invoked suggesting a role for many endogenous substances such as oestrogens, progesterone, cortisol, relaxin, oxytocin, adrenergic and cholinergic secretions, cyclic nucleotides and calcium ions. In most, if not all, theories of parturition currently being considered, prostaglandins play an integral part.

Conversion of arachidonic acid to prostaglandins increases rapidly after 100 days gestation, in sheep cotyledons (Rice, Wong & Thorburn, 1988) and similarly PGE_2 production by the chorioallantois and chorioamnion of the pig increases markedly after 90 days gestation up to term (around 115 days in the pig) (Rice et al., 1989). There is a similar pattern in the rabbit (Elliot et al., 1984). It is not clear what regulates the placental PGE_2 synthesis during the last third of gestation but the fetal pituitary hormones have been suggested, and particularly the gonadotrophins (Thorburn, 1991). It is proposed that in sheep the increased PGE_2 during the last third of gestation by the fetal trophoblast activates the fetal hypothalamic–pituitary–adrenal axis leading to an increase in fetal cortisol concentrations. High cortisol levels can increase placental 17α-hydroxylase activity leading to a decrease in maternal progesterone concentrations and an increase in maternal oestrogen concentrations. The increase in the oestrogen/progesterone ratio results in increased $PGF_{2\alpha}$ release from the placenta which can give rise to increased uterine activity and parturition (Thorburn, 1991).

A 48-hour period of food withdrawal from a ewe significantly increases fetal plasma PGE_2 concentrations (Fowden et al., 1987). This increase in PGE_2 is associated with a decrease in plasma glucose concentrations. From about day 130 onwards 2 days of food restriction can induce the ewe to go into premature labour (Fowden & Silver, 1983). Similarly, partial occlusion of the uterine arterial supply in sheep can give rise to reduced placental blood flow and hypoxaemia in the fetus, and to increased placental output of PGE_2 (Hooper et al., 1990). The PGE_2 concentrations remain elevated while uterine blood flow is restricted. Maternal hyperthermia can also increase secretion of PGE_2 (Andrianakis et al., 1989). The fetus may exert an influence on the timing of parturition in a manner necessary for well-being and survival. This influence may work via prostaglandins. From this stems the hypothesis that the growth pattern of the fetus represents a genetically programmed 'clock' which acts by stimulating placental PGE_2 production leading to maturation of key organ systems in the fetus and finally parturition (Thorburn, 1991).

Conclusions

In this chapter we have reviewed the synthesis and function of prostaglandins in relation to uterine activity. Since the 1960s, when interest in prostaglandins was primarily focused on reproduction, there is overwhelming evidence for their role in myometrial function and parturition. This is reflected in the many therapeutic applications of prostaglandins in obstetrics and gynaecology. They have many actions at the cellular and subcellular levels and their effects on nucleic acid replication and translation are as yet largely unknown. Prostaglandins and their metabolites provide a complex interaction of intracellular signalling systems closely linked with membrane receptors and ion channels. Inevitably there are more questions than answers. More knowledge of the control of prostaglandin production and catabolism at the molecular level, will help to explain the mechanisms of parturition.

References

Abdel-Latif, A. A. (1986) Calcium-mobilizing receptors, polyphosphoinositides, and the generation of second messengers. *Pharmacology Reviews*, **38**, 227–72.

Abel, M. H. & Kelly, R. W. (1979). Differential production of prostaglandins within the human uterus. *Prostaglandins*, **18**, 821–8.

Acarregui, M. I., Shyder, J. M., Mitchell, M. D. & Mendelson, C. R. (1990). Prostaglandins regulate surface protein A (SP-A) gene expression in human fetal lung *in vitro*. *Endocrinology*, **127**, 1105–11.

Aitken, M. A., Rice, G. E. & Brennecke, S. P. (1990). Gestational tissue phospholiopase A2 messenger RNA content and the onset of spontaneous labour in the human. *Reproduction and Fertility Developments*, **2**, 575–80.

Andrianakis, P., Walker, D. W., Ralph, M. M. & Thorburn, G. D. (1989). Effect of inhibiting prostaglandin synthesis in pregnant sheep with 4-amino antipyrine under normothermic and hyperthermic conditions. *American Journal of Obstetrics and Gynecology*, **161**, 241–7.

Arkinstall, S. J. & Jones, C. T. (1990). Pregnancy suppresses G protein coupling to phosphoinositide hydrolysis in guinea pig myometrium. *American Journal of Physiology*, **259**, E57–65.

Ashford, M. L. J., Khan, R. N. & Smith, S. K. (1991). Single channel recording of a K^+-selective channel in pregnant dispersed human myometrial cells. *Journal of Physiology (London)*, **438**, 104P.

Bala, G. A., Thakur, N. R. & Bleasdale, J. E. (1990). Characterization of the major phosphoinositide-specific phospholipase C of human amnion. *Biology of Reproduction*, **43**, 704–11.

Baraban, J. M., Gould, R. J., Peroutka, S. J. & Snyder, S. H. (1985). Phorbol ester effects on neurotransmission: interaction with neurotransmitters and calcium in smooth muscle. *Proceedings of the National Academy of Sciences, USA*, **82**, 604

Bauknecht, T. K., Krabe, B., Rechenbach, U., Zahradnik, H. P. & Breckwoldt, M. (1980). Distribution of prostaglandin E2 and prostaglandin F2α receptors in human myometrium. *Acta Endocrinologica*, **98**, 446–50.

Belardetti, F., Campbell, W., Flack, J. R., Demontis, G. & Rosolowsky, M. (1988). Products of heme-catalyzed transformation of the arachidonate derivative 12-HPETE open S-type $K+$ channels in aplysia. *Neuron*, **3**, 497–505.

Benham, C. D., Bolton, T. B., Lang, R. J. & Takewaki, T. (1986). Calcium-activated potassium channels in single smooth muscle cells of rabbit jejunum and guinea-pig mesenteric artery. *Journal of Physiology (London)*, **371**, 45–67.

Bennett, C. F., Balcarek, J. M., Varrichio, A. & Crooke, S. T. (1988). Molecular cloning and complete amino-acid sequence of form-I phosphoinositide-specific phospholipase C. *Nature*, **334**, 268–70.

Berridge, M. J. (1984). Inositol triphosphate and diacylglycerol as second messengers. *Biochemical Journal*, **54**, 205–35.

Berridge, M. J. & Irvine, R. F. (1984). Inositol triphosphate, a novel second messenger in cellular signal transduction. *Nature*, **312**, 315–21.

Bleasdale, J. E. & Johnston, J. M. (1984). Prostaglandins and human parturition: regulation of arachidonic acid mobilization. In *Reviews in Perinatal Medicine*. Ed. E. M. Scarpelli and D. V. Cosmi. Alan R. Liss, New York.

Brass, L. F. & Laposata, M. (1987). Diacylglycerol causes Ca release from the platelet dense tubular system: Comparisons with Ca release caused by inositol 1,4,5-triphosphate. *Biochemical and Biophysical Research Communications*, **142**, 7–14.

Brayden, J. E. & Nelson, M. T. (1992). Regulation of arterial tone by activation of calcium-dependent potassium channels. *Science*, **256**, 532–5.

Breuiller-Fouche, M., Doualla-Bell Kotto Maka, F., Geny, B. & Ferre, F. (1991). Alpha-1 adrenergic receptor: binding and phosphoinositide breakdown in human myometrium. *Journal of Pharmacological Experimental Therapy*, **258**, 82–7.

Calder, A. A. & Embrey, M. P. (1973). Prostaglandins and the unfavourable cervix. *Lancet*, **ii**, 1322–3.

Carsten, M. E. (1973). Prostaglandins and cellular calcium transport in the pregnant human uterus. *American Journal of Obstetrics and Gynecology*, **117**, 824–32.

Carsten, M. E. (1974a). Hormonal regulation of myometrial calcium transports. *Gynecology Investigations*, **5**, 269–75.

Carsten, M. E. (1974b). Prostaglandins and oxytocin: their effects on uterine smooth muscle. *Prostaglandins*, **5**, 33–40.

Carsten, M. E. & Miller, J. D. (1977). Effects of prostaglandin and oxytocin on calcium release from a uterine microsomal fraction. *Journal of Biological Chemistry*, **252**, 1576–81.

Carsten, M. E. & Miller, J. D. (1981). Prostaglandin E2 receptor in the myometrium: distribution in subcellular fractions. *Archives of Biochemistry and Biophysics*, **212**, 700.

Carsten, M. E. & Miller, J. D. (1985). Ca^{2+} release by inositol triphosphate from Ca^{2+}-transporting microsomes derived from uterine sarcoplasmic reticulum. *Biochemical and Biophysical Research Communications*, **130**, 1027–31.

Carsten, M. E. & Miller, J. D. (1987). A new look at uterine muscle contraction: current development. *American Journal of Obstetrics and Gynecology*, **157**, 1303–15.

Carsten, M. E. & Miller, J. D. (1990). Calcium control mechanisms in the myometrial cell and the role of the phosphoinositide cycle. In *Uterine Function Molecular and Cellular Aspects*. Ed. M. E. Carsten and J. D. Miller, Plenum Press, New York.

Chan, W. Y. (1983). Uterine and placental prostaglandins and their modulation of oxytocin sensitivity and contractility in the parturient uterus. *Biology of Reproduction*, **29**, 680–8.

Chan, W. Y. (1987). Enhanced prostaglandin synthesis in the parturient rat uterus and its effects on myometrial oxytocin receptor concentrations. *Prostaglandins*, **34**, 888–902.

Chan, W. Y., Berezin, I., Daniel, E. E., Russel, K. C. & Hruby, V. J. (1991). Effects of inactivation of oxytocin receptor and inhibition of prostaglandin synthesis on uterine oxytocin receptor and gap junction formation and labor in the rat. *Canadian Journal of Physiology and Pharmacology*, **69**, 1262–7.

Chan, W. Y. & Chen, D. L. (1992). Myometrial oxytocin receptors and prostaglandin in the parturition process of the rat. *Biology of Reproduction*, **46**, 58–64.

Christensen, N. J. & Green, K. (1983). Bioconversion of arachidonic acid in human pregnant reproductive tissues. *Biochemical Medicine*, **30**, 162–80.

Clark, M. A., Chen, M. J., Crooke, S. T. & Bomalaski, J. S. (1988). Tumour necrosis factor (catechin) induces phospholipase A2 activity and synthesis of a phospholipase A2-activating protein in endothelial cells. *Biochemical Journal*, **250**, 125–32.

Cockcroft, S. & Gomperts, B. D. (1985). Role of guanine nucleotide-binding in the activation of polyphosphoinositide phosphodiesterase. *Nature (London)*, **314**, 534–6.

Csapo, A. (1970). The diagnostic significance of the intrauterine pressure. *Obstetric and Gynecology Survey*, **25**, 403–35.

Dale, H. H. (1906). On some physiologic actions of ergot. *Journal of Physiology (London)*, **34**, 163–205.

Delfert, D. M., Hill, S., Pershadsingh, H. A., Sherman, W. R. & McDonald, J. M. (1986). myo-Inositol 1,4,5-triphosphate mobilizes Ca^{2+} from isolated adipocyte endoplasmic reticulum but not from plasma membranes. *Biochemical Journal*, **236**, 37–44.

Diamond, J. & Hartle, D. K. (1976). Cyclic nucleotide levels during carbachol-induced smooth muscle contractions. *Journal of Cyclic Nucleotide Phosphoprotein Research*, **2**, 179–83.

Diamond, J. (1983). Lack of correlation between cyclic GMP elevation and relaxation of nonvascular smooth muscle by nitroglycerin, nitroprusside, hydroxylamine and sodium azide. *Journal of Pharmacology Experimental Therapy*, **225**, 422–6.

Di Renzo, G. C., Venincasa, M. D. & Bleasdale, J. E. (1984a). The identification and characterization of α-adrenergic receptors in human amnion tissue. *American Journal of Obstetrics and Gynecology*, **148**, 398–405.

Di Renzo, G. C., Anceschi, M. M. & Bleasdale, J. E. (1984b). β-Adrenergic stimulation of prostaglandin production in human amnion. *Prostaglandins*, **27**, 37–49.

Dokhac, L., Mokhtari, A. & Harbon, S. (1986). A re-evaluated role for cyclic AMP in uterine relaxation. Differential effect of isoproterenol and forskolin. *Journal of Pharmacology Experimental Therapy*, **239**, 236–42.

Domnie, J., Poyser, N. I. & Wunderlich, M. (1974). Levels of prostaglandins in human endometrium during the menstrual cycle. *Journal of Physiology (London)*, **236**, 465–72.

Dubin, N. H., Ghodaonkar, R. B. & King, T. M. (1979). Role of prostaglandin production in spontaneous and oxytocin-induced uterine contractile activity in *in vitro* pregnant rat uteri. *Endocrinology*, **105**, 47–51.

Dutar, P. & Nicoll, R. A. (1988). Stimulation of phosphatidylinositol (PI) turnover may mediate the muscarinic suppression of the M-current in hippocampal pyramidal cells. *Neuroscience Letters*, **85**, 89–94.

Elliot, W. J., McLaughlin, L. L., Bloch, M. H. & Needleman, P. (1984). Arachidonic acid metabolism by rabbit fetal membranes of various gestational ages. *Prostaglandins*, **27**, 27–36.

Engstrom, T., Atke, A. & Vilhardt, H. (1988). Oxytocin receptors and contractile responses of the myometrium after long term infusion of prostaglandin $F_{2\alpha}$, indomethacin, oxytocin and an oxytocin antagonist in rats. *Regulatory Peptides*, **20**, 65–72.

Ewald, D. A., Williams, A. & Levitan, I. B. (1985). Modulation of single Ca^{2+}-dependent K^+-channel activity by protein phosphorylation. *Nature*, **315**, 503–6.

Fowden, A. L. & Silver, M. (1983). The effect of the nutritional state on uterine prostaglandin F metabolite concentrations in the pregnant ewe during late gestation. *Quarterly Journal of Experimental Physiology*, **68**, 337–49.

Fowden, A. L., Harding, R., Ralph, M. M. & Thorburn, G. D. (1987). The nutritional regulation of plasma prostaglandin E concentrations in the fetus and pregnant ewe during late gestation. *Journal of Physiology (London)*, **394**, 1–12.

Fulle, H.-J., Hoer, D., Lache, W., Rosenthal, W., Schultz, G. & Oberdisse, E. (1987). *In vitro* synthesis of 32p-labelled phosphatidylinositol 4,5-biphosphate and its hydrolysis by smooth muscle membrane-bound phospholipase C. *Biochemical and Biophysical Research Communications*, **145**, 673–9.

Fuse, I. & Tai, H. H. (1987). Stimulation of arachidonate release and inositol-1,4,5-triphosphate formation are mediated by distinct G-proteins in human platelets. *Biochemical and Biophysical Research Communications*, **146**, 659–65.

Fuse, I., Iwanga, T. & Tai, H. H. (1989). Phorbol ester, 1,2-diacylglycerol, and collagen induce inhibition of arachidonic acid incorporation into phospholipids in human platelets. *Journal of Biological Chemistry*, **264**, 3890–5.

Garrioch, D. B. (1978). The effect of indomethacin on spontaneous activity in the isolated human myometrium and on the response to oxytocin and prostaglandins. *British Journal of Obstetrics and Gynaecology*, **85**, 47–52.

Ghodgaonkar, R. B., Dubin, N. H , Blake, D. A. & King, T. M. (1979). 13,14-Dihydro-15-keto-prostaglandin F2α concentrations in human plasma and amniotic fluid. *American Journal of Obstetrics and Gynecology*, **134**, 265–9.

Giannopoulos, G., Jackson, K., Kredentser, J. & Tulchinsky, D. (1985). Prostaglandin E and F2α receptors in human myometrium during the menstrual cycle and in pregnancy and labour. *American Journal of Obstetrics and Gynecology*, **153**, 904–10.

Goldberg, N. D., Haddox, M. K., Hartle, D. K. & Hadden, J. W. (1973). The biological role of cyclic 3′,5′-guanosine monophosphate. Proceedings of the Fifth International Congress Pharmacology, Basel, Karger. **5**, 146–55.

Green, K., Bygdeman, M., Toppozada, M. & Wiqvist, N. (1974). The role of prostaglandin F2α in human parturition: endogenous plasma levels of 15-keto-13,14-dihydro-prostaglandin F2α. *American Journal of Obstetrics and Gynecology*, **120**, 25–31.

Green, K. A., Foster, R. W. & Small, R. C. (1991). A patch-clamp study of K⁺-channel activity in bovine isolated tracheal smooth muscle cells. *British Journal of Pharmacology*, **102**, 871–8.

Guillemette, G., Balla, T., Baukal, A. J., Spat, A. & Catt, K. J. (1987). Intracellular receptors for inositol 1,4,5-triphosphate in angiotensin II target tissues. *Journal of Biological Chemistry*, **262**, 1010–15.

Hamberg, M. (1974). Quantitative studies on prostaglandin synthesis in man. III. Excretion of the major metabolite of prostaglandin F1 and F2 during pregnancy. *Life Sciences*, **14**, 247–54.

Hensby, C. N., Seed, M. P., Williams, K. I. & Antipolis, S. (1986). Effects of oxytocic drugs on prostaglandin synthesis by human pregnant endometrium. *British Journal of Pharmacology [Suppl.]*, **86**, 806P.

Hoffman, G. E., Rao, C. H. V., Barrows, G. H. & Sanfilippo, J. S. (1983). Topography of human uterine prostaglandin E and F2α receptors and their profiles during pathological states. *Journal of Clinical Endocrinology Metabolism*, **57**, 360–6.

Hooper, S. B., Coulter, C. C., Deayton, J. M., Harding, R. & Thorburn, G. D. (1990). Fetal endocrine responses to prolonged hypoxemia in sheep. *American Journal of Physiology*, **259**, R703–8.

Horton, E. W. & Poyser, N. I. (1976). Uterine luteolytic hormone: a physiological role for prostaglandin F2α. *Physiology Review*, **56**, 595–651.

Karim, S. M. M. & Devlin, J. (1967). Prostaglandin content of amniotic fluid during pregnancy and labour. *Journal of Obstetrics and Gynaecology of the British Commonwealth*, **74**, 230–4.

Karim, S. M. M., Trussell, R. R., Patel, R. C. & Hillier, K. (1968). Response of pregnant human uterus to prostaglandin F2α-induction of labour. *British Medical Journal*, **4**, 621–3.

Karim, S. M. M. & Filshie, G. M. (1970). Therapeutic abortion using prostaglandin F2α. *Lancet*, **1**, 157–9.

Keirse, M. J. N. C. (1978). Biosynthesis and metabolism of prostaglandins in the pregnant human uterus. *Advances Prostaglandin Thromboxane Research*, **87**, 4–11.

Keirse, M. J. N. C. (1989). Treatment of postpartum uterine hypotonia with prostaglandins. *Eicosanoids Fatty Acids*, **7**, 25–30.

Keirse, M. J. N. C. (1990). Eicosanoids in human pregnancy and parturition. In *Eicosanoids in Reproduction*. Ed. M. D. Mitchell, CRC Press, Florida.

Keirse, M. J. N. C., Hicks, B. R., Mitchell, M. D. & Turnbull, A. C. (1977a). Increase of the prostaglandin precursor arachidonic acid, in amniotic fluid during spontaneous labour. *British Journal of Obstetrics and Gynaecology*, **84**, 937–40.

Keirse, M. J. N. C., Mitchell, M. D. & Turnbull, A. C. (1977b). Changes in prostaglandin F and 13,14-dihydro-15-keto-prostaglandin concentrations in amniotic fluid at the onset of and during labour. *British Journal of Obstetrics and Gynaecology*, **84**, 743.

Khan, R. N., Smith, S. K., Morrison, J. & Ashford, M. L. J. (1992). Single Ca^{2+}-activated K channels recorded from human cultured myometrial cells. *Journal of Physiology (London)*, **446**, 555P.

Kihira, M., Matsuzawa, K., Tokuno, H. & Tomita, T. (1990). Effects of calmudulin antagonists on calcium-activated potassium channels in pregnant rat myometrium. *British Journal of Pharmacology*, **100**, 353–9.

Kim, D. & Clapham, D. E. (1989). Potassium channels in cardiac cells activated by arachidonic acid and phospholipids. *Science*, **244**, 1174–6.

Kurachi, Y., Ito, H., Sugimoto, T., Shimuzu, T., Miki, I. & Ui, M. (1989). Arachidonic acid metabolites as intracellular modulators of the G protein-gated cardiac K^{+} channel. *Nature*, **337**, 555–7.

Lanman, J. T., Herod, L. & Thau, R. (1972). Premature induction of labour with dilinoleyl lecithin in rabbits. *Pediatric Research*, **6**, 701–4.

Lanman, J. T., Herod, L. & Thau, R. (1974). Phospholipids and fatty acids in relation to the premature induction of labour in rabbits. *Pediatric Research*, **8**, 1–4.

Levitan, I. B. (1988). Modulation of ion channels in neurons and other cells. *Annual Review of Neuroscience*, **11**, 119–36.

Litime, M. H., Pointis, G., Brueiller-Fouche, M., Cabrol, D. & Ferre, F. (1989). Disappearance of beta-adrenergic response of human myometrial adenylate cyclase at the end of pregnancy. *Journal of Clinical Endocrinology Metabolism*, **69**, 1–6.

Lumsden, M. A., Brown, A. & Baird, D. T. (1984). Prostaglandin production from homogenates of separated glandular epithelium and stroma from human endometrium.

Prostaglandins, **28**, 485–96.

Luukkainen, T. U. & Csapo, A. I. (1963). Induction of premature labour in the rabbit after pretreatment with phospholipids. *Fertility and Sterility*, **14**, 65–71.

Mahon, W. A., Reid, D. W. J. & Day, R. A. (1967). The *in vivo* effects of beta-adrenergic stimulation and blockage on the human uterus at term. *Journal of Pharmacology Experimental Therapy*, **156**, 178–80.

Markiewicz, L. & Gurpide, E. (1988). C-19 adrenal steroids enhance prostaglandin F2α output by human endometrium *in vitro*. *American Journal of Obstetrics and Gynecology*, **159**, 500–4.

Mitchell, M. D. (1986). Pathway of arachidonic acid metabilism with specific application to the fetus and mother. *Seminars in Perinatology*, **10**, 242–54.

Moonen, P., Klok, G. & Keirse, M. J. N. C. (1984). Increase in concentrations of prostaglandin endoperoxide synthase and prostacyclin synthase in human myometrium in late pregnancy. *Prostaglandins*, **28**, 309–21.

Moonen, O., Klok, G. & Keirse, M. J. N. C. (1985). Immunohistochemical localization of prostaglandin endoperoxide synthase and prostacyclin synthase in pregnant human myometrium. *European Journal of Obstetrics, Gynecology and Reproductive Biology*, **19**, 151–8.

Moonen, P., Klok, G. & Keirse, M. J. N. C. (1986). Distribution of prostaglandin endoperoxide synthase and prostacyclin synthase in the late pregnant uterus. *British Journal of Obstetrics and Gynaecology*, **93**, 255–9.

Nakla, S., Skinner, K., Mitchell, B. F. & Challis, J. R. G. (1986). Changes in prostaglandin transfer across human fetal membranes obtained after spontaneous labour. *American Journal of Obstetrics and Gynecology*, **155**, 1337–41.

Nathanielsz, P. W., Abel, M. & Smith, G. W. (1973). Hormonal factors in parturition in the rabbit. In *Foetal and Neonatal Physiology*. Ed. K. S. Comline, K. W. Cross, G. S. Dawes *et al.* Cambridge University Press, Cambridge.

Ogawa, Y., Herod, L. & Thau, R. (1970). Phospholipids and the onset of labour in rabbits. *Gynecological Investigations*, I, 240–6.

Okazaki, T., Okita, J. R., MacDonald, P. C. & Johnston, J. M. (1978). Initiation of human parturition. X. Substrate specificity of phospholipase A2 in human fetal membranes. *American Journal of Obstetrics and Gynecology*, **130**, 432–8.

Okazaki, T., Sagawa, N., Bleasdale, J. E., Okita, J. R., MacDonald, P. C. & Johnston, J. M. (1981*a*). Initiation of human parturition. XIII. Phospholipase C, phospholipase A2 and diacylglycerol lipase activities in fetal and decidua vera tissues from early and late gestation. *Biology of Reproduction*, **25**, 103–9.

Okazaki, T., Casey, M. L., Okita, J. R., MacDonald, P. C. & Johnston, J. M. (1981*b*). Initiation of human parturition. XII. Biosynthesis and metabolism of prostaglandins in human fetal membranes and uterine decidua. *American Journal of Obstetrics and Gynecology*, **139**, 373–81.

Okazaki, T., Ban, C. & Johnston, J. M. (1984). The identification and characterization of protein kinase C activity in fetal membranes. *Archives of Biochemistry and Biophysics*, **229**, 27–32.

Okita, J. R., MacDonald, P. C., Johnston, J. M. (1982*a*). Mobilization of arachidonic acid from specific glycerophospholipids of human fetal membranes during early labour. *Journal of Biological Chemistry*, **257**, 14029–34.

Okita, J. R., MacDonald, P. C. & Johnston, J. M. (1982*b*). Initiation of human paturition.

XIV. Increase in the diacylglycerol content of amnion during parturition. *American Journal of Obstetrics and Gynecology*, **142**, 432–5.

Ordway, R. W., Walsh, J. V. Jr & Singer, J. J. (1989). Arachidonic acid and other fatty acids directly activate potassium channels in smooth muscle cells. *Science*, **244**, 1176–9.

Pfaffinger, P. J. & Siegelbaum, S. A. (1990). K^+ channel modulation by G proteins and second messengers. In *Channels: Structure, Function, Classification and Therapeutic Potential*. Ed. N. S. Cook. Ellis Horwood Press, Hemel Hempstead.

Pickles, V. R., Hall, W. J., Best, F. A. & Smith, G. N. (1965). Prostaglandins in endometrium and menstrual fluid from normal and dysmenorrhoeic subjects. *Journal of Obstetrics and Gynaecology of the British Commonwealth*, **72**, 185–92.

Piper, I., Minshall, E., Downing, S. J., Hollingsworth, M. & Sadrei, H. (1990). Effects of several potassium channel openers and glibenclamide on the uterus of the rat. *British Journal of Pharmacology*, **101**, 901–7.

Rhee, S. G., Suh, P. G., Ryu, S. H. & Lee, S. Y. (1989). Studies of phospholipid-specific phospholipase C. *Science*, **244**, 546–50.

Rice, G. E., Wong, M. H. & Thorburn, G. D. (1988). Gestational changes in prostaglandin synthase activity of ovine cotyledonary microsomes. *Journal of Endocrinology*, **118**, 265–70.

Rice, G. E., Christensen, P., Dantzer, V. & Skadhauge, E. (1989). Gestational profile of prostaglandin E2 synthesis by porcine placenta and fetal membranes. *Eicosanoids*, **2**, 235–40.

Roseblade, C. K., Sullivan, M. H. F., Khan, H., Lumb, M. R. & Elder, M. G. (1990). Limited transfer of prostaglandin E2 across the fetal membrane before and after labour. *Acta Obstetrica Gynecologica Scandinavica*, **69**, 399–403.

Ruzycky, A. L. & Crankshaw, D. J. (1988). Role of inositol phospholipid hydrolysis in the initiation of agonist-induced contractions of rat uterus: effects of domination of 17-β-estradiol and progesterone. *Canadian Journal of Physiology and Pharmacology*, **66**, 10–17.

Sagawa, N., Bleasdale, J. E. & Di Renzo, G. C. (1983). The effects of polyamines and amino glycosides on phosphatidylinositol-specific phospholipase C from human amnion. *Biochimica et Biophysica Acta*, **752**, 153–61.

Saida, K. & van Breemen, C. (1987). GTP requirement for inositol 1,4,5-triphosphate-induced Ca^{2+} release from sarcoplasmic reticulum in smooth muscle. *Biochemical and Biophysical Research Communications*, **144**, 1313–16.

Satoh, K., Yasumizu, T., Fukuoka, H. *et al.* (1979). Prostaglandin F2α metabolite levels in plasma, amniotic fluid, and urine during pregnancy and labour. *American Journal of Obstetrics and Gynecology*, **133**, 886–90.

Schartz, F., Markiewicz, L. & Gurpide, E. (1987). Differential effects of estradiol, arachidonic acid and A-23187 on prostaglandin F2α output by epithelial and stromal cells of human endometrium. *Endocrinology*, **120**, 1465–71.

Scherey, M. P., Read, A. M. & Steer, P. J. (1987). Stimulation of phospholipid hydrolysis and arachidonic acid mobilization in human decidua cells by phorbol ester. *Biochemical Journal*, **246**, 705–13.

Scherey, M. P., Cornford, P. A., Read, A. M. & Steer, P. J. (1988). A role for phosphoinositide hydrolysis in human uterine smooth muscle parturition. *American Journal of Obstetrics and Gynecology*, **159**, 964–70.

Schieman, W. P. & Buxton, I. L. O. (1991). Adenosine A1-receptor coupling to phosphoinositide metabolism in pregnant guinea pig myometrium. *American Journal of*

Physiology, **261**, E665–72.

Schultz, M. F., Schwarz, B. E., MacDonald, P. C. & Johnston, J. M. (1975). Initiation of human parturition. II. Identification of phospholipase A2 in fetal chorioamnion and uterine decidua. *American Journal of Obstetrics and Gynecology*, **123**, 650–3.

Schwarz, B. E., Schultz, E. M., MacDonald, P. C. & Johnston, J. M. (1975). Initiation of human parturition. III. Fetal membrane content of prostaglandin E2 and F2α precursor. *Obstetrics and Gynecology*, **46**, 564–8.

nger, J. J. & Walsh, J. V. (1987). Characterization of calcium-activated potassium channels in single smooth muscle cells using the patch-clamp technique. *Pfügers Archives*, **408**, 98–111.

mith, J. B., Smith, L. & Higgins, B. L. (1985). Temperature and nucleotide dependance of calcium release by myo-inositol 1,4,5-triphosphate in cultured vascular smooth muscle cells. *Journal of Biological Chemistry*, **260**, 14413–16.

mith, S. K., Abel, M. H., Kelly, R. W. & Baird, D. T. (1981a). Prostaglandin synthesis in the endometrium of women with ovular dysfunctional uterine bleeding. *British Journal of Obstetrics and Gynaecology*, **88**, 434–42.

Smith, S. K., Abel, M. H., Kelly, R. W. & Baird, D. T. (1981b). A role for prostacyclin (PG12) in excessive menstrual bleeding. *Lancet*, **i**, 552–4.

Storey, D. J., Shears, S. B., Kirk, C. J. & Mitchell, R. H. (1984). Stepwise enzymatic dephosphorylation of inositol 1,4,5-triphosphate to inositol in liver. *Nature*, **312**, 374–6.

Tagaki, S., Yoshida, T., Togo, Y. *et al.* (1976). The effects of intramyometrial injection of prostaglandin F2a on severe postpartum haemorrhage. *Prostaglandins*, **12**, 565–79.

Takuwa, Y., Takuwa, N. & Rasmussen, H. (1986). Carbachol induces a rapid and sustained hydrolysis of phosphoinositide in bovine tracheal smooth muscle measurements of the mass of polyphosphoinositides, 1,2-diacylglycerol, and phosphatidic acid. *Journal of Biological Chemistry*, **261**, 14670–5.

Tanfin, Z. & Harbon, S. (1987). Heterologous regulations of cAMP responses in pregnant rat myometrium. Evolution from a stimulatory to an inhibitory prostaglandin E2 and prostacyclin effect. *Molecular Pharmacology*, **32**, 249–57.

Thorburn, G. D. (1979). Physiology and control of parturition. Reflection on the past ideas for the future. *Animal Reproduction*, **2**, 1–27.

Thorburn, G. D. (1991). The placenta, prostaglandins and parturition: A review. *Reproduction and Fertility Developments*, **3**, 277–94.

Trautmann, A. & Marty, A. (1984). Activation of Ca-dependent K$^+$ channels by carbamoylcholine in rat lacrimal glands. *Proceedings of the National Academy of Sciences USA*, **81**, 611–15.

Van Dongen, A. M. J., Codina, J., Olate, J. *et al.*, (1988). Newly identified brain potassium channels gated by the guanine nucleotide binding protein G_0. *Science*, **242**, 1433–7.

Vane, J. R. & Williams, K. I. (1973). The contribution of prostaglandin production to contractions of the isolated uterus of the rat. *British Journal of Pharmacology*, **48**, 629–39.

Vesin, M. F. & Harbon, S. (1974). The effects of epinephrine, prostaglandins, and their antagonists on adenosine cyclic 3′,5′ monophosphate concentrations and motility of the rat uterus. *Molecular Pharmacology*, **10**, 457–73.

Villar, A., D'Ocon, D. & Anselmi, E. (1985). Calcium requirement of uterine contraction induced by PGE1: Importance of intracellular calcium stores. *Prostaglandins*, **30**, 491–6.

Von Euler, U. S. (1934). Zur Kenntnis derpharmakologischen Wirkungen von nativsekreten and extrakten mannlicher accessorischer Geschlechtsdrusen. *Archive in Experimental*

Pharmakologie, **175**, 78–84.

Von Euler, U. S. (1936). On the specific vasodilating and plain muscle stimulating substances from accessory genital glands in man and certain animals (prostaglandin and vesiglandin). *Journal of Physiology (London)*, **88**, 213–34.

Welsh, C., Dubyak, G. & Douglas, J. G. (1988). Relationship between phospholipase C activation and prostaglandin E2 and cyclic adenosine monophosphate production in rabbit tubular epithelial cells. Effects of angiotensin, bradykinin and arginine vasopressin. *Journal of Clinical Investigations*, **81**, 710–19.

Wijkander, J. & Sundler, R. (1989). A role for protein kinase C mediated phosphorylation in the mobilization of arachidonic acid in mouse macrophages. *Biochimica et Biophysica Acta*, **1010**, 78–87.

Williams, D. L., Katz, G. M., Roy-Contacin, L. & Reuben, J. P. (1988). Guanosine-5′-monophosphate modulates gating of high conductance Ca^{2+}-activated K^{+}-channels in vascular smooth muscle cells. *Proceedings of the National Academy of Sciences USA*, **83**, 7119–23.

Wilson, T. (1990). Phospholipases in human parturition. *Reproduction and Fertility Developments*, **2**, 511–21.

Wilson, T., Liggins, C. C. & Whittaker, D. J. (1988). Oxytocin stimulates the release of arachidonic acid and prostaglandins $F_{2\alpha}$ from human decidual cells. *Prostaglandins*, **35**, 8771–80.

Yang, J. C., Triner, L., Vulliemoz, Y., Verosky, M. & Ngai, S. H. (1973). Effects of halothane on the cyclic 3′,5′-adenosine monophosphate (cyclic AMP) system in rat uterine muscle. *Anesthesiology*, **38**, 244–50.

Zakar, T. & Olson, D. M. (1989). Stimulation of human amnion prostaglandin E2 production by activators of protein kinase C. *Journal of Clinical Endocrinology Metabolism*, **67**, 915–23.

Zuckerman, H., Reis, U. & Rubinstein, I. (1974). Inhibition of human premature labour by indomethacin. *Obstetrics and Gynecology*, **44**, 787–92.

11

Relaxin

G. D. BRYANT-GREENWOOD

Introduction

It is more than six decades since relaxin was first shown to cause a modification of the pubic symphysis necessary for the successful birth of live young (Hisaw, 1926). Additional biological actions of relaxin in pregnancy – the inhibition of myometrial contraction and the promotion of cervical softening – were described later (Krantz, Bryant & Carr, 1950; Graham & Dracy, 1952). One or more sites in the female reproductive tract are the primary sources of relaxin during pregnancy. Although the major site of systemic relaxin production during pregnancy varies between species, this fails to follow any logical pattern according to the dependency of the species upon the ovary for pregnancy maintenance. The male reproductive tract is also capable of local relaxin production, but relaxin does not appear in the systemic circulation.

Historically, research on relaxin has been driven by the pharmaceutical industry, despite the fact that no clear endocrinopathy is related to increased or decreased relaxin production. The attempts in the 1950s to use impure preparations of pig relaxin to stop premature labour in women, gave the hormone a suspect reputation from which it is only now recovering. Indeed, it was audacious in 1980 to use pig relaxin, albeit highly purified and topically applied, to dilate the cervices of women in late pregnancy (MacLennan *et al.*, 1980). These and subsequent pioneering clinical trials (Evans *et al.*, 1983; MacLennan *et al.*, 1986a) caused a resurgence of interest. The successful elucidation of the gene sequences for the two human relaxins H1 and H2 (Hudson *et al.*, 1983, 1984) then allowed the development of recombinant H2 relaxin which is now in clinical trial. Even with the homologous hormone available, the elucidation of its role(s) in human pregnancy and parturition, as well as the study of its autocrine/paracrine actions at these and other stages of the reproductive cycle in both men and women, are still largely unexplored (Bryant-Greenwood, 1991a). The roles of systemic relaxins and those produced for local action have also be to investigated. A novel interaction was recently proposed for relaxins in the guinea-pig, between the uterine (systemic) source and the mammary gland (paracrine) source (Bryant-Greenwood *et al.*, 1991).

Until relatively recently the uterus was considered to be merely a target tissue for systemic ovarian relaxin. We are now beginning to appreciate that it is much more than this, and it is therefore necessary to discuss briefly in this chapter several other reproductive tissues and their relationship with the uterus. Because work on human relaxins is still in its infancy, the many gaps in our knowledge will be identified to indicate directions for future work.

The sources of human relaxins in women

The pig corpus luteum produces and stores large amounts of relaxin. This allowed development of methods for the isolation of purified relaxin (Sherwood & O'Byrne, 1974), followed rapidly by the description of its primary amino acid sequence and its classification as a member of the insulin family (Bryant-Greenwood, 1982; Sherwood, 1988). However, the rich source and high plasma levels prepartum in this species overshadowed the importance of the lower concentrations found in other tissues and species. It is now apparent that the porcine corpus luteum is an exception and that the corpora lutea of most other species produce considerably less relaxin during pregnancy. The pig studies also contributed to the dogma that in any one species there is a single major tissue source of systemic or circulating relaxin. The necessity to explore tissues other than the corpus luteum is strongly emphasized in the human.

The multiple sites of relaxin production in the human are listed in Table 1, together with the likely mode of delivery to their putative target tissues. Methods for the detection of relaxin mRNAs and peptides in human tissues have become increasingly sensitive and it is likely that other tissues will be added to this list. It has also become apparent that most of the sites of production in the pregnant state are also sites of production during the menstrual cycle (Table 1).

The ovary

The human corpus luteum of pregnancy, like that of the sow, was shown to be a site of relaxin storage and secretion, using a porcine relaxin RIA (Weiss, O'Byrne & Steinetz, 1976). Samples from the ovarian vein draining the corpus luteum contained a four-fold higher concentration of relaxin than plasma from the contralateral ovary or in peripheral venous samples. Extracts of human corpora lutea obtained at term were shown to have biological activity, but the levels in

Table 1. *Sources and putative target tissues of human relaxins in the cyclic and pregnant female*

Tissue	Delivery	Putative target
Ovary: follicle (theca) corpus luteum	Autocrine/paracrine Endocrine	Intra-ovarian Myometrium, cervix, mammary gland
Endometrium/decidua	Autocrine/paracrine	Endometrium/decidua, amnion, chorion, cervix, myometrium
Placenta	Autocrine/paracrine	Decidua, amnion, chorion, cervix, myometrium
Breast	Autocrine/paracrine Exocrine	Breast, neonate

this tissue during the cycle were too low to be detected with the porcine relaxin RIA (O'Byrne *et al.*, 1978). Similarly, immunocytochemical detection with antisera to porcine relaxin was successful only in the corpus luteum of pregnancy (Mathieu, Rahier & Thomas, 1981). With more sensitive techniques, immunolocalization has been achieved at both the light and electron microscope levels and the results verified with an antibody to human relaxin (Stoelk *et al.*, 1991). The homologous human reagents allowed the development of an ELISA system of sufficient sensitivity to detect relaxin in the systemic circulation of luteal phase women (Stewart *et al.*, 1990). Relaxin production by the cyclic corpus luteum was shown unequivocally when mRNA for the hormone was detected in this tissue (Ivell *et al.*, 1989; Hansell, Bryant-Greenwood & Greenwood, 1991).

In the pig the preovulatory follicle is capable of relaxin production, as shown by RIA, immunocytochemistry, Northern analysis and *in situ* hybridization histochemistry. These data were extrapolated to the human where it was first detected by RIA and immunolocalization and shown in both the tissue and fluid of stimulated human follicles (Wathes *et al.*, 1986; Yki-Jarvinen *et al.*, 1984). Recent studies with a monoclonal antibody to human relaxin show that, as in the pig, it is localized to the theca interna cells (Lee *et al.*, unpublished observations).

The development of the first homologous human relaxin RIA clearly showed the absence of the prepartum ovarian relaxin surge which had been identified in other species (Bell *et al.*, 1987). Since the endocrine events occurring in women at this time differ greatly from those in most other mammals it is not surprising that the significance of relaxins within the uterus should be considerably different in the human.

Intra-uterine tissue sources

An extra-ovarian relaxin source is essential for isolation and characterization, since human ovaries are not generally available. In the 1960s the decidua basalis was identified as a possible site of relaxin production, but this was not generally accepted because a less than homogeneous porcine relaxin preparation was used to generate the antiserum used for immunolocalization (Dallenbach & Dallenbach-Hellweg, 1964). Bigazzi was one of the first to recognize the human decidua as an endocrine tissue and to suggest that relaxin was one of its products (Bigazzi *et al.*, 1980). Two other laboratories were working concurrently on the placenta and decidua as sources of human relaxin (Fields & Larkin, 1981; Yamamoto *et al.*, 1981). There were major difficulties in applying the procedure developed for pig and rat tissue to the low levels present in human tissues. Some believed that there were extraluteal human relaxin sources, others were more sceptical (Sherwood, 1988). We used a number of porcine relaxin antisera to immunolocalize relaxin in the human parietal decidua, decidua basalis and the chorionic cytotrophoblast of the chorion laeve (Koay *et al.*, 1985). The syncytiotrophoblast of the placenta showed variable staining, a finding confirmed by others using antibodies to human relaxin (Sakbun *et al.*, 1990). However, immunocytochemistry cannot distinguish between hormone produced and that sequestered from another source. In an attempt to make this distinction, we raised an antibody to a synthetic segment of the connecting peptide of human relaxin and used this for immuno-localizations (Sakbun, Koay & Bryant-Greenwood, 1987). This antibody was able to recognize intracellular preprorelaxin, prorelaxin and/or its connecting peptide and could therefore identify cells producing the hormone. That human relaxin was indeed a product of these tissues was further verified by the isolation and detection of mRNA by Northern analysis using a 48 mer oligoprobe (Sakbun *et al.*, 1990). This study showed that the decidua parietalis was the primary intrauterine relaxin source, but that the placental basal plate (decidua basalis), chorionic cytotrophoblast of the chroion laeve and the placental trophoblast were additional sources. The relaxin mRNA derived from the placenta was slightly smaller in size than that derived from the decidua, whilst the placental basal plate containing both fetal and maternal cells showed both sizes of mRNA. When the poly (A) + tails of mRNAs from decidua and placenta were enzymatically removed, the size differences remained, suggesting that the truncation of placental relaxin mRNA is probably located in the 5′ or 3′ untranslated regions. It would not be surprising if there were different transcription initiation sites or different polyadenylation sites for the decidual and placental relaxins. Their complete nucleotide sequences have not been reported, but preliminary data in our laboratory suggest that their transcribed sequences are identical.

A collaborative study with Dr E. M. Rutanen was undertaken to identify the

cells involved in relaxin synthesis throughout the menstrual cycle and to follow
these into pregnancy. This study used antibodies to human relaxin provided by
Genentech Inc. Relaxin predominates in the epithelial cells lining the glands and
the uterine lumen in the proliferative phase of the cycle. The intensity of this
stain increased through the secretory phase and into pregnancy. The stromal
cells of the proliferative phase endometrium stained weakly for relaxin but this
intensified by the late secretory phase and early pregnancy when it was strongest
in the decidual cells of the zona compacta region. The cyclic endometrium also
appear to be a source of relaxin mRNA. The relative contributions of the
endometrium and ovaries to the plasma relaxin levels in the menstrual cycle is
not known. However, women without ovaries, enrolled in an IVF programme
and who became pregnant, do not have detectable relaxin in their sera (Emmi
et al., 1991). This suggests that circulating relaxin in pregnancy originates mainly
from the corpus luteum; endometrial relaxin is produced, acts and is inactivated
locally.

The production of relaxin by the placental trophoblast was first suggested by
immunolocalization (Fields & Larkin, 1981). However, results were inconsistent
(Koay *et al.*, 1985; Sakbun *et al.*, 1990), a problem which appears to be confined
to the placenta. The mRNA levels in this tissue are much less variable, suggesting
that the difficulty is in the detection of the protein.

The breast

Immunocytochemical localization demonstrates relaxin in normal, cystic and
neoplastic breast tissue (Mazoujian & Bryant-Greenwood, 1990). Evidence for
the expression of the relaxin genes in these tissues has recently been obtained in
this laboratory (Tashima *et al.*, unpublished observations). It is possible that
relaxin has an autocrine/paracrine function and that it may have a role in the
neonate via its transfer in the milk (Eddie *et al.*, 1989). On the other hand, a
systemic role cannot be excluded since circulating relaxin is detectable in lactating
women, although the levels are lower than those of milk.

Human relaxins: genes and peptides

Genes

The coding regions of a human preprorelaxin gene was first determined using a
genomic clone probed with a cDNA to porcine relaxin (Hudson *et al.*, 1983).
This sequence was thought to be the only human relaxin gene and was
subsequently called H1 relaxin. The structure included an intron in a position

Table 2. *The percentage homologies between the H1 and H2 relaxins at the nucleotide and derived amino acid levels for each of the peptide regions, A and B chains and the C-peptide*

Peptide region	Nucleotides %	Amino acids %
Signal peptide	94.7	84.0
B-chain	94.8	87.5
C-peptide	91.3	84.6
A-chain	77.8	62.5
Overall homology	90.6	82.2

similar to one of the introns in the human insulin gene and provided evidence that the two hormones arose by gene duplication from a common ancestor. A cDNA library made to RNA isolated from a human corpus luteum of pregnancy was subsequently probed with cDNAs corresponding to exon I and exon II of the human relaxin H1 gene and a second human relaxin gene was identified with a different sequence; this was called human relaxin H2 (Hudson *et al.*, 1984). The homologies between the H1 and H2 relaxins at the nucleotide and derived amino acid levels are summarized for each of the peptide regions in Table 2. The greatest homology lies in the B chain with 94.8% and 87.5% respectively. This suggests that the H1 and H2 relaxins may have similar or overlapping biological activities since replacement of the two arginine residues in the mid B chain (B13 and B17) by an uncharged isosteric amino acid caused loss of biological activity in the H2 relaxin (Schwabe & Bullesbach, 1990). The similarities between the H1 and H2 relaxins are sufficient to suggest that these genes arose by duplication subsequent to the separation from the insulin gene. However, the differences in the primary amino acid sequences of the processed hormones (Fig. 1) may be sufficient for them to have differences in their receptor binding properties. Such differences have not yet been studied, since the genetically engineered H1 peptide is not currently available. The relatively small amounts needed could be met by chemical synthesis (Bullesbach & Schwabe, 1991).

The occurrence of two genes for relaxins may be restricted to the human. Early work on the H2 relaxin gene showed that it is transcribed and translated in the human corpus luteum (Hudson *et al.*, 1984). Northern analysis of mRNA identified two relaxin mRNA species, 2 kb and 1 kb, with the 1 kb message dominating in pregnancy, whereas there was more of the larger 2 kb in the late luteal phase.

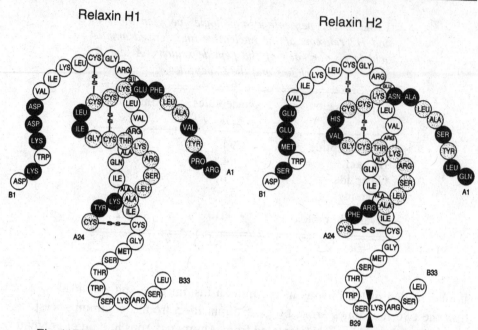

Fig. 1. The covalent structures of the processed hormones, human relaxin H1 (A24, B33) and human relaxin H2 (A24, B29/33) predicted from the nucleotide sequences of the two human relaxin genes. The amino acids shown in black are different in the two hormones, and the amino acids of the A chain are shown shaded for clarity. (Adapted from Kemp & Niall, Vit & Horm, 1984, **41**, 79–115.)

The development of the polymerase chain reaction (PCR) technique allowed the detection of the expression of the H1 relaxin gene in intra-uterine tissues. This, coupled with the specificity of the restriction enzymes (Hpa1 will only cut H2 relaxin and Hpa2 will only cut H1 relaxin), allowed our laboratory to show that the H1 relaxin gene was not a pseudogene. We confirmed that the corpus luteum expresses only the H2 relaxin gene while both H1 and H2 relaxin genes are expressed in the decidua and placenta (Hansell *et al.*, 1991). However, current antibodies cannot distinguish these two gene products. The presence of either or both of the translated peptides in these tissues has not yet been unequivocally demonstrated.

Peptides

Relaxin is a member of the insulin and insulin-like growth factor family of hormones, based on structure rather than function, since there is little sequence homology other than the conserved cysteine residues which form identical inter- and intra-chain disulphide bridges (Stults *et al.*, 1990). The human prohormone has an amino-terminal signal sequence which allows secretion of the peptide and a relatively long (104 amino acids) connecting peptide which is thought to play a role in its folding. However, correct folding can be achieved with a much smaller connecting peptide, which raises the question of whether there is a second biologically active peptide present within this sequence. The prohormone is processed, by enzymes as yet unidentified, to form a 6000 dalton peptide consisting of two peptide chains, the smaller A chain (24 amino acids) and the longer B chain (33 amino acids) with two interchain disulphide bridges and one intrachain disulphide bridge in the A chain, shown in Fig. 1.

The interest in the clinical use of human relaxin for the dilatation of the cervix stimulated the production of chemically synthesized H2 relaxin, made available by Genentech Inc. Recently they have succeeded in producing recombinant H2 relaxin using novel technologies for the production of the two chains and subsequent chemical recombination. This hormone is available to investigators willing to abide by approved research protocols. Much is now known of the physico-chemical and biological properties of recombinant H2 relaxin. The precise assignment of the disulphide linkages has been established for the recombinant peptide and compared with those of the native H2 relaxin isolated from the human corpus luteum (Canova-Davis, Baldonado & Teshima, 1990). The biological activity of the full-length hormone A24 B33 as well as its shorter analogue A24 B29 (Fig. 1) were shown to be equipotent in the mouse interpubic ligament bioassay, and to be of potency equal to native porcine relaxin (Johnston *et al.*, 1985). Most recently, the chemically synthesized and recombinant H2 relaxins have been shown to be equipotent, and of comparable bioactivity to native human relaxin isolated from human corpora lutea in an assay which measures the secretion of cAMP from human uterine endometrial cells *in vitro* (Canova-Davis *et al.*, 1991). However, the full amino acid sequence analysis of native H2 relaxin is still not known because of the very small quantities which can be isolated from any tissue source. This task has been made especially difficult because of the blocked pyroglutamic acid at the terminus of the A chain. The native hormone has, however, been shown to be 4 residues shorter in the B-chain, indicated in Fig. 1. This has no effect on its biological activity and the recombinant form is of this size. What may be more significant is that in solution the H2 hormone self-associates to form dimers (Shire, Holladay & Rinderknecht, 1991). This is a reversible change but upon dissociation there may be a significant change in the tyrosine environment but this is not accompanied by any significant changes in secondary structure. Preliminary studies using crystallized H2 relaxin for X-ray diffraction have confirmed this dimerization. This appears to be unique to the human structure and has important implications for those investigators assessing the biological activities of this peptide *in vivo* or *in vitro*.

Table 3. *The effect of pig relaxin and H2 recombinant human relaxin on pig and human myometrial quiescence* in vitro

	Pig myometrium	Human myometrium
Pig relaxin	+ +	—
Recombinant (H2) human relaxin	+ +	Equivocal

A novel chemical synthesis of H2 relaxin has also been reported by Bullesbach & Schwabe (1991) who combined solid-phase peptide synthesis with a novel thiol-protecting group strategy which allows perfect alignment of the disulphide bonds. Synthesis of H1 relaxin is also theoretically possible; authentic samples of H1 relaxin are needed in order to compare the physico-chemical properties and biological activities of H1 relaxin with the H2 peptide.

The biological actions of human relaxins

Relaxin has two major but surprisingly disparate biological actions which have formed the basis of the classical biological assays: rapid inhibition of myometrial activity, and a slow effect on connective tissue remodelling in the reproductive tract. We have suggested that these allow relaxin a key role in the synchronization of events at parturition. Other biological functions such as an effect upon uterine glycogen accumulation have been shown in animals.

The myometrium

Porcine relaxin acts on the myometrium of its homologous species as well as that of rodents, both *in vivo* and *in vitro*. However, the porcine hormone appears to have little or no effect on human myometrial contractility when the muscle is taken from either non-pregnant or pregnant women (MacLennan *et al.*, 1986*b*) (Table 3). Recombinant H2 relaxin was able to inhibit completely the contractions of pig uterine muscle *in vitro*, whereas it had a marginal effect on the human myometrium, even when added at 10-fold the concentration needed to show its activity in the pig model. When the human myometrial sample had been exposed *in vivo* to oestrogen, human relaxin *in vitro* attenuated its spontaneous contractility (MacLennan & Grant, 1991). However, there was no synergistic effect of treatment of the muscle strip with progesterone prior to its treatment with relaxin, though such treatment does have an effect on myometrium from other non-human species (MacLennan & Grant, 1991). Similar results have been reported from another laboratory with human myometrial strips taken from both the fundus and isthmus of the uterus during spontaneous or stimulated contraction (Peterson *et al.*, 1991).

These data raise the question of whether the human myometrium is capable of responding *in vivo* to human relaxin and whether this tissue possesses relaxin receptors. The difficulty of these studies is that it is not possible to control the endocrine environment of the myometrium before it is removed from the woman.

The mechanisms by which relaxin may cause uterine quiescence have only been examined in rodents. Porcine relaxin causes a decrease in myosin light chain kinase phosphorylation and myosin light chain kinase activity (Sanborn, 1986). Similar studies are needed for human relaxins H1 and H2 with human myometrium.

The endometrium/decidua

Human uterine-derived cells have been used to study responses to exogenous relaxin *in vitro*. Usually, the cells are kept *in vitro* for extended periods making it difficult to relate the effects to the possible *in vivo* response. No obvious biological role for relaxin in the uterus has emerged. However, relaxin probably acts in an autocrine/paracrine manner; its actions are likely to be steroid-hormone dependent; and cAMP may be a component of the action of relaxin. More than one target cell type may be involved and this may change with the reproductive cycle.

The interrelationships between relaxin and other endometrial peptides (prolactin, IGF-1, IGFBP-1) have been studied *in vitro*. Porcine relaxin in combination with medroxyprogesterone acetate (MPA) and oestrogen causes an increase in the production of prolactin by endometrial stromal cells over a period of 5 days (Huang *et al.*, 1987). The dependence upon exogenous steroid would be expected since most bioassays for relaxin depend upon prior oestrogen priming and the relaxin receptor is upregulated by oestrogen treatment *in vivo* in the rat and pig (Bryant-Greenwood, 1982) by endometrial stromal cells in long term culture. MPA plus oestrogen treatment also enhances the action of relaxin on prolactin production (Rosenberg, Mazella & Tseng, 1991). The receptors on decidual cells for relaxin are distinct from those for insulin and IGF-1 (Thrailkill *et al.*, 1990); thus the three structurally related peptides may represent a system of autocrine/paracrine regulatory control in this tissue.

A dose-related effect of human relaxin on cAMP production by endometrial cells, cultured for between 13 and 22 passages has been used as a bioassay for the recombinant hormone (Fei *et al.*, 1990). However, most work on the stimulation of cAMP by relaxin has been on rodent cells and there is no consensus as to whether cAMP is an obligatory second messenger system for this hormone. Results may vary with the species from which the hormone and cells are derived, the cell type and conditions for culture. There is certainly scope for involvement of alternative second messengers for the relaxins.

It is difficult to design a system for testing the effect of one hormone upon a single uterine cell type without imposing a number of limitations. We have attempted to devise a system, based upon the cell immunoblot assay for rat pituitary prolactin, by dispersing term decidual cells and quantitating the secretion of relaxin by immunohistochemical staining in individual cells. The basement membrane which surrounds each cell is disrupted and their connections with tissue macrophages are altered. In time-course experiments we have found that relaxin is secreted by 15 minutes and the release represents *de novo* synthesis rather than cell leakage or death. Both porcine and human relaxins cause an increase in intracellular accumulation and the extracellular secretion of relaxin: prolactin added to these cells had no effect on relaxin secretion (to be published). Single-cell systems capable of quantitation by computerized densitometry may allow screening of a range of pregnancy hormones which may be involved in the control of the secretion of relaxin by the decidua.

The cervix and fetal membranes

The mouse interpubic ligament bioassay for relaxin is based upon collagenolytic activity. We take the view that relaxin produced locally within the reproductive tract can direct local collagen remodelling (Bryant-Greenwood, 1982). Porcine relaxin applied locally to the human cervix in late pregnancy can enhance dilatation and shorten labour (MacLennan *et al.*, 1980). There is no pre-partum ovarian relaxin surge in pregnant women and women without ovaries undergo normal labour and delivery. Thus a locally produced relaxin may be involved in the remodelling of the cervical connective tissues. We have also proposed that intra-uterine relaxin is involved in the loss of amniotic collagen which allows the stretching and expansion of the fetal membranes in the last weeks of pregnancy (Bryant-Greenwood, 1991*a,b*). There is a wide range of materials which might be involved in cervical and fetal membrane collagenolysis. The interplay of the proteases with tissue inhibitors and activators lends itself to multicomponent control. We have immunolocalized the major collagens, enzymes and inhibitors in the amnion, chorion and decidua (Bryant-Greenwood, 1991*a,b*). Differences in the amount of components such as tissue plasminogen activator before and after labour as detected by immunocytochemistry are reflected in the amounts of mRNA in the tissues (to be published). Similar studies might be conducted in rodents. The collagenolytic activity of human relaxin is not confined to reproductive tissues since it has been shown to increase the secretion of procollagenase and decrease its inhibitor (TIMP) released by dermal fibroblasts *in vitro* (Unemori & Amento, 1990). The changes were reflected at both the mRNA and protein levels.

Relaxin treatment also down-regulated the secretion of collagen types I and III with an increase in collagen matrix turnover and decreasing overall tissue collagen. We propose that relaxin reduces the collagen content of the amnion and chorion in late pregnancy, and that this might also be the mechanism by which relaxin causes enhanced cervical dilatation.

The relaxin receptor

It is difficult to label relaxin so that it retains its receptor-binding ability. Emphasis on the production of a biologically active tracer using either ^{32}P (Osheroff *et al.*, 1990) for human relaxin or ^{125}I (Yang *et al.*, 1992) for porcine relaxin should now allow studies to proceed. At an early stage we were successful in examining the rat myometrial relaxin receptor using conventional techniques (Bryant-Greenwood, 1982). Later evaluation of receptor binding with highly purified porcine relaxin label has shown specific binding in the pubic symphysis, ovary, uterus and brain of the mouse (Yang *et al.*, 1992). A ^{32}P labelled human relaxin has also been used in the rat to demonstrate specific binding to the uterus, cervix and brain (Osheroff & Phillips, 1991). Studies using human relaxin on human tissues are also needed. Some years ago we were able to show specific binding of a labelled porcine relaxin to membrane preparations from human amnion and chorion (Bryant-Greenwood, 1991*b*); these studies are being repeated with the human hormone and more refined labelling techniques. Concurrent studies with labelled human relaxins H1 and H2 are also necessary in order to determine whether these hormones have unique receptors or share a single receptor. Such studies must be performed before attempts can be made to isolate the relaxin receptor(s). Knowledge of the receptor sequence(s) will allow development of the necessary probes and permit study of even the low density receptors necessary for autocrine and paracrine actions in human reproductive tissues.

Acknowledgements

The work in my laboratory was made possible by financial support from the National Institutes of Health (HD-24314, RR-03061, GM07683 and GM08125) and the dedication of Mrs S. Yamamoto, post-doctoral fellows, graduate and undergraduate students over a 20-year period and the continuous support of my husband, Dr F. C. Greenwood. The author was limited by the editors to 50 references and apologizes for any omissions.

References

Bell, R. J., Eddie, L. W., Lester, A. R., Wood, E. C., Johnston, P. D. & Niall, H. D. (1987). Relaxin in human pregnancy serum measured with an homologous RIA. *Obstetrics and Gynecology*, **69**, 585–9.

Bigazzi, N., Nardi, E., Bruni, P. & Petrucci, F. (1980). Relaxin in human decidua. *Journal of Clinical Endocrinology Metabolism*, **51**, 939–41.

Bryant-Greenwood, G. D. (1982). Relaxin as a new hormone. *Endocrine Reviews*, **3**, 62–90.

Bryant-Greenwood, G. D. (1991a). The human relaxins: consensus and dissent. *Molecular Cell Endocrinology*, **79**, C125–32.

Bryant-Greenwood, G. D. (1991b). Human decidual and placental relaxins. *Reproduction and Fertility Developments*, **3**, 385–9.

Bryant-Greenwood, G. D., Tashima, L., Greenwood, F. C., Taylor, E. & Peaker, M. (1991). Endometrial relaxin: effects of mastectomy in the cyclic and pregnant guinea pig. *Endocrinology*, **129**, 2119–25.

Bullesbach, E. E. & Schwabe, C. (1991). Total synthesis of human relaxin and human relaxin derivatives by solid-phase synthesis and site-directed chain combination. *Journal of Biological Chemistry*, **266**, 10754–61.

Canova-Davis, E., Baldonado, I. P. & Teshima, G. M. (1990). Characterization of chemically synthesized human relaxin by high performance liquid chromatography. *Journal of Chromatography*, **508**, 81–96.

Canova-Davis, E., Kessler, T. J., Lee, P. J. *et al.* (1991). Use of recombinant DNA derived human relaxin to probe the structure of the native protein. *Biochemistry*, **30**, 6006–13.

Dallenbach, F. D. & Dallenbach-Hellweg, G. (1964). Immunohistological studies of the localization of relaxin in human placenta and decidua. *Archive Pathology, Anatomy and Physiology*, **337**, 301–26.

Eddie, L. W., Sutton, B., Fitzgerald, S., Bell, R. J., Johnston, P. D. & Tregear, G. W. (1989). Relaxin in paired samples of serum and milk from women after term and pretern delivery. *American Journal of Obstetrics and Gynecology*, **161**, 970–3.

Emmi, A. M., Skurnick, J., Goldsmith, L.T. *et al.* (1991). Ovarian control of pituitary hormone secretion in early human pregnancy. *Journal of Clinical Endocrinology & Metabolism*, **72**, 1359–63.

Evans, M. I., Dougan, M. N., Moawad, A. H., Evans, W. J., Bryant-Greenwood, G. D. & Greenwood, F. C. (1983). Ripening of the human cervix with porcine ovarian relaxin. *American Journal of Obstetrics and Gynecology*, **147**, 410–14.

Fei, D. T. W., Gross, M. C., Lofgren, J. L., Mora-Worms, M. & Chen, A. B. (1990). Cyclic AMP response to recombinant human relaxin by cultured human endometrial cells, a specific and high through put *in vitro* bioassay. *Biochemical and Biophysical Research Communications*, **170**, 214–22.

Fields, P. A. & Larkin, L. H. (1981). Purification and immunohistochemical localization of relaxin in the human term placenta. *Journal of Clinical Endocrinology & Metabolism*, **52**, 79–85.

Graham, E. F. & Dracy, A. E. (1952). The effects of relaxin on the cow's cervix. *Journal of Dairy Science*, **35**, 499–505.

Hansell, D. J., Bryant-Greenwood, G. D. & Greenwood, F. C. (1991). Expression of the human relaxin H1 gene in the decidua, trophoblast and prostate. *Journal of Clinical Endocrinology & Metabolism*, **72**, 899–904.

Hisaw, F. L. (1926). Experimental relaxation of the pubic ligament of the guinea pig. *Proceedings of Experimental Biology and Medicine*, **23**, 661–3.

Huang, J. R., Tseng, L., Bischof, P. & Janne, O. A. (1987). Regulation of prolactin production by progestin, estrogen and relaxin in human endometrial stromal cells. *Endocrinology*, **121**, 2011–17.

Hudson, P., Haley, J., John, M. *et al.* (1983). Structure of a genomic clone encoding biologically active human relaxin. *Nature*, **301**, 628–31.

Hudson, P., John, M., Crawford, R. *et al.* (1984). Relaxin gene expression in human ovaries and the predicted structure of a human preprorelaxin by analysis of cDNA clones. *EMBO Journal*, **3**, 2333–9.

Ivell, R., Hunt, N., Khan-Dawood, F. & Dawood, F. (1989). Expression of the human relaxin gene in the corpus luteum of the menstrual cycle and prostate. *Molecular Cell Endocrinology*, **66**, 251–5.

Johnston, P. D., Burnier, J., Chen, S. *et al.* (1985). Structure/function studies on human relaxin. In *Peptides: Structure and Function*. Ed. C. M. Deber, V. J. Hruby and K. D. Kopple, pp. 683–6. Proceedings of the 9th American Peptide Symposium. Pierce Chem. Co. Rockford, IL.

Koay, E. S. C., Bagnell, C. A., Bryant-Greenwood, G. D., Lord, S. B., Cruz, A. C. & Larkin, L. H. (1985). Immunocytochemical localization of relaxin in human decidua and placenta. *Journal of Clinical Endocrinology & Metabolism*, **60**, 859–63.

Krantz, J. C., Bryant, H. H. & Carr, C. J. (1950). The action of aqueous corpus luteum extract upon uterine activity. *Surgical Gynecology Obstetrics*, **90**, 372–6.

MacLennan, A. H., Green, R., Bryant-Greenwood, G. D., Greenwood, F. C. & Seamark, R. F. (1980). Ripening of the human cervix and induction of labour with purified porcine relaxin. *Lancet*, **i**, 220–3.

MacLennan, A. H., Green, R., Grant, P. & Nicolson, R. (1986a). Ripening of the human cervix and induction of labor with intracervical purified porcine relaxin. *Obstetrics and Gynecology*, **68**, 598–601.

MacLennan, A. H., Grant, P., Ness, D. & Down, A. (1986b). Effect of porcine relaxin and progesterone on rat, pig and human myometrial activity *in vitro*. *Journal of Reproductive Medicine*, **31**, 43–9.

MacLennan, A. H. & Grant, P. (1991). Human relaxin *in vitro* response of human and pig myometrium. *Journal of Reproductive Medicine*, **36**, 630–4.

Mathieu, P., Rahier, J. & Thomas, K. (1981). Localization of relaxin in human gestational corpus luteum. *Cell Tissue Research*, **219**, 213–16.

Mazoujian, G. & Bryant-Greenwood, G. D. (1990). Relaxin in breast-tissue. *Lancet*, **335**, 298–9.

O'Byrne, E. M., Flitcraft, J. F., Sawyer, W. I., Hochman, J., Weiss, G. & Stinetz, B. G. (1978). Relaxin bioactivity and immunoactivity in human corpora lutea. *Endocrinology*, **102**, 1641–4.

Osheroff, P. L. & Phillips, H. S. (1990). Autoradiographic localization of relaxin binding sites in rat brain. *Proceedings of the National Academy of Sciences, USA*, **88**, 6413–17.

Osheroff, P. L., Ling, V. T., Vandlen, R. L., Cronin, M. J. & Lofgren, J. A. (1990). Preparation of biologically active ^{32}P-labeled human relaxin. *Journal of Biological Chemistry*, **265**, 9396–401.

Peterson, L. K., Svane, D., Uldbjerg, N. & Forman, A. (1991). Effects of human relaxin on isolated rat and human myometrium and utero placental arteries. *Obstetrics and Gynecology*, **78**, 757–62.

Rosenberg, M., Mazella, J. & Tseng, L. (1991). Relative potency of relaxin, insulin-like growth factors and insulin on the prolactin production in progestin-primed human endometrial stromal cells in long-term culture. *Annals of NY Academy of Sciences*, **622**, 138–44.

Sakbun, V., Koay, E. S. C. & Bryant-Greenwood, G. D. (1987). Immunocytochemical localization of prolactin and relaxin C-peptide in human decidua and placenta. *Journal of Clinical Endocrinology & Metabolism*, **65**, 339–43.

Sakbun, V., Ali, S. M., Greenwood, F. C. & Bryant-Greenwood, G. D. (1990). Human relaxin in the amnion, chorion, decidua-parietalis, basal plate and placental trophoblast by immunocytochemistry and Northern analysis. *Journal of Clinical Endocrinology & Metabolism*, **70**, 508–14.

Sanborn, B. M. (1986). Role of relaxin in uterine function. In *The Physiology and Biochemistry of the Uterus in Pregnancy and Labor*. Ed. G. Huzar, pp. 225–38. CRC Press, Boca Raton, Florida.

Schwabe, C. & Bullesbach, E. E. (1990). Relaxin. *Comparative Biochemistry and Physiology*, **96B**, 15–21.

Sherwood, O. D. & O'Byrne, E. M. (1974). Purification and characterization of porcine relaxin. *Archives in Biochemistry and Biophysics*, **160**, 185–96.

Sherwood, O. D. (1988). Relaxin. In *The Physiology of Reproduction*. Ed. E. Knobil and J. Neill, pp. 585–673, Raven Press, New York.

Stewart, D. R., Celniker, A. C., Taylor, C. A., Cragun, J. R., Overstreet, J. W. & Lasley, B. L. (1990). Relaxin in the peri-implantation period. *Journal of Clinical Endocrinology & Metabolism*, **70**, 1771–3.

Shire, S. J., Holladay, L. A. & Rinderknecht, E. (1991). Self-association of human and porcine relaxin as assessed by analytical ultracentrifugation and circular dichroism. *Biochemistry*, **30**, 7703–11.

Stoelk, E., Chegini, N., Lei, Z. M., Rao, Ch. V., Bryant-Greenwood, G. D. & Sanfilippo, J. (1991). Immunocytochemical localization of relaxin in human corpora lutea: cellular and subcellar distribution and dependence on reproductive state. *Biology of Reproduction*, **44**, 1140–7.

Stults, J. T., Bourell, J. H., Canova-Davis, E. *et al.* (1990). Structural characterization by mass spectrometry of native and recombinant human relaxin. *Biochemical Environment Mass Spectroscopy*, **19**, 655–64.

Thrailkill, K. M., Clemmons, D. R., Busby, W. H. & Handwerger, S. (1990). Differential regulation of insulin-like growth factor binding protein from human decidual cells by IGF-1, insulin and relaxin. *Journal of Clinical Investigation*, **86**, 878–83.

Unemori, E. N. & Amento, E. P. (1990). Relaxin modulates synthesis and secretion of procollagenase and collagen by human dermal fibroblasts. *Journal of Biological Chemistry*, **265**, 681–5.

Wathes, D. C., Wardle, P. G., Rees, J. M. *et al.* (1986). Identification of relaxin immunoreactivity in human follicular fluid. *Human Reproduction*, **1**, 515–17.

Weiss, G., O'Byrne, E. M. & Steinetz, B. G. (1976). Relaxin: a product of the corpus luteum of pregnancy. *Science*, **194**, 948–9.

Yamamoto, S., Kwok, S., Greenwood, F. C. & Bryant-Greenwood, G. D. (1981). Relaxin purification from human placental basal plates. *Journal of Clinical Endocrinology & Metabolism*, **51**, 601–4.

Yang, S. U., Rembiesa, B., Bullesbach, E. E. & Schwabe, C. (1992). Relaxin receptors in mice: demonstration of ligand binding in symphysial tissue and uterine membrane fragments. *Endocrinology*, **130**, 179–85.

Yki-Jarinen, H., Wahlstrom, T., Tenhunen, A., Koskimies, A. I. & Seppala, M. (1984). The occurrence of relaxin in hyperstimulated preovulatory follicles collected in an *in vitro* fertilization program. *Journal of* in vitro *Fertility and Embryo Transplants*, **1**, 180–2.

12

Oxytocin in human parturition

T. CHARD

Oxytocin is widely used for the artificial induction of labour. Many therefore assume that an increase in maternal levels of endogenous oxytocin might be responsible for the onset of spontaneous labour. Two decades of research have failed to confirm this simple view. The reality is more complex, involving an interplay of maternal, uterine, placental and fetal factors.

Uterine activity during pregnancy and labour

The control of uterine activity must be considered in relation to the development of that activity during pregnancy and labour. There have been extensive studies on the human because examination of uterine activity is essential in the diagnosis of disorders in late pregnancy and during labour. In early pregnancy, uterine activity is minimal. Thereafter there is a progressive evolution of activity, although there has been disagreement as to the timing, rate, and nature of the change. Caldeyro-Barcia & Sereno (1961) and Csapo & Sauvage (1968) maintained that the process accelerates in the last 4 to 8 weeks of pregnancy, shading almost imperceptibly into the onset of labour. According to Caldeyro-Barcia and Sereno, this activity effaces the cervix. Once the cervical os is fully taken up, it can dilate and true labour begins. By contrast, Theobald (1969) always maintained that there is a rapid evolution of activity from a state of relative quiescence in a matter of days or hours before the onset of labour.

To understand the mechanism of the onset of labour it is important to know which of the these alternatives is correct. If uterine activity evolves gradually, then the control factors must follow a similar pattern with a slowly increasing stimulus, or slowly decreasing inhibition. By contrast, if evolution is abrupt, then this may represent the attainment of a threshold or the intervention of a new factor. More recent studies suggest that a compromise between these two alternatives may be correct. There is an increase in the frequency of uterine contractions around the 36th week of gestation, but the major acceleration is not

268

seen until the last 24 hours before delivery (Newman, Gill & Katz, 1986; Zahn, 1984).

Secretion of oxytocin

General aspects of the secretion and action of oxytocin have been well reviewed by Mohr, Meyerhof & Richter (1992). Oxytocin is synthesized in magnocellular and parvocellular neurons of the paraventricular nucleus of the hypothalamus (Swanson & Sawchenko, 1983). The magnocellular neurons terminate in the posterior pituitary gland and are the main source of circulating oxytocin; the parvocellular neurons terminate in other areas of the brain and spinal cord and are the source of oxytocin in cerebrospinal fluid. Oxytocin from the parvocellular neurons may play an important role in memory and behavioural functions (Richard, Moos & Freund-Mercier, 1991). There is also some evidence for paracrine secretion of oxytocin. High levels of oxytocin mRNA have been shown in the decidua with much lower levels in the membranes and placenta (Chibbar, Miller & Mitchell, 1993) (Zingg, Lefebvre and Giaid, 1993).

As with all hypothalamic hormones, oxytocin is released discontinuously, and serial measurements reveal sharply fluctuating levels in the circulation. Oxytocin is a particularly striking example of this phenomenon: the concentration in blood may vary tenfold or more over a relatively short period of sampling. This process has been described as 'spurt' release and is illustrated diagrammatically in Fig. 1. Rapid serial sampling over a period of seconds or minutes, rather than hours, is the only procedure by which oxytocin can be accurately quantitated (Gibbens & Chard, 1976; Dawood, 1983; McNeilly *et al.*, 1983; Fuchs *et al.*, 1991). Similar spurt release may also be seen in cerebrospinal fluid (Challinor, Cameron & Amico, 1992).

Oxytocin and vasopressin circulate as free peptide in the bloodstream. The principal sites of clearance are the kidneys and the liver (Ginsburg, 1968); small amounts of hormone are excreted in urine (Frandsen & Jensen, 1971). The half-life of either oxytocin or vasopressin in the human has been variously estimated from 2.7 to 17 minutes (Dawood, 1983; Ginsburg, 1968; Gonzalez-Panizza, Sica-Blanco & Mendez-Bauer, 1961; Chard *et al.*, 1970; Gibbens, Boyd & Chard, 1972). When oxytocin infusion is continued at a fixed rate, blood oxytocin levels increase and reach a plateau in approximately 40 minutes. The clearance rate of oxytocin is the same in the pregnant as the non-pregnant woman (17.4 ± 9.2 ml/kg), and similar to that in men (17.6 ± 2.1 ml/kg) (Amico, Seitchik & Robinson, 1984; Leake, Weitzman & Fisher, 1980) despite the existence during pregnancy of high blood levels of the placenta enzyme, cysteine aminopeptidase (oxytocinase) which can split the oxytocin molecule between the tyrosine residue and the N-terminal haemicysteine residue (Fig. 2).

T. Chard

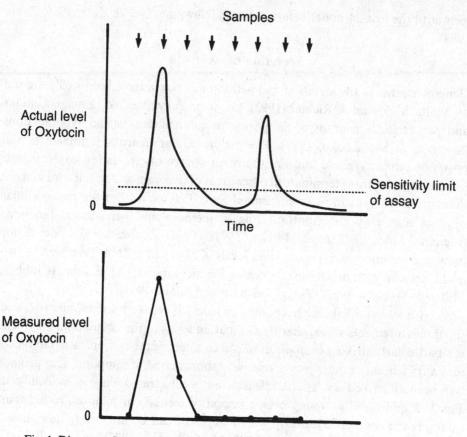

Fig. 1. Diagram of spurt release of oxytocin. The peaks, which may last a minute or less, can easily be missed even by close serial sampling.

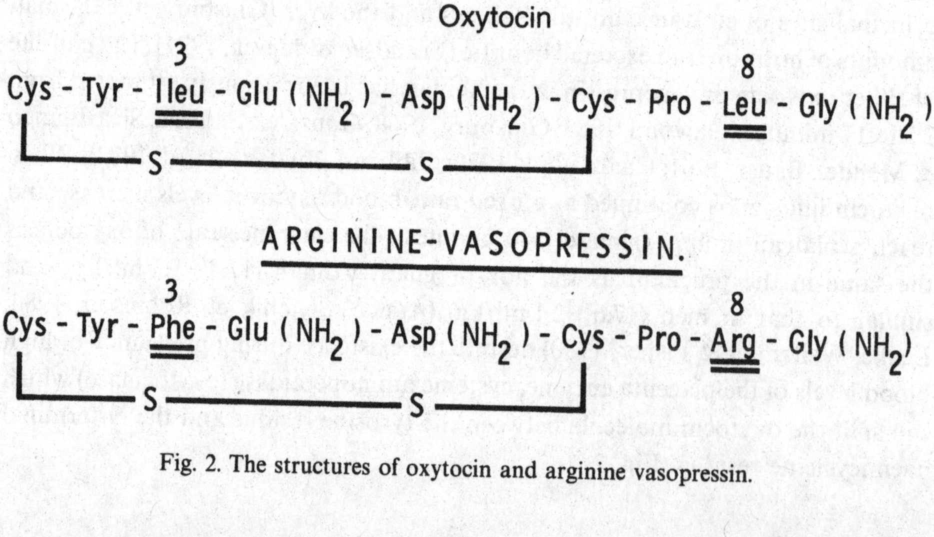

Oxytocin

Cys - Tyr - Ileu - Glu (NH$_2$) - Asp (NH$_2$) - Cys - Pro - Leu - Gly (NH$_2$)

ARGININE-VASOPRESSIN.

Cys - Tyr - Phe - Glu (NH$_2$) - Asp (NH$_2$) - Cys - Pro - Arg - Gly (NH$_2$)

Fig. 2. The structures of oxytocin and arginine vasopressin.

Control of oxytocin release

The release of oxytocin by the neurohypophysis is controlled by two neural mechanisms. The first is a neuroendocrine reflex originating from touch stimulation of the nipple. The second is the reflex arising from stretch receptors in the lower genital tract: this is known as Ferguson's reflex (Ferguson, 1941). Spurt release of oxytocin during stimulation of the cervix in women has been shown by some (Chard & Gibbens, 1983) but not all workers (Thornton, Davison & Baylis, 1989). This reflex may be responsible for the surge of oxytocin that occurs during the expulsive phase of labour in a variety of species including man. In agreement with this is the fact that oxytocin levels in the second stage of labour are reduced in women with epidural analgesia (Goodfellow *et al.*, 1983).

Oxytocin release can be stimulated by administration of prostaglandins (Gillespie, Brummer & Chard, 1972; Fuchs *et al.*, 1983). Release is also stimulated by dopamine, the effect being blocked by the dopamine antagonist haloperidol (Clarke & Lincoln, 1975). Certain vagally mediated stimuli, such as nausea, aversion and food intake, also cause oxytocin secretion (Verbalis *et al.*, 1986). Gastrointestinal peptide hormones including cholecystokinin (Verbalis *et al.*, 1986) and vasoactive intestinal polypeptide (Ottenen *et al.*, 1984), which are also present in the brain, stimulate the release of oxytocin, and might function as endogenous regulators of oxytocin release. Oxytocin secretion is inhibited by opiates (Bicknell, 1985; Dyer, 1988; Russell *et al.*, 1989; Falke, 1991; Neumann, Russell & Landgraf, 1991; Lindow *et al.*, 1992). This may represent a natural mechanism by which delivery can be delayed if the environment is unfavourable. In turn, oxytocin can inhibit ACTH/cortisol secretion (Chiodera *et al.*, 1991).

Oxytocin and parturition

Once spontaneous labour has begun, the human myometrium is exquisitely sensitive to oxytocin. The mechanism of action of oxytocin on the myometrium is considered in detail elsewhere in this volume.

Many obstetricians assume that circulating oxytocin, released from the maternal pituitary, plays an important role in the initiation and maintenance of labour. Quite reasonably, this assumption is based on the routine use of oxytocin the the therapeutic induction of labour (for review see Owen & Hauth, 1992). However, this constitutes only indirect evidence that it is involved in spontaneous labour.

The early authors who described the uterine-stimulating effects of posterior pituitary extracts made no specific comments on its possible physiological role. By the 1930s, however, a number of workers were performing experimental studies on the relationship between the posterior pituitary gland and parturition in animals. The evidence that has been assembled since that time can be divided into two parts: indirect evidence in which situations have been studied that might demonstrate a relationship between oxytocin and parturition; and direct evidence in which oxytocin levels have been measured in the circulation before and during parturition (Chard, 1989).

Indirect evidence that oxytocin is involved in human parturition

Pregnancy and diabetes insipidus

There have been at least 80 published cases of pregnancy associated with diabetes insipidus. The general conclusion is that neither the onset nor the maintenance of labour is abnormal in most cases of diabetes insipidus. The occasional exceptions can be explained by the fact prolonged pregnancy and labour are not uncommon in subjects with no endocrine abnormality. However, a normal labour in a woman with diabetes insipidus does not exclude the involvement of maternal oxytocin. The deficiency might not be absolute, and the reserve capacity for the production of oxytocin may be substantial; it is notable that lactation and milk ejection is normal in such women. Furthermore, normal levels of oxytocin have been reported in women with diabetes insipidus (Sende *et al.*, 1976; Shangold *et al.*, 1983). Congenital diabetes insipidus in animals is associated with normal or even elevated oxytocin levels, showing that the synthesis and secretion of the two neurohypophysial hormones may be independent under some circumstances (Balment, Brimble & Forsling, 1982).

Association of milk ejection with parturition

The most specific physiologic and pharmacologic effect of oxytocin is an increase in intramammary pressure leading to ejection of milk. An increase in pressure *in vivo*, in the absence of other factors, would therefore be good evidence for the release of endogenous oxytocin. This 'bioassay' has been used as an index of circulating oxytocin during labour. Gunther (1948) reported on the occurrence of milk ejection during labour; however, most clinical experience suggests that milk ejection during labour is unusual. Cobo (1968) could not find any increase in intramammary pressure during labour, recorded via cannulae placed in the mammary ducts. At the same time, an increase in pressure could be induced by the injection of 2 mU of oxytocin. These findings argue against the existence of any sharp increase in maternal oxytocin levels during human labour. However, labour in women is associated with a marked increase in plasma catecholamines and prostaglandins, both of which might act peripherally to inhibit the action of oxytocin on the mammary gland. Seoud & colleagues (1993) have shown that electrical breast stimulation can cause uterine contractions at term, and that this process is associated with a release of oxytocin.

Influence of alcohol and other blocking agents on myometrial activity

Alcohol depresses the function of the neurohypophysis. Fuchs and colleagues (Fuchs *et al.*, 1963, 1967; Zlatnik & Fuchs, 1972) advocated the use of alcohol for the inhibition of preterm labour, the effect being attributed to inhibition of oxytocin release from the maternal pituitary. Ethanol can suppress the spurt release of oxytocin during human term labour (Gibbens & Chard, 1976), and a similar phenomenon has been observed in preterm labour (Fuchs *et al.*, 1982). Alcohol may also have a direct effect on the uterine muscle (Gimeno *et al.*, 1971; Fuchs & Fuchs, 1981; Schrok *et al.*, 1989) but this may only be significant at levels that exceed therapeutic blood alcohol levels. Ethanol increases the threshold sensitivity to oxytocin (Lauersen, Wilson & Fuchs, 1981). Studies on the possible effects of ethanol on prostaglandin-induced uterine activity have yielded conflicting results (Karim & Sharma, 1971; Lauersen *et al.*, 1973).

Analogues of oxytocin with antagonist activity inhibit the uterine contractions in premature labour (Akerlund *et al.*, 1987). This provides further confirmation that oxytocin plays a major role in spontaneous myometrial contractility, but not that an increase in oxytocin secretion was primarily responsible for the contractions.

Effect of oxytocin on the uterus at different stages of pregnancy

The sensitivity of the human myometrium to oxytocin changes during pregnancy, but the exact pattern has been the subject of dispute. The arguments follow lines similar to those already discussed on the development of spontaneous uterine activity. Caldeyro-Barcia & Sereno (1961) maintained that there is a progressive increase in the sensitivity of the uterus throughout pregnancy, reaching a plateau at the 36th week. However, as first noted by Theobald, Robards & Suter (1969) and later agreed by Caldeyro-Barcia's group and others, there is a further and major increase in myometrial sensitivity at or shortly before the onset of labour (Csapo & Sauvage, 1968; Caldeyro-Barcia & Theobald, 1968).

Indirect estimation of oxytocin levels

Prior to the availability of direct assays for oxytocin, several investigators attempted to estimate the levels of circulating oxytocin in human labour from

Table 1. *Levels of circulating oxytocin in human labour, estimated from the rate of infusion required to produce contractions identical with those of spontaneous labour*

Rate of infusion (mU/min)	Estimated level (μU/ml)	Reference
2 (first stage)	0.07	Theobald *et al.*, 1969
8 (second stage)	2.5[a]	Caldeyro-Barcia & Sereno, 1961
	3	Saameli, 1963
3–16	4	Gonzalez-Panizza *et al.*, 1961
	4–20[a]	Mantell & Liggins, 1970

[a] Estimated from a volume of distribution of 4 l and a half-life of 5 min.

the rate of infusion required to produce contractions identical with those of spontaneous labour (Fuchs, 1978; Gonzalez-Panizza, Sica-Blanco & Mendez-Bauer, 1961; Saameli, 1963; Theobald, 1969; Mantell & Liggins, 1970) (Table 1). There was substantial disagreement as to what could be regarded as 'physiological' rates of infusion. In addition, the contractions produced by intravenous oxytocin in late pregnancy are not guaranteed to be identical to those of normal, early labour. However, the general conclusion from these studies was that circulating oxytocin levels would not exceed 10 μU/ml of plasma in human labour. The rate of infusion needed to induce labour in most women near term (2 to 7 mU/min) would not, given the volume of distribution and half-life of oxytocin, yield plasma levels in excess of 10 μU/ml.

Direct evidence that oxytocin is involved in parturition

Methods of measurement of circulating oxytocin

Circulating oxytocin levels during labour have been studied by both bioassay and radioimmunoassay. Biological assays have been reviewed by Chard & Forsling (1976). The lower detection limits of biological assays are of the order 1 to 5 μU/ml. Most studies using bioassay found high levels during the second stage, and some found high levels during the first stage. However, all methods of oxytocin bioassay lack specificity, since many substances can mimic the effect of oxytocin in causing smooth muscle contraction. These substances occur in normal plasma and some may result from the processing of the blood sample.

There have been many descriptions of radioimmunoassays (RIA) for oxytocin. The sensitivity of these is similar to, although not better than, that of the best bioassays. Their chief advantage is that they are relatively specific, especially when associated with extraction procedures. However, different antisera may yield discrepant results, perhaps due to the presence of oxytocin–vasotocin-like peptides in pregnancy women (Amico *et al.*, 1986). Oestrogen induces an oxytocin-like peptide that is recognized as oxytocin by some antisera but not others (Mantell & Liggins, 1970). Furthermore, the radioimmunoassay measures only a particular sequence of amino acids and may therefore detect fragments of the oxytocin molecule that are not biologically active. The extent of this dissociation has been studied in detail in a number of experimental situations (Chard, 1973), but does not appear to present a serious problem in most physiological circumstances.

Measurement of circulating oxytocin levels in the mother

The published data from assay procedures using generally acceptable RIA methodology are summarized in Table 2 (early measurements of circulating oxytocin by both bioassay and radioimmunoassay often yielded apparent high levels that were clearly impossible by other criteria). Non-specificity can affect RIA as well as bioassays, especially those that do not use an extraction procedure. Human pregnancy plasma poses a special challenge: interfering substances may be present and extraction procedures are necessary, even with the best antibodies (Robinson, 1980). It is interesting to note that most studies using a non-extraction RIA yielded a similar pattern: a progressive rise in oxytocin levels during pregnancy with no further change during labour (Table 2). This would be the expected result if, as seems likely, the assay is primarily measuring the enzyme oxytocinase.

From the information presented in Table 2, the following conclusions can be drawn. There is probably a continuous low level of spurt release of oxytocin in all women. The overall levels of oxytocin may increase progressively during pregnancy, although examination of the original data suggests that this increase, if it occurs at all, is small. The frequency of the spurts (and hence the mean levels of oxytocin) increases with the onset of labour and reaches a maximum at the time of delivery (Fig. 3) (Gibbens & Chard, 1976; Fuchs *et al.*, 1991). Spurt release of oxytocin has also been observed in animals during parturition (Fuchs, 1985). There is no obvious direct relationship between the timing of the spurts and that of the uterine contractions. The total amount of oxytocin release must be small, because there is no obvious increase in urine oxytocin levels during labour (Boyd & Chard, 1973). The oxytocin release is inhibited by regional anaesthesia (Vasicka *et al.*, 1978) and by opiates (Lindow *et al.*, 1992).

Recent evidence indicates local synthesis of oxytocin by the decidua in both the rat and the human (Zingg, Lefebvre & Giail, 1993; Chibbar, Miller & Mitchell, 1993).

Table 2. *Some studies on human parturition using direct measurement of oxytocin in the mother by radioimmunoassay. Earlier studies on this topic were reviewed in detail by Chard (1972)*

Reference	Findings
Gibbens & Chard, 1976	Progressive increase in the frequency of detectable values ('spurts') during labour reaching maximum in second stage.
Vasicka et al., 1978	Progressive increase during pregnancy, surge during cervical dilatation and vaginal distension.
Leake et al., 1981a	No increase during pregnancy or early labour, increase during expulsive phase.
Sellers et al., 1981	Progressive increase during pregnancy, no change during labour.
Fuchs et al., 1982	Increase during premature labour, reduced by ethanol treatment.
Dawood, 1983	Positive results during pregnancy, progressive increase during labour.
Fuchs et al., 1983	Increased levels during first stage of labour compared with non-labouring controls, levels during oxytocin-induced labour similar to that during spontaneous labour.
Goodfellow et al., 1983	Increase between full dilatation of the cervix and crowning of head, no increase in presence of epidural analgesia
Nagata et al., 1983; 1987	Levels higher in spontaneous labour than in labour induced by amniotomy or prostaglandin administration
Otsuki et al., 1983a	Progressive increase during pregnancy, no increase in first stage of labour.
De Geest et al., 1985	Progressive increase during pregnancy, no increase in first stage of labour.
Burd et al., 1987	Pulsatile release of oxytocin during first stage of labour in some but not all subjects.
Padayachi et al., 1988	Increase during pregnancy, no change during labour.
Thornton & Davison, 1988	Highest levels during third stage of labour.
Oosterbaan & Swaab, 1989	Increase during labour, levels correlated with those in amniotic fluid.
Fuchs et al., 1991	Oxytocin released in spurts, frequency increased in spontaneous labour (1.2/30 min before labour; 4.2/30 min in first stage; 6.7/30 min in second and third stages).
Stock, Bremme & Uvnas-Moberg, 1991	Progressive increase during pregnancy.
Lindow et al., 1992	Oxytocin secretion in first stage of labour is inhibited by morphine but not naloxone.
Thornton, Davison & Baylis, 1992	Low levels throughout labour in most subjects; occasional women show a large surge immediately before delivery.

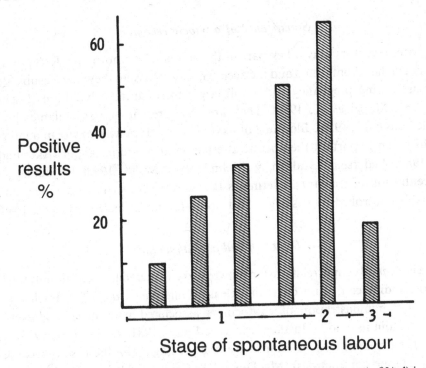

Fig. 3. The frequency of positive results (oxytocin level greater than 1 μU/ml) in serial samples from women during spontaneous labour (modified from Gibbens & Chard, 1976).

Significance of maternal oxytocin release in women

Intermittent release of oxytocin may have a greater effect on the uterus than a continuous release of the same amount of hormone. Thus spurt release could be highly effective as a uterine stimulant (Pavlou *et al.*, 1978; Odem, Work & Dawood, 1988; Cummiskey & Dawood, 1990).

Whether or not maternal (or fetal) oxytocin could be a primary stimulus for the initiation of spontaneous labour remains uncertain. The problem, as with so many factors which have been evaluated in relation to the onset of labour, is to determine whether changing levels of a compound preceded contractions and might therefore be the primary stimulus to uterine activity, or whether the changing levels were the result of the contractions and therefore play only a secondary role in the process of labour. This point is well illustrated by the elegant study of MacDonald and Casey (1993) showing that accumulation of prostaglandins in amniotic fluid is an *after-effect* of uterine contractions and not, as many believe, the primary stimulus.

Significance of oxytocin receptors

Oxytocin receptors play a key part in the action of the hormone. Receptors are present in the myometrium and the decidua; in both tissues they show a substantial increase during pregnancy and a still larger increase in early labour (Fuchs *et al.*, 1982; Maggi *et al.*, 1990). They are also present in the fetal membranes (Benedetto *et al.*, 1990). Blockade of oxytoxin receptors with oxytocin analogues might be an important therapeutic alternative in pre-term labour (Akerlund *et al.*, 1987; Andersen, Lyndrup & Melin, 1989); Melin, 1993. In animals, the concentration of receptors determines the uterine sensitivity to oxytocin and is probably controlled by oestrogen and progesterone levels (Fuchs *et al.*, 1983).

Oxytocin and prostaglandins

There is a complex interrelationship between oxytocin and prostaglandins. Infused prostaglandins can cause oxytocin release (Gillespie *et al.*, 1972; Fuchs *et al.*, 1983) and administration of oxytocin is associated with increased levels of prostaglandin in blood (Husslein, Fuchs & Fuchs, 1981; Fuchs *et al.*, 1983). The latter phenomenon may be indirect (i.e. the prostaglandin increase is secondary to the uterine contractions) (MacDonald & Casey, 1993) but could also result from receptor-mediated stimulation of prostaglandin synthesis by oxytocin (Chan, Powell & Hruby, 1982). In addition, oxytocin can stimulate prostaglandin release by the membranes and decidua *in vitro* (Fuchs, Husslein & Fuchs, 1981; Pasetto *et al.*, 1992).

Release of oxytocin by the fetal posterior pituitary in labour

Oxytocin is present in the human fetal pituitary at 14 weeks gestation and the amount increases progressively up to term (Khan-Dawood & Dawood, 1984). In early pregnancy there is a high vasopressin to oxytocin ratio, which decreases as pregnancy advances (Burford & Robinson, 1982). Processing of the oxytocin prohormone is much less efficient in the fetus than in the adult (Altstein *et al.*, 1988). In addition to oxytocin and vasopressin, human fetal blood also contains arginine vasotocin and other related peptides (Ervin *et al.*, 1988). The human fetus releases substantial amounts of oxytocin (and vasopressin) in association with the process of labour (Chard *et al.*, 1971) (Table 3). High concentrations of both hormones are found in human umbilical arterial and venous blood collected at the time of delivery (Fig. 4). The concentrations are higher in the umbilical artery than in the umbilical vein, indicating that the hormones originate from the fetus itself. The highest levels are found at the time of vaginal delivery, the lowest at Caesarean section when the patient is not in labour, and intermediate

Table 3. *Some studies on the release of oxytocin by the human fetal pituitary in relation to parturition*

Reference	Findings
Chard *et al.*, 1971	Umbilical oxytocin (and vasopressin) levels higher than mother, arteriovenous difference, progressive increase associated with labour.
Vasicka *et al.*, 1978	Levels higher than maternal and possibly related to fetal hypoxia
Leake *et al.*, 1981*b*	Umbilical arteriovenous difference.
Sellers *et al.*, 1981	Umbilical arteriovenous difference, higher levels than mother during labour.
Fuchs *et al.*, 1982	Umbilical levels higher than mother during early labour and preterm labour.
Dawood, 1983	Umbilical arteriovenous difference, progressive increase associated with labour, oxytocin present in amniotic fluid and fetal urine.
Otsuki *et al.*, 1983*b*	Umbilical oxytocin absent in four cases of anencephaly.
Swaab & Oosterbaan, 1983	Umbilical oxytocin absent in some but not all anencephalics, amniotic fluid oxytocin identical in anencephalics and controls.
De Geest *et al.*, 1985	Umbilical levels higher than maternal, higher in spontaneous delivery than at elective Caesarean section.
Fuchs, 1985	Umbilical levels higher than maternal, umbilical arteriovenous difference present in very early labour and in preterm labour.
Pochard & Lutz-Bucher, 1986	Umbilical arteriovenous difference, progressive increase in levels during labour.
Kuwabara *et al.*, 1987	Umbilical oxytocin levels at delivery similar to maternal, higher in spontaneous delivery than at elective Caesarean section.
Padayachi *et al.*, 1988	Umbilical levels higher than maternal, arteriovenous difference.
Oosterbaan & Swaab, 1989	Umbilical arteriovenous difference, levels higher than maternal and increase during labour.
Thornton, Murray & Baylis, 1993	Umbilical arteriovenous difference; difference increased by epidural analgesia but not pethidine; no difference in levels between Caesarean section before and during labour.

concentrations are found at Caesarean section carried out during labour (Chard *et al.*, 1971; Dawood, 1983). The release appears to be associated with the process of labour and is maximal during the expulsive phase. There is little or no release of fetal oxytocin during labour in rhesus monkeys (Hirst *et al.*, 1993).

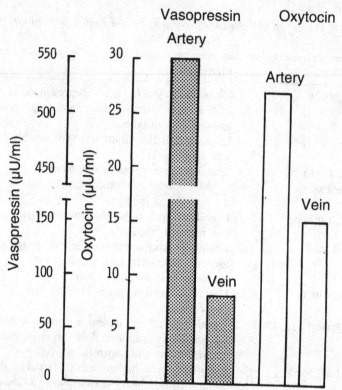

Fig. 4. Levels of oxytocin (open bars) and vasopressin (shaded bars) in the umbilical artery and vein at the time of spontaneous delivery (modified from Chard *et al.*, 1971).

Significance of fetal oxytocin release during labour

The primary stimulus to the activation of the human fetal pituitary is not known. It is possible that anoxia might be a common denominator, but there is no direct evidence for this. The significance of the release is also uncertain. However, oxytocin can cross the placenta (Noddle, 1964) and oxytocin in the umbilical circulation might be able to stimulate uterine activity. It is directed at the area of the myometrium, the placental site, which is responsible for the normal quiescence of the uterus during pregnancy. There is also a vasoconstrictor effect of both oxytocin and vasopressin and a reduction in uterine blood flow may stimulate uterine activity. Fetal release of oxytocin cannot be essential for uterine activity, since normal deliveries occur with an anencephalic fetus, which lacks a posterior pituitary and in which neither oxytocin nor vasopressin can be detected in the umbilical circulation (Otsuki *et al.*, 1983a,b). If fetal release of oxytocin plays a role, it may be as a signal from the fetus that alters the balance of other factors in favour of uterine contractions.

Conclusions

Numerous studies conclude (1) oxytocin is secreted in short-lasting spurts; therefore levels measured at infrequent intervals do not give accurate information on the amounts of oxytocin secreted during labour; (2) there is little or no evidence for an increase in maternal oxytocin secretion at the onset of labour; (3) during labour there is a progressive increase in oxytocin secretion with a maximum during the expulsive phase; (4) fetal secretion of oxytocin (and vasopressin) also increases markedly during labour, but the timing of this increase is still uncertain; (5) there is an increase in human uterine oxytocin receptors at term, making the uterus responsive to very small amounts of oxytocin. Thus the onset of labour in the human could be explained by an increase in oxytocin receptors, rendering the myometrium sensitive to a fixed circulating concentration of oxytocin (maternal and/or fetal). As a secondary result of uterine contractions there is an increase in secretion of both maternal and fetal oxytocin, and this increase might play an important part in the expulsive phase of labour.

References

Akerlund, M., Carlsson, A. M., Melin, P. & Trojnar, J. (1985). The effect on human uterus of two newly developed competitive inhibitors of oxytocin and vasopressin. *Acta Obstetrica et Gynecologica Scandinavica*, **64**, 499–504.

Akerlund, M., Stromberg, P., Hauksson, A., Andersen, L. F., Lyndrup, J. & Melin, P. (1987). Inhibition of uterine contractions of premature labour with an oxytocin analogue. Results from a pilot study. *British Journal of Obstetrics and Gynaecology*, **94**, 1040–4.

Altstein, M., Whitnall, M. H., House, S., Keys, S. & Gainer, H. J. (1988). An immunochemical analysis of oxytocin and vasopressin prohormone processing *in vivo*. *Peptides*, **9**, 87–105.

Amico, J. A., Ervin, M. G., Finn, F. M., Leake, R. D., Fisher, C. A. & Robinson, A. G. (1986). The plasma of pregnant women contains a novel oxytocin-vasotocin-like peptide. *Metabolism*, **35**, 586–601.

Amico, J. A., Seitchik, J. & Robinson, A. G. (1984). Studies of oxytocin in plasma of women during hypocontractile labor. *Journal of Clinical Endocrinology and Metabolism*, **58**, 274–9.

Andersen, L. F., Lyndrup, J. & Melin, P. (1989). Oxytocin receptor blockage: a new principle in the treatment of preterm labour. *American Journal of Perinatology*, **6**, 196–9.

Balment, R. J., Brimble, M. J. & Forsling, M. L. (1982). Oxytocin release and renal actions in normal and Brattleboro rats. *Annals of the New York Academy of Sciences*, **394**, 241–52.

Benedetto, M. T., De-Cicco, F., Rossiello, F., Nicosia, A. L., Lupi, G. & Dell-Acqua, S. (1990). Oxytocin receptor in human fetal membranes at term and during labour. *Journal of Steroid Biochemistry*, **35**, 205–8.

Bicknell, R. J. (1985). Endogenous opioid peptides and hypothalamic neuroendocrine neurones. *Journal of Endocrinology*, **107**, 436–46.

Boyd, N. R. H. & Chard, T. (1973). Human urine oxytocin levels during pregnancy and labor. *American Journal of Obstetrics and Gynecology*, **115**, 827–9.

Burd, J. M., Davison, J., Weightman, D. R. & Baylis, P. H. (1987). Evaluation of enzyme inhibitors of pregnancy associated oxytocinase: application to the measurement of plasma immunoreactive oxytocin during human labor. *Acta Endocrinologica*, **114**, 458–64.

Burford, G. D. & Robinson, I. C. A. F. (1982). Oxytocin, vasopressin and neurophysins in the hypothalamoneurohypophysial system of the human fetus. *Journal of Endocrinology*, **95**, 403–8.

Caldeyro-Barcia, R. & Sereno, J. A. (1961). The response of the human uterus to oxytocin throughout pregnancy. In *Oxytocin*. Ed R. Caldeyro-Barcia and H. Heller, pp. 177–200. Pergamon Press, New York.

Caldeyro-Barcia, R. & Theobald, G. W. (1968). Sensitivity of the pregnancy human uterus to oxytocin. *American Journal of Obstetrics and Gynecology*, **102**, 1181.

Challinor, S. M., Cameron, J. L. & Amico, J. Al (1992). Pulses of oxytocin in the cerebrospinal fluid of Rhesus monkeys. *Hormone Research*, **37**, 230–5.

Chan, W. Y., Powell, A. M. & Hruby, V. L. (1982). Antioxytocic and anti-prostaglandin releasing effects of oxytocin antagonists in pregnancy rats and pregnancy human myometrial strips. *Endocrinology*, **111**, 48–53.

Chard, T. (1972). The posterior pituitary in human and animal parturition. *Journal of Reproduction and Fertility*, **16**, 121–38.

Chard, T. (1973). The radioimmunoassay of oxytocin and vasopressin. *Journal of Endocrinology*, **58**, 143–60.

Chard, T. (1989). Fetal and maternal oxytocin in human parturition. *American Journal of Perinatology*, **6** (2), 145–52.

Chard, T., Boyd, N. R. H., Edwards, C. R. W. & Hudson, C. N. (1971). Release of oxytocin and vasopressin in the human fetus during labour. *Nature*, **234**, 352.

Chard, T., Boyd, N. R. H., Forsling, M. L., McNeilly, A. S. & Landon, J. (1970). The development of a radioimmunoassay for oxytocin: the extraction of oxytocin from plasma and its measurement during parturition in human and goat blood. *Journal of Endocrinology*, **48**, 223–34.

Chard, T. & Forsling, M. L. (1976). Bioassay and radioimmunoassay of oxytocin and vasopressin. In *Hormones in Human Blood*. Ed. H. N. Antoniades, pp. 488–516, Harvard University Press, Cambridge.

Chard, T. & Gibbens, G. L. D. (1983). Spurt release of oxytocin during surgical induction of labor in women. *American Journal of Obstetrics and Gynecology*, **147**, 678–80,

Chibbar, R., Miller, F. D. & Mitchell, B. F. (1993). Synthesis of oxytocin in amnion, chorion, and decidua may influence the timing of human parturition. *Journal of Clinical Investigation*, **91**, 185–92.

Chiodera, P., Salvarani, C., Bacchi-Modena, A., Spallanzani, R., Cigarini, C., Alboni, A., Gardini, E. & Coiro, V. (1991). Relationship between plasma profiles of oxytocin and adrenocorticotropin hormone during suckling or breast stimulation in women. *Hormone Research*, **35**, 119–23.

Clarke, G. & Lincoln, D. W. (1975). Evidence for a dopaminergic component in the milk-ejection reflex of the rat. *Journal of Endocrinology*, **67**, 32P–3P.

Cobo, E. (1968). Uterine and milk ejecting activities during human labor. *Journal of Applied Physiology*, **24**, 317–25.

Csapo, A. & Sauvage, J. (1968). The evolution of uterine activity during human pregnancy. *Acta Obstetrica et Gynecologica Scandinavica*, **47**, 181–91.

Cummiskey, K. C. & Dawood, M. Y. (1990). Induction of labour. *American Journal of Obstetrics and Gynecology*, **163**, 1868–74.

Dawood, M. Y. (1983). Neurohypophysial hormones. In *Endocrinology of Pregnancy*. Ed. F. Fuchs and A. Klopper, pp. 204–28, Harper & Row, New York.

De Geest, K., Thiery, M., Piron-Possuyt, G. & Vanden Driessche, R. (1985). Plasma oxytocin in human pregnancy and parturition. *Journal of Perinatal Medicine*, **13**, 3–13.

Dyer, R. G. (1988). Oxytocin and parturition – new complications. *Journal of Endocrinology*, **116**, 167–8.

Ervin, M. G., Amico, J. A., Leake, R. D., Ross, M. G., Robinson, A. G. & Fisher, D. A. (1988). Arginine vasotocin and a novel oxytocin-vasotocin-like material in plasma and human newborns. *Biology of the Neonate*, **53**, 17–22.

Falke, N. (1991). Modulation of oxytocin and vasopressin release at the level of the neurohypophysis. *Progress in Neurobiology*, **36**, 465–84.

Ferguson, J. K. W. (1941). A study of the motility of the intact uterus at term. *Surgery, Gynaecology and Obstetrics*, **73**, 359–66.

Frandsen, P. & Jensen, S. E. (1971). Excretion of oxytocin and vasopressin in human urine. *Acta Endocrinologica (Copenhagen)*, **66**, 540–5.

Fuchs, A. R. (1978). Hormonal control of myometrial function during pregnancy and parturition. *Acta Endocrinologica (Copenhagen)*, **89** (Suppl. 121), 1–70.

Fuchs, A. R. (1985). Oxytocin in animal parturition. In *Oxytocin. Clinical and Laboratory Studies*. Ed. J. A. Amico and A. G. Robinson, pp. 207–235, Excerpta Medical International Congress Series, Amsterdam.

Fuchs, A. R. & Fuchs, F. (1981). Ethanol for prevention of preterm birth. *Seminars in Perinatology*, **5**, 236–51.

Fuchs, A. R., Fuchs, F., Husslein, P., Soloff, M. S. & Fernstrom, M. J. (1982). Oxytocin receptors and human parturition: a dual role for oxytocin in the initiation of labor. *Science*, **215**, 1396–8.

Fuchs, A. R., Goeschen, K., Husslein, P., Rasmussen, A. B. & Fuchs, F. (1983). Oxytocin and the initation of labor. III. Plasma levels of oxytocin and 13,14-dihydro-15-keto-prostaglandin F2alpha during spontaneous oxytocin induced labor. *American Journal of Obstetrics and Gynecology*, **144**, 753–60.

Fuchs, A. R., Husslein, L., Sumulong, L., Micha, J. P., Dawood, M. Y. & Fuchs, F. (1982). Plasma levels of oxytocin and 13,14-dihydro-15-keto-PGF2alpha in preterm labor and the effect of ethanol and ritodrine. *American Journal of Obstetrics and Gynecology*, **144**, 753–60.

Fuchs, A. R., Husslein, P. & Fuchs, F. (1981). Oxytocin and the initiation of human parturition. II. Stimulation of prostaglandin production in human decidua by oxytocin. *American Journal of Obstetrics and Gynecology*, **141**, 694–7.

Fuchs, A. R., Husslein, P., Koffler, E., Grunberger, W., Rasmussen, A. & Rehnstrom, J. (1983). Effect of cervical application of prostaglandin (PG)E2 on plasma 13,14-dihydro-15-keto-PGF2 alpha and oxytocin in pregnant women at term. *British Journal of Obstetrics and Gynaecology*, **90**, 612–17.

Fuchs, A. R., Olsen, P. & Petersen, K. (1965). Effect of distention of uterus and vagina on uterine motility and oxytocin release in puerperal rabbits. *Acta Obstetrica et Gynecologica Scandinavica*, **50**, 239–48.

Fuchs, A. R., Peryasamy, S., Alexandrova, M. & Soloff, M. S. (1983). Correlation between oxytocin receptor concentration and responsiveness to oxytocin in pregnancy rat myometrium: effects of ovarian steroids. *Endocrinology*, **113**, 742–9.

Fuchs, A. R., Romero, R., Keefe, D., Parra, M., Oyarzun, E. & Behnke, E. (1991). Oxytocin secretion and human parturition: pulse frequency and duration increase during spontaneous labor in women. *American Journal of Obstetrics and Gynecology*, **165**, 1515–23.

Fuchs, A. R. & Wagner, G. (1963). Effect of alcohol on release of oxytocin. *Nature*, **198**, 92–4.

Fuchs, F. (1973). Initiation of labor – facts and fancies. In *Endocrine Factors in Labour*. Ed A. Kloppper and J. Gardner, pp. 1–24, Cambridge University Press, Cambridge.

Fuchs, F. (1985). The role of maternal and fetal oxytocin in human parturition. In *Oxytocin. Clincal and Laboratory Studies*. Ed J. Amico and A. G. Robinson, pp. 236–56, Excerpta Medica International Congress Series, Amsterdam.

Fuchs, R., Fuchs, A. R., Poblete, V. F. & Rizk, A. (1967). Effect of alcohol on threatened premature labor. *American Journal of Obstetrics and Gynecology*, **99**, 627–33.

Fuchs, A. R. & Wagner, G. (1963). Effect of alcohol on release of oxytocin. *Nature*, **198**, 92–4.

Gibbens, D., Boyd, N. R. H. & Chard, T. (1972). Spurt release of oxytocin during human labour. *Journal of Endocrinology*, **43**, iv.

Gibbens, G. L. D. & Chard, T. (1976). Observations on maternal oxytocin release during human labour and the effect of intravenous alcohol administration. *American Journal of Obstetrics and Gynecology*, **126**, 243–6.

Gillespie, A., Brummer, C. & Chard, T. (1972). Oxytocin release by infused prostaglandin. *British Medical Journal*, **1**, 543.

Gimeno, M. A. R., Bedners, A. S., De Vastik, F. J. K. & Gimeno, A. L. (1971). Effect of ethanol on the motility of isolated ray myometrium. *Archives of Pharmacodynamics and Therapeutics*, **191**, 213–17.

Ginsburg, M. (1968). Production, release, transportation and elimination of the neuro-hypophysial hormones, in *Neurohypophysial Hormones and Similar Polypeptides. Handbook of Experimental Pharmacology*. Ed. B. Berde, pp. 286–38]71, Springer-Verlag, Berlin.

Gonzalez-Panizza, V. H., Sica-Blanco, Y. & Mendez-Bauer, C. (1961). The fate of injected oxytocin in the pregnancy women near term. In *Oxytocin*. Ed R. Caldeyro-Barcia and H. Heller, pp. 347–51, Pergamon Press, London.

Goodfellow, C. F., Hull, M. G. R., Swaab, D. F., Dogterom, J. & Buijs, R. M. (1983). Oxytocin deficiency at delivery with epidural analgesia. *British Journal of Obstetrics and Gynaecology*, **90**, 214–19.

Gunther, M. (1948). The posterior pituitary and labour. *British Medical Journal*, **1**, 567–9.

Hirst, J. J., Haluska, G. J., Cook, M. J. & Novy, M. J. (1993). Plasma oxytocin and nocturnal uterine activity: maternal but not fetal concentrations increase progressively during late pregnancy and delivery in rhesus monkeys. *American Journal of Obstetrics and Gynecology*, **169**, 415–22.

Husslein, P., Fuchs, A. R. & Fuchs, F. (1981). Oxytocin and initiation of human parturition. I. Prostaglandin release during induction of labor by oxytocin. *American Journal of Obstetrics and Gynecology*, **141**, 688–93.

Karim, S. M. M. & Sharma, S. D. (1971). The effect of ethyl alcohol on prostaglandins E1 and F2alpha induced uterine activity in pregnancy women. *Journal of Obstetrics and Gynaecology of the British Commonwealth*, **78**, 251–6.

Khan-Dawood, F. S. & Dawood, M. Y. (1984). Oxytocin content in human fetal pituitary cells. *American Journal of Obstetrics and Gynecology*, **148**, 420–3.

Kuwabara, S., Takeda, M., Mizuno, M. & Sakamoto, S. (1987). Oxytocin levels in maternal and fetal plasma, amniotic fluid, and neonatal plasma and urine. *Archives of Gynecology and Obstetrics*, **241**, 12–23.

Lauersen, N. H., Raghavan, K. S., Wilson, K. H., Fuchs, F. & Niemann, W. H. (1973). Effect of prostaglandin F2alpha, oxytocin and ethanol on the uterus of the pregnant baboon. *American Journal of Obstetrics and Gynecology*, **115**, 912–18.

Lauersen, N. H., Wilson, K. H. & Fuchs, F. (1981). The inhibitory effect of ethanol on oxytocin-induced labor at term. *Journal of Reproductive Medicine*, **26**, 547–50.

Leake, R. D., Weitzman, R. E. & Fisher, D. A. (1980). Pharmacokinetics of oxytocin in the human subject. *Obstetrics and Gynecology*, **56**, 701–4.

Leake, D. R., Weitzman, R. E. & Fisher, D. A. (1981a). Oxytocin concentrations during the neonatal period. *Biology of the Neonate*, **39**, 127–31.

Leake, R. D., Weitzman, R. E., Glatz, T. H. & Fisher, D. A. (1981b). Plasma oxytocin concentrations in men, nonpregnant women and pregnant women before and during spontaneous labor. *Journal of Clinical Endocrinology and Metabolism*, **53**, 730–3.

Lindow, S. W., van der Spuy, Z., Hendricks, M. S., Rosselli, A. P., Lombard, C. & Leng, G. (1992). The effect of morphine and naloxone administration on plasma oxytocin concentrations in the first stage of labour. *Clinical Endocrinology*, **37**, 349–53.

MacDonald, P. C. & Casey, M. L. (1993). The accumulation of prostaglandins (PG) in amniotic fluid is an after effect of labour and not indicative of a role for PGE-2 or PGF-2α in the initiation of human parturition. *Journal of Clinical Endocrinology and Metabolism*, **76**, 1332–9.

Maggi, M., Del Carlo, P., Fantoni, G., Gianni, S., Torris, C., Casparis, D., Massi, G. & Serio, M. (1990). Human myometrium during pregnancy contains and responds to V1 vasopressin receptors as well as oxytocin receptors. *Journal of Clinical Endocrinology and Metabolism*, **70**, 1142–54.

Mantell, C. D. & Liggins, G. C. (1970). The effect of ethanol on the myometrial response to oxytocin in women at term. *Journal of Obstetrics and Gynaecology of the British Commonwealth*, **77**, 976–81.

Melin, P. (1993). Oxytocin antagonists and their therapeutic use. *Regulatory Peptides*, **45**, 285–8.

McNeilly, A. S., Robinson, I. C. A. F., Houston, M. J. & Howie, P. W. (1983). Release of oxytocin and prolactin in response to suckling. *British Medical Journal*, **286**, 257–9.

Mohr, E., Meherhof, W. & Richter, D. (1992). The hypothalamic hormone oxytocin: from gene expression to signal transduction. *Review of Physiology, Biochemistry and Pharmacology*, **121**, 31–48.

Moos, F. & Richard, P. H. (1975). Importance de la liberation d'oxytocine induite par la dilatation vaginale (reflexe de Ferguson) et la stimulation vagale (reflex vagopituitaire) chez la ratte. *Journal of Physiology (Paris)*, **70**, 307–32.

Nagata, I., Kato, K., Makimura, N., Uesato, T., Seki, K. & Kikuchi, Y. (1983). Comparison of plasma oxytocin levels during spontaneous labor induced by amniotomy, prostaglandin F2alpha and prostaglandin E2. *American Journal of Obstetrics and Gynecology*, **147**, 259–67.

Nagata, I., Seki, K., Uesato, T., Sunaga, H., Furuya, K., Makimura, N. & Kato, K. (1987). Changes in plasma oxytocin, prostaglandin E1, and 13,14-dihydro-15-keto-prostaglandin F2alpha during labor induced by prostaglandin E2 or F2alpha and spontaneous labor. *Acta Obstetrica et Gynecologica Scandinavica*, **39**, 1627–33.

Neumann, I., Russell, J. A. & Landgraf, R. (1992). Endogenous opioids regulate intracerebral oxytocin release during parturition in a region-specific manner. In *Progress in Brain Research*. Ed. A. Ermisch, R. Landgraf and H. J. Ruhle, pp. 55–8, Elsevier Science Publishers BV, Amsterdam.

Newman, R. B., Gill, P. J. & Katz, M. (1986). Uterine activity during pregnancy in ambulatory pateints. Comparison of singleton and twin gestations. *American Journal of Obstetrics and Gynecology*, **154**, 530–1.

Noddle, B. A. (1964). Transfer of oxytocin from the maternal to the foetal circulation of the ewe. *Nature*, **203**, 414–17.

Odem, R. R., Work, B. A. & Dawood, M. Y. (1988). Pulsatile oxytocin for induction of labor: a randomized prospective controlled study. *Journal of Perinatal Medicine*, **16**, 31–7.

Oosterbaan, H. P. & Swaab, D. F. (1989). Amniotic oxytocin and vasopressin in relation to human fetal development. *Early Human Development*, **19**, 253–62.

Otsuki, Y., Tanizawa, O., Yamaji, K., Fujita, M. & Kurachi, K. (1983a). Fetomaternal plasma oxytocin levels in normal and anencephalic pregnancies. *Acta Obstetrica et Gynecologica Scandinavica*, **62**, 235–7.

Otsuki, Y., Yamaji, K., Fujita, M., Takagi, T. & Tanizawa, O. (1983b). Serial plasma oxytocin levels during pregnancy and labor. *Acta Obstetrica et Gynecologica Scandinavica*, **62**, 15–18.

Ottensen, B., Hansen, B., Fahrenkrug, J. & Fuchs, A. R. (1984). Vasoactive intestinal polypeptide (VIP) stimulates oxytocin and vasopressin release from the neurohypophysis. *Endocrinology*, **115**, 1648–51.

Owen, J. & Hauth, J. C. (1992). Oxytocin for the induction or augmentation of labor. *Clinics in Obstetrics and Gynaecology*, **35**, 464–75.

Padayachi, T., Norman, R. J., Dhavaraj, K., Kemp, M. & Joubert, S. M. (1988). Serial oxytocin levels in amniotic fluid and maternal plasma during normal and induced labour. *British Journal of Obstetrics and Gynaecology*, **95**, 888–93.

Pasetto, N., Zicari, A., Piccione, E., Lenti, L., Pontieri, G. & Ticconi, C. (1992). Influence of labour and oxytocin on in vitro leukotriene release by human fetal membranes and uterine decidua at term gestation. *American Journal of Obstetrics and Gynecology*, **166**, 1500–6.

Pavlou, C., Barker, G. H., Roberts, A. & Chamberlain, G. V. P. (1978). Pulsed oxytocin infusion in the induction of labour. *British Journal of Obstetrics and Gynaecology*, **85**, 96–100.

Pochard, J. L. & Lutz-Bucher, B. (1986). Vasopressin and oxytocin levels in human noenates. *Acta Paediatrica Scandinavica*, **75**, 774–8.

Richard, P., Moos, F. & Freund-Mercier, M. (1991). Central effects of oxytocin. *Physiology Reviews*, **71**, 331–70.

Robinson, I. C. A. F. (1980). The development and evaluation of a sensitive and specific radioimmunoassay for oxytocin in unextracted plasma. *Journal of Immunoassay*, **1**, 323–47.

Russell, J. A., Gosden, R. G., Humphreys, E. M., Cutting, R., Fitzsimmons, N., Johnson, V., Liddle, S., Scott, S. & Stirland, J. A. (1989). Interruption of parturition in rats by morphine: a result of inhibition of oxytocin secretion. *Journal of Endocrinology*, **121**, 521–36.

Saameli, K. (1963). An indirect method for the estimation of oxytocin blood concentrations and half-life in pregnant women near term. *American Journal of Obstetrics and Gynecology*, **85**, 186–92.

Sadowsky, D. W., Martel, J., Cabalum, T., Poore, M. G. & Nathanielsz, P. W. (1992). Oxytocin given in a pulsatile manner to the ewe at 120 and 140 days' gestational age increases fetal sheep plasma cortisol. *American Journal of Obstetrics and Gynecology*, **166**. 200–5.

Schrok, A., Fidi, C., Low, M. & Baumgarten, K. (1989). Low-dose ethanol for inhibition of preterm uterine activity. *American Journal of Perinatology*, **8**, 191–5.

Sellers, S. M., Hodgson, H. T., Mountford, L. A., Mitchell, M. D., Anderson, A. B. M. & Turnbull, A. C. (1981). Is oxytocin involved in parturition? *British Journal of Obstetrics and Gynaecology*, **88**, 725–9.

Sende, P., Pantelakis, N., Susuki, K. & Bashore, R. (1976). Plasma oxytocin determinations in pregnancy with diabetes insipidus. *Obstetrics and Gynecology*, **48**, 38S–51S.

Seoud, M. A. F., Sayigh, R., Khayat, H., Ali, L. A. & Azoury, R. S. (1993). Electrical breast stimulation: oxytocin, prolactin and uterine response. *Journal of Reproductive Medicine*, **38**, 438–42.

Shangold, M. M., Freeman, R., Kumaresan, P., Feder, A. S. & Vasicka, A. (1983). Plasma oxytocin concentrations in a pregnant woman with total vasopressin deficiency. *Obstetrics and Gynecology*, **61**, 662–7.

Stock, S., Bremme, K. & Uvnas-Moberg, K. (1991). Plasma levels of oxytocin during the menstrual cycle, pregnancy and following treatment with HMG. *Human Reproduction*, **8**, 1056–62.

Swaab, D. F. & Oosterbaan, H. P. (1983). Exclusion of the fetal brain as the main source of rat and human amniotic fluid oxytocin. *British Journal of Obstetrics and Gynaecology*, **90**, 1160–7.

Swanson, L. W. & Sawchenko, P. E. (1983). Hypothalamic integration: organisation of the paraventricular and supraoptic nuclei. *Annual Review of Neuroscience*, **6**, 269–324.

Theobald, G. W. (1969). Oxytocin reassessed. *Obstetrical and Gynaecological Survey*, **23**, 109–16.

Theobald, G. W., Robards, M. F. & Suter, T. (1969). Changes in myometrial sensitivity to oxytocin in man during the last six weeks of pregnancy. *Journal of Obstetrics and Gynaecology of the British Commonwealth*, **76**, 385–90.

Thornton, S. & Davison, J. M. (1988). Plasma oxytocin during third stage of labour: comparison of natural and active management. *British Medical Journal*, **297**, 167–9.

Thornton, S., Davison, J. M. & Baylis, P. H. (1989). Amniotomy-induced labour is not mediated by endogenous oxytocin. *British Journal of Obstetrics and Gynaecology*, **96**, 945–8.

Thornton, S., Davison, J. M. & Baylis, P. H. (1992). Plasma oxytocin during the first and second stages of spontaneous human labour. *Acta Endocrinologica*, **126**, 425–9.

Thornton, S., Murray, B. J. & Baylis, P. H. (1993). The effect of early labour, maternal analgesia and fetal acidosis on fetal plasma oxytocin concentrations. *British Journal of Obstetrics and Gynaecology*, **100**, 425–9.

Vasicka, A., Kumaresan, P., Han, G. S. & Kumaresan, M. (1978). Plasma oxytocin in initiation of labor. *American Journal of Obstetrics and Gynecology*, **130**, 263–73.

Verbalis, J. G., McCann, M. J., McHale, C. M. & Stricker, E. M. (1986). Oxytocin secretion in response to cholecystokinin and food: differentiation of nausea from satiety. *Science*, **232**, 1417–19.

Zahn, V. (1984). Uterine contractions during pregnancy. *Journal of Perinatal Medicine*, **12**, 107–12.

Zingg, H. H., Lefebvre, D. L. & Giaid, A. (1993). Uterine oxytocin gene expression: a novel framework for oxytocin action. *Regulatory Peptides*, **45**, 43–6.

Zlatnik, F. J. & Fuchs, F. (1972). A controlled study of ethanol in threatened premature labour. *American Journal of Obstetrics and Gynecology*, **112**, 610–12.

13

The cervix during pregnancy

A. A. CALDER

Through the course of a woman's life, the uterine cervix may do many things. During her reproductive years it transmits a monthly flow of menses and produces a peri-ovulatory secretion of mucus. It can accept and transport semen, a function vital for conception and it is capable of being 'capped' to prevent conception. It may be subject to displacements such as prolapse or diseases, most importantly cancers which may even end her life. Surgical dilatation may be necessary for termination of pregnancy, while failure to remain competent may lead to premature expulsion of the pregnancy. However, the paramount function is to remain securely closed for the normal duration of pregnancy and then to dilate widely, quickly and efficiently to permit passage of the offspring during parturition. This latter drama, perhaps the command performance of the cervix, will probably occur on only a very few occasions, occupying a few hours in the course of a lifetime. These functions are crucial for efficient and successful propagation of the species.

The physiological mechanisms which regulate these functions, although not yet fully elucidated, are steadily becoming clearer. Much of the confusion and uncertainty which has surrounded this subject can be attributed to a basic failure to define the cervix in anatomical and structural terms, a deficiency which only began to be rectified with the contribution of Danforth fewer than 50 years ago (Danforth, 1947). No single contribution has approached this in importance for the understanding of the human cervix and, like many another important advance in the history of medicine, Danforth's work was initially greeted with scepticism, at times bordering on ridicule.

The great cervix controversy

While *competence* of the cervix – the capacity to remain firmly closed for the greater part of pregnancy – has long been recognized as essential to a successful outcome, the means whereby this is accomplished remains far from clear. There has been a widely held presumption that the uterus is a sort of sac designed to contain the growing conceptus and then expel the mature fetus. As such it has been viewed as essentially a muscular structure, the two main parts of which were the corpus, whose contractility was required for expulsion, and the cervix, whose contractility was necessary for containment. Traditional anatomical teaching complicated this simple picture by the concept of the *isthmus* which, following the work of Aschoff (1905), became an established component of uterine anatomy. For the past 90 years, the isthmus has been considered to be that part of the non-pregnant uterus lying between the corpus and the cervix. Its boundaries were defined only by landmarks within the lumen of the uterus, namely the anatomical internal os where the uterine cavity is seen to constrict down to the diameter of the endocervical canal and the (lower) histological internal os which marked the microscopic point of transition from endocervical mucosa to 'isthmic mucosa' (which more closely resembled endometrium). The original illustration from Aschoff's second publication is reproduced as Fig. 1 (Aschoff, 1906).

Present-day clinicians have been brought up with the concept of a 'lower uterine segment' which is said to develop from the isthmus during pregnancy. This part of the uterus is considered to stretch and widen as pregnancy advances in order to accommodate the fetal head as it presents towards the pelvis. An important practical implication of this concept is that, should the placenta be implanted within this 'lower segment', there is a high likelihood of haemorrhage during the ante-partum or intra-partum period.

These concepts of 'isthmus' and 'lower uterine segment' have been uncritically accepted for decades but may now be usefully challenged. To begin with it seems quite unsatisfactory to define a portion of the uterus entirely on the basis of surface landmarks within the lumen. To do so is comparable with saying that Oxfordshire is that part of England which lies between the towns of Goring and Lechlade on the river Thames. It becomes even more unsatisfactory when one recognizes, as did Danforth, that Aschoff's landmarks of an anatomical and histological internal os are so imprecise.

In his 1947 paper, Danforth described his original studies on the anatomy of the uterus which led him to the conclusion: 'Therefore, it is believed that the concept of the isthmus uteri as a separate, distinct entity should be eliminated and that, rather, the uterus should be considered as being composed of two major parts, corpus and cervix, according to whether the fundamental structure is chiefly muscular or chiefly fibrous'. He based this conclusion on his finding that the transition from fibrous to muscular tissue in the lower part of the uterus is generally quite abrupt and that the area of the uterus traditionally described as the isthmus (hard to define though it was) 'is an indefinite variable segment

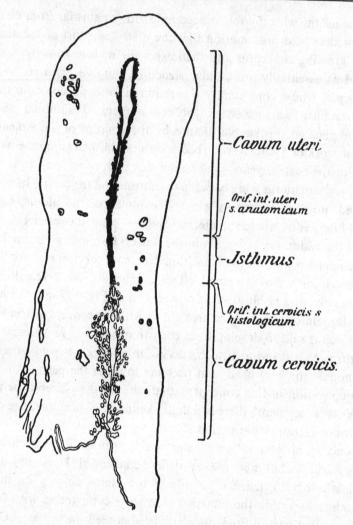

-Cavum uteri

Orif. int. uteri
s. anatomicum

-Isthmus

Orif. int. cervicis s
histologicum

-Cavum cervicis.

Fig. 1. Original drawing reproduced from the work of Aschoff (1906) to illustrate his concept of the uterine isthmus lying between his two separately defined ora of the cervix: *Anatomicium and Histologicum*.

composed principally of smooth muscle ... is bounded below by the fibrous cervix, and which above blends imperceptibly with the remainder of the uterine musculature'. He concluded this iconoclastic contribution with the view that the isthmus should be considered as part of the corpus (just as the fundus is part of the corpus) stopping just short of suggesting that the concept of an isthmus might be eliminated altogether.

Danforth's findings were supported the following year by his fellow Americans Schwarz & Woolf (1948) but there followed a series of transatlantic challenges.

Nixon of University College Hospital (Nixon, 1951) with the support of Hughesden also of UCH (Hughesden, 1952) and C. P. Wendell-Smith of St Bartholomew's Hospital (Wendell-Smith, 1954) mounted a highly critical assault on the Danforth thesis. They accused him of suggesting 'entirely false inferences' and of having been misled and let down by artefact and inadequate methods of examination. Nixon attempted to refute Danforth's view with recordings which seemed to demonstrate independent contractile properties of the cervix. Danforth (1954) countered by accusing Nixon of a *non sequitur* and of drawing 'entirely illogical' conclusions. In essence, Danforth accepted the capacity of the cervix to contract, but stressed that this was in no way incompatible with his claim that the cervix was *predominantly* composed of fibrous tissue.

Hughesden's findings were that the outermost quarter of the cervix was muscular and the inner three-quarters collagenous which may not seem too much at odds with the Danforth concept. However, the main point of contention was Hughesden's claim that the muscle was of greater functional importance than the connective tissue; Wendell-Smith's paper on the 'lower uterine segment' reinforced this view.

Danforth returned to the offensive with his rebuttal of 1954 (Danforth, 1954), a rejoinder which he was later to reflect may have been 'a caustic reply' and 'a fine example of overkill' (Danforth, 1980) but thereafter the matter seems to have been allowed to rest. During the intervening 40 years, however, the concepts of 'uterine isthmus' and 'lower uterine segment' have remained prominent in the thinking and teaching of obstetricians and gynaecologists. However, from a physiological standpoint, if not an anatomical one, the need to understand the function of the cervix during pregnancy and labour in terms of connective tissue biology rather than smooth muscle physiology has steadily gained currency.

Perhaps all concerned would have benefited from studying the contribution from the father of the anatomy of the pregnant uterus William Hunter. '*Ad cervicem uteri, fimbrae musculosae, in fasciculos collecti, nullae conspicientur*' wrote Hunter in his *Magnum Opus The Anatomy of the Human Gravid Uterus* in 1774. 'At the cervix, no distinct bundles of muscle fibres are to be seen.' This wonderful atlas, engraved by Sir Robert Strange from the drawings by Jan van Rymsdyke of Hunter's original anatomical dissections, gave a remarkable insight into the uterus during pregnancy more than two centuries ago, an insight which has scarcely been improved upon to this day, despite the sophistication of modern techniques of diagnostic imaging. What better illustration could we have of the clinical problem of *placenta praevia* than plate XII from Hunter's atlas (Fig. 2). Hunter bequeathed virtually all his estate to the University of Glasgow including the original chalk illustrations by van Rymsdyke. Of further interest are many of the original dissections; these survive within the Department of Anatomy.

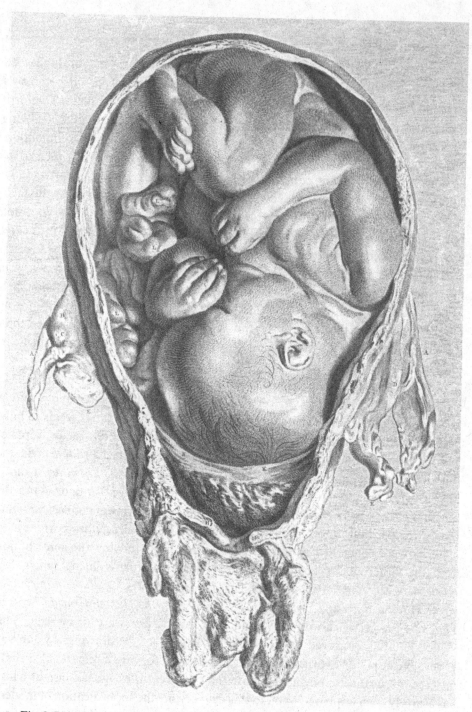

Fig. 2. Plate XII from *The Anatomy of the Human Gravid Uterus*, William Hunter (1774). This illustrated Hunter's dissection of a woman who 'died of a flooding in the ninth month of pregnancy'. It shows the situation of the placenta 'at the inside of the mouth of the womb under the child's head and detached from the womb, the occasion of the fatal haemorrhage'. Hunter goes on to observe 'as parturition approached the dilatation of these parts occasioned a separation which was necessarily followed by an haemorrhage'. This represents a classic description of a major degree of *placenta praevia*.

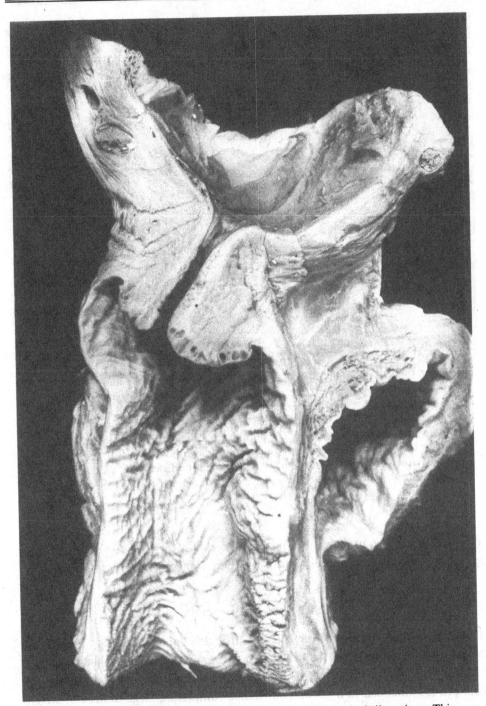

Fig. 3. A photograph of one of William Hunter's anatomical dissections. This shows 'the cervix uteri in the ninth month of pregnancy'. Hunter described it as 'a side view of the cervix uteri in its short state also of the vagina and bladder'. (From the Hunterian Anatomical Museum, University of Glasgow, by kind permission of Professor R. J. Scothorne.)

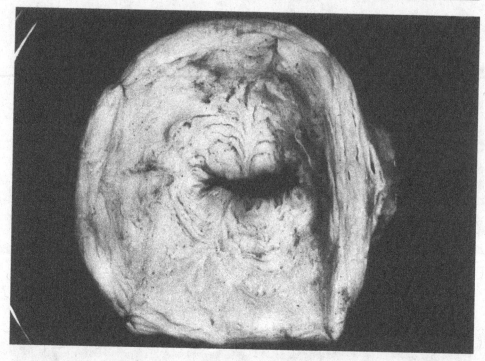

Fig. 4. Photograph of another of Hunter's dissections 'the cervix and os uteri in the last month of pregnancy'. The mucosal pattern of the cervix, forming the *plicae palmatae* (literally palm like folds) is clearly seen and shows the progress of effacement or 'taking up' of the cervix in late pregnancy, this mucosa having hitherto occupied the endocervical canal. The fibromuscular junction described in the text will by this stage have demonstrated a centrifugal migration towards the periphery of the specimen. (From the Hunterian Anatomical Museum in the Anatomy Department of the University of Glasgow by kind permission of Professor R. H. Scothorne.)

Photographs of two of these specimens are reproduced as Figs. 3 and 4 and these give a fascinating view of the anatomy of the human cervix in late pregnancy.

Structure of the cervix

The main formed element of the cervical stroma is collagen, fibrils of which are bound together into dense bundles. It is these which confer on the cervix the rigidity which characterizes its non-pregnant and early pregnant condition. The collagen is embedded in a ground substance comprising large molecular weight proteoglycan complexes containing a variety of glycosaminoglycans (GAGs). In cervical tissue the most abundant GAGs are chondroitin and its epimer, dermatan sulphate (von Maillot *et al.*, 1979; Uldbjerg, Ekman & Malstrom,

1983*a*). As well as forming the ground substance of the tissue, proteoglycans invest collagen fibrils with their protein cores attaching to the collagen (Scott & Orford, 1981). The relationship between the GAG side chains and the collagen fibrils is important in orientating the latter and conferring on the cervix its mechanical strength (Lindahl & Hook, 1978; Golichowski, 1980). Qualitative changes in the proteoglycans and their constituent GAGs are responsible for altering the binding of collagen and for facilitating collagen breakdown.

The major cellular component of cervical connective tissue is the fibroblast. These cells appear to be responsible for the synthesis of both collagen and ground substance. The cervix also contains elastin fibres (Leppert & Yu, 1990) but this is six- or seven-fold less abundant than is the collagen component. Where the role of collagen seems likely to confer rigidity on the tissue, elastin may be responsible for the element of the elasticity; this assists in closing the cervix after delivery and thereafter returning it to its non-pregnant configuration.

The presence of muscle within the cervical tissue, and the controversy relating to its functional role, have already been discussed. While opinion has undoubtedly moved towards the view that the connective tissue in the cervix is functionally more important than the muscle component, it would nevertheless be facile to suggest that the muscle in the cervix is present to no purpose. It is unquestionably capable of both spontaneous and drug induced contractility (Nixon, 1951; Hillier & Karim, 1970). It seems unlikely, both on the basis of the low concentration of muscle and also its spatial arrangement within the cervix, that it fulfils any sort of muscular sphincter mechanism. However, it may, as Hughesden (1952) claimed, have a role in transmitting a longitudinal pull onto the cervix from the contracting corpus. More likely is the possibility that its role is restricted to protecting important blood vessels during labour and perhaps also bringing about prompt closure of the cervix following delivery.

Normal cervical function in pregnancy

Conception

The cervix, and, in particular, the plug of mucus which occupies its canal are considered important in the uptake from the vagina of semen and its onward transmission to the expectant ovum. It is generally accepted that the situation and direction of the cervix in the upper dilated portion of the vagina leads to immersion of the external os in the seminal pool which collects in the posterior vaginal fornix (Elstein & Chantler, 1991). The diameter of the external os and cervical canal show cyclical alterations favouring the passage of sperm during the preovulatory phase of the cycle. The uptake of sperm cells into the cervical mucus is thought to protect them from the hostile environment of the vagina, and from being phagocytosed, and there may be a nutritive contribution from the mucus to assist with the energy requirements of sperm. The process of sperm capacitation may also occur, at least in part, within cervical mucus (Lambert, Overstreet & Morales, 1985). It is thus important that the cervix and its mucus should perform these functions efficiently if normal fertility is to be attained. The concept of hostile cervical mucus, whether due to immunological or biochemical abnormalities, is often proposed as a cause of subfertility. Further problems may arise from structural abnormalities in the cervix, whether congenital or acquired.

Maintenance of pregnancy

The most obvious role of the cervix in pregnancy is to remain closed thereby holding the developing conceptus within the uterine cavity. In view of this, it may seem surprising that one of the earliest clinical signs of pregnancy is a softening of the cervical tissue. A pelvic examination in early pregnancy reveals an increase in vascularity which confers an obvious colour change and softening in the consistency of the cervix. This is rather surprisingly accompanied by an *increase* is the internal diameter of the endocervical canal during the first trimester to as much as one centimetre (Johnstone *et al.*, 1974). This could be the result of radial hypertrophy although this has not been quantified. There does not, however, appear to be any dramatic change in the length of the endocervical canal during the first half of pregnancy (Calder, 1981). The overall length of the cervix remains constant at around 4.5 centimetres in the non-pregnant condition and throughout the first half of pregnancy.

The increasing softness of the early pregnant cervix accords with measures of compliance of the cervix at that time. Anthony *et al.* (1982) employed an electronic device in order to measure the forces required to bring about short-term dilatation of the cervix up to 8 millimetres in pregnant and non-pregnant subjects (Fig. 5). In nulliparous subjects, the presence of a first trimester pregnancy leads to a reduction of approximately one-third in the force required for such surgical dilatation and a reduction of one quarter in multiparas.

Despite these changes, the cervix continues to resist dilatation, remaining competent and fulfilling its role as gatekeeper of the uterus until the later stages of pregnancy. It would appear to have two principal functions. The first is mechanical: remaining closed in order to retain the growing amniotic sac within the uterine cavity. The second is to block the entry of pathogenic organisms or other noxious influences through the endocervical canal. In this second role it relies on the *operculum* or mucus plug which not only acts as a physical block but also possesses anti-bacterial properties. Studies of the ultrastructure of the cervix show little change in the composition of the stroma through the first and

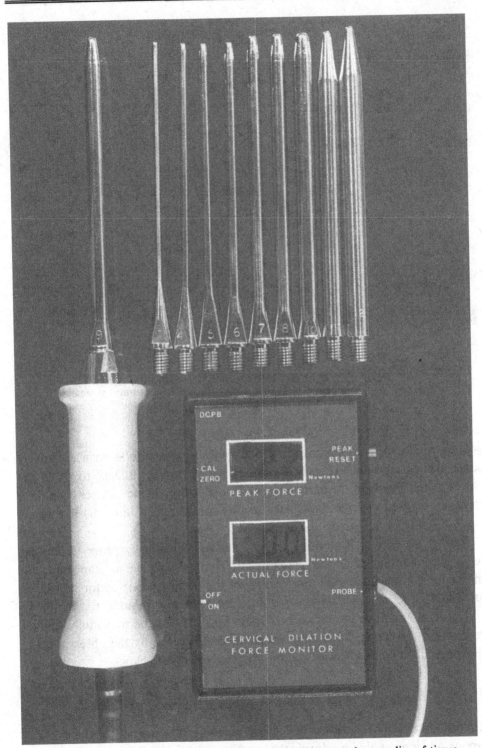

Fig. 5. Electronic force measuring device employed to conduct studies of tissue compliance during surgical dilatation.

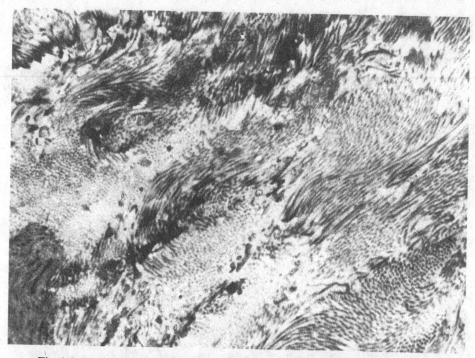

Fig. 6. An electron micrograph of cervical stroma during the first half of pregnancy. Collagen fibres are abundant and well organized while the ground substance is relatively sparse.

second trimesters, with a preponderance of highly organized collagen in a relatively scant ground substance (Fig. 6). Although it has proved difficult to study the cervix histologically in the more advanced stages of pregnancy, it seems unlikely that any marked change takes place in this configuration until the five or six weeks leading up to parturition (*prelabour*).

Among the factors responsible for maintaining pregnancy progesterone has long been considered to be pre-eminent. It may also be as important for maintaining the competence and rigidity of the uterine cervix as for its role as an inhibitor of myometrial contractility. Progesterone inhibits the action of collagenase within the uterine corpus (Jeffrey *et al.*, 1971) and may fulfil a similar role within the cervix. Such an assumption is supported by the observation of the cervical softening effect of the antiprogesterones (see below).

Late pregnancy – cervical ripening

The remarkable phenomenon of cervical ripening is a prelude to the onset of labour, and is most obvious during the last five or six weeks of pregnancy although

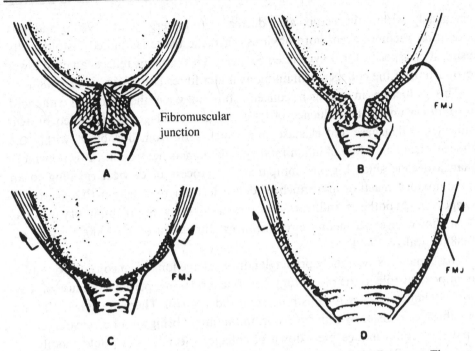

Fig. 7. Diagrammatic representation of the process of cervical effacement. The fibromuscular junction shows centrifugal migration from around the original internal cervical os resulting in a reduction in the length of the cervix as a prelude to dilatation. (From Danforth & Hendrick, 1977, with permission.)

it may have its origins even earlier. Ripening refers to the increased softening, distensibility, effacement and early dilatation which can be readily detected by digital pelvic examination. The most obvious component of the process is a change in shape, from a long, closed barrel-like structure to a thin saccular configuration. This remarkable change from a structure with a length of three or four centimetres to one of virtually no length is known as effacement. It is illustrated in Fig. 7 and may be seen happening in Hunter's specimen shown as Fig. 3. This would probably correspond to part (*b*) of Fig. 7 (Danforth & Hendrick, 1977).

Such a radical change in the shape of the cervix before the onset of labour would be impossible were it not for profound alterations in the biomechanical properties of cervical tissue. These changes include a reduction in collagen concentration, an increase in water content and a change in GAG composition (Calder & Greer, 1992). The cervical connective tissue at term shows widely scattered and dissociated fibrils of collagen and a marked increase in the ground substance when compared to the non-pregnant or early pregnant cervix (Danforth, Buckingham & Roddick, 1960). The concentration of collagen measured biochemically within the cervix also decreases (Uldbjerg *et al.*, 1983*b*) and this alteration becomes even more obvious when the tissue is studied histologically using stains specific for polymerized collagen. This perhaps reflects an even lower proportion of the collagen remaining as intact fibres (Junqueira *et al.*, 1980).

This reduction in collagen concentration may be the result of enhanced breakdown under the influence of lytic enzymes. Collagen is degraded by two enzymes, collagenase and elastase, and which arise from fibroblasts within the tissue or from an influx of inflammatory cells such as neutrophils. It is now more than a decade since Liggins compared the process of cervical ripening to an inflammatory reaction and much evidence has emerged within that period to support his hypothesis. Infiltration of cervical tissue with inflammatory cells has been shown in experimental circumstances (Junquiera *et al.*, 1980; Rath *et al.*, 1988; Chwalisz, 1988).

Prostaglandins, especially prostaglandin E_2, have long been considered to play an important role in the physiology of cervical ripening, perhaps because of their proven clinical efficacy for this purpose (Calder, 1980). There are essentially two possible mechanisms by which prostaglandins might bring about cervical ripening. First they could induce breakdown of collagen. Second they could modify the binding of collagen and the hydration of tissue by altering the composition of the proteoglycan complexes. Treatment with prostaglandin E_2 reduces collagen concentration (Ekman, Malmstrom & Uldbjergn, 1086) but it is not clear whether this is the result of collagen breakdown. Szalay and colleagues (1981) have reported an increase in collagenase activity following the administration of PGE_2 while others (Ellwood *et al.*, 1981; Rath *et al.*, 1987) have shown no such change. Rath and colleagues supported their findings by showing an absence of collagen degradation products following prostaglandin therapy. The alternative explanation, namely that prostaglandins act by altering the ground substance, is supported by the studies of several groups (Norstrom, 1984; Cabrol *et al.*, 1987) while Johnston *et al.* (1993) have demonstrated that PGE_2 administration in late pregnancy provokes a rise in circulating levels of chondroitin sulphate similar to those seen in spontaneous labour. This supports the concept that PGE_2 may induce a breakdown in the proteoglycan complex.

Other naturally occurring substances may influence this process. Reference has already been made to the inhibitory role of progesterone while oestrogens such as oestradiol may favour cervical ripening, perhaps by stimulating prostaglandin production within the tissues (Horton & Poyser, 1976).

There is strong theoretical evidence for a role of relaxin in human cervical ripening. It is known to provoke increased collagenase activity (von Maillot *et al.*, 1977) perhaps via a mitogenic effect of fibroblasts which are known to have relaxin receptors (McMurty, Floerscheim & Bryant-Greenwood, 1980). However,

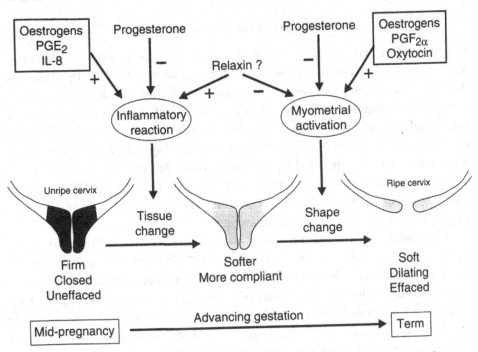

Fig. 8. Schematic representation of the process of cervical ripening and the biological factors which may control this process.

an unequivocal role for this hormone in human cervical ripening remains to be demonstrated.

Our own group has reported production of interleukin-8 by the human cervix (Barclay *et al.*, 1993). Interleukin-8 is the neutrophil attracting or activating peptide (NAP-1) and may be responsible for bringing about the influx of neutrophils into cervical tissue (Junqueira *et al.*, 1980; Rath *et al.*, 1988). It is possible that the role of prostaglandin E_2 in promoting cervical ripening may be the result of synergistic interaction with interleukin-8 (Colditz, 1990). Thus prostaglandin E_2 may act by dilating and increasing the permeability of cervical blood vessels; this allows interleukin-8 to draw neutrophils into the substance of the tissue and stimulate them to degranulate and release their collagenolytic enzymes. These concepts are summarized in Fig. 8.

Abnormalities of cervical function

The cervix fulfils two equally important and opposite roles: to remain shut for the duration of gestation and to open efficiently during parturition. Failure of the first may produce the clinical phenomenon of cervical incompetence, failure of the second is usually the result of absence of normal cervical ripening.

Cervical incompetence

Failure of the cervix to remain closed for the normal duration of pregnancy may lead either to spontaneous abortion in the second trimester or to premature delivery. The aetiology of cervical incompetence is obscure, but there may be congenital or acquired deficiencies in the cervix. Danforth (1980) suggested that there might be an excess of muscle while Leppert and Yu (1990) proposed an excess of elastin. A failure of normal cervical development may sometimes be responsible. This is supported by the observation that cervical incompetence is often found in women whose mothers were exposed to diethylstilboestrol in early pregnancy (Novy, Hammond & Nichols, 1990). Other cases may be the result of obstetric injury or gynaecological surgery.

Traditionally such cases have been treated by cervical cerclage. The recent report from the MRC/RCOG working party (1993) has concluded that the operation may be beneficial. The study included 1292 women whose obstetricians were uncertain whether to recommend cerclage or not. The subjects were randomized to cerclage or no cerclage. The conclusion was that the operation had been beneficial in only 1 case in 25 of the study population but at the price of increased complications (albeit it might be expected to perform better in women in whom the obstetricians were convinced of its benefit). This clinical condition has always been difficult to diagnose. Efforts are continuing to find a more reliable clinical index such as the use of ultrasound (Calder, 1981) or the use of measurements of cervical resistance between pregnancies (Anthony, Calder & Macnaughton, 1982) using the device illustrated in Fig. 5.

Failure of cervical ripening

The process of cervical ripening is normally gradual and progressive in the last five or six weeks of pregnancy. Bishop, whose scoring system is used to assess cervical ripeness (Bishop, 1964) showed in his original study that the degree of cervical ripeness was inversely correlated with the delay before the onset of spontaneous labour. An unripe cervix at term is particularly ominous in primigravid women. The onset of labour may be delayed and artificial induction will often lead to a difficult and complicated labour with a high level of fetal and maternal complications including maternal pyrexia, Caesarean section and birth asphyxia (Calder, 1980). In most instances, cervical ripening goes hand in hand with the onset of parturition, reflecting the synchrony between corpus and cervix. Failure of cervical ripening is probably therefore synonymous with failure of the onset of labour. There are sporadic reports in the literature of spontaneous annular detachment of the cervix during labour (Ingraham & Taylor, 1947) which points to the possibility that these two processes are not always intimately linked.

Cervical softening

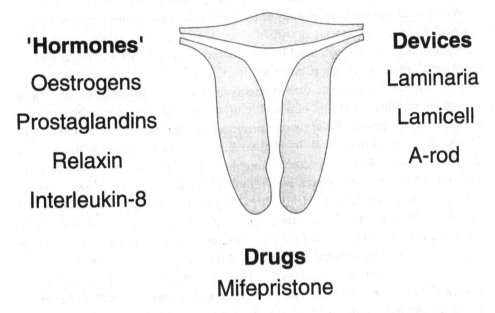

'Hormones'

Oestrogens

Prostaglandins

Relaxin

Interleukin-8

Devices

Laminaria

Lamicell

A-rod

Drugs

Mifepristone

Fig. 9. Schematic representation of the therapeutic options for cervical softening.

From a clinical standpoint, there is a need to avoid methods of inducing labour which do not, at the same time, address the question of cervical ripening.

Cervical therapy

Therapy to ripen the cervix may improve the clinical outcome either if the cervix has failed to ripen normally at term or if there is a need to interrupt the pregnancy at an earlier gestation. A variety of naturally occurring substances, mechanical devices and drugs have been directed towards this clinical objective (Fig. 9). At term pregnancy the agent of choice is prostaglandin E_2 administered locally within the genital tract in a gel (Calder & Greer, 1992). Alternative therapies such as oestrogens have been explored but have not gained an established place. Relaxin showed some early promise (MacLennan, 1981) but recent experience with recombinant human preparations has proved disappointing (Brennand, J. B. *et al.*, unpublished observations). In early pregnancy the choice of a cervical softening agent has been between prostaglandin analogues such as gemeprost or intracervical devices such as laminaria, 'Lamicell' or 'the A-rod'. These techniques increase cervical compliance and reduce the surgical effort required to produce dilatation. It is hard to find definite evidence that such techniques reduce the morbidity of termination of pregnancy, but clinicians feel more comfortable when cervical dilatation is accomplished without undue effort.

Where interruption of pregnancy at later gestation calls for induction of labour, cervical ripening is associated with a consistent reduction in the incidence of complications such as prolonged labour, maternal pyrexia, fetal hypoxia and the need for Caesarean section (Calder & Greer, 1992).

The most exciting recent development concerns the antiprogesterone agent mifepristone. This is the first of a family of compounds which interfere with the action of progesterone. Mifepristone produces cervical softening throughout the course of gestation (Radestad, Bygdeman & Green, 1988; Rodger & Baird, 1990; Frydman *et al.*, 1991). These compounds hold great promise for improving the outcome of clinical procedures which depend on a soft cervix. Their mode of action is not as yet entirely clear, although one possibility is inhibition of the metabolic breakdown of endogenous prostaglandins (Kelly & Bukman, 1990). They are already used for medical interruption of early pregnancy, and at later stages when a specific cervical effect is desirable (prior to surgical dilatation or as a prelude to myometrial stimulation). The duration and quantity of uterine contractility is much reduced. There has been little experience with these agents as an adjunct to labour induction at term, but the early indications are extremely promising.

Conclusions

The uterine cervix plays a crucial role in the maintenance of pregnancy and process of parturition. The mechanisms whereby the cervix remains closed through the course of gestation prior to rapid dilatation over a very few hours during labour have not yet been fully elucidated. A complete understanding of these processes depends on recognition of the fibrous nature of cervical tissue and on knowledge of the roles of muscle and collagen, steroid hormones and prostaglandins, inflammatory cells and lytic enzymes.

References

Anthony, G. S., Calder, A. A. & Macnaughton, M. C. (1982). Cervical resistance in patients with previous spontaneous mid-trimester abortion. *British Journal of Obstetrics and Gynaecology*, **89**, 1046–9.

Anthony, G. S., Fisher, J., Coutts, J. R. T. & Calder, A. A. (1982). Forces required for surgical dilatation of the pregnant and non-pregnant human cervix. *British Journal of Obstetrics and Gynaecology*, **89**, 913–16.

Aschoff, L. (1905). Zur Cervix Frage: Machtag zu der Arbeit der Herrn Dr Hohmieier. *Monatschrift für Geburtschülfe und Gynäkologie*, **22**, 611.

Aschoff, L. (1906). *Zeitschrift für Geburtschülfe und Gynäkologie*, **58**, 328.

Barclay, C. G., Brennand, J. E., Kelly, R. W. & Calder, A. A. (1993). Interleukin-8 production by the human cervix. *American Journal of Obstetrics and Gynecology*, (in press).

Bishop, E. H. (1964). Pelvic scoring for elective induction. *Obstetrics and Gynecology*, **24**, 266–8.

Cabrol, D., Dubois, P., Sedbon, E. *et al.* (1987). Prostaglandin E_2-induced changes in the distribution of glycosaminoglycans in the isolated rat uterine cervix. *European Journal of Obstetrics and Gynecology*, **26**, 359–65.

Calder, A. A. (1980). Pharmacological management of the unripe cervix in the human. In *Dilatation of the Uterine Cervix*. Ed. F. Naftolin and P. G. Stubblefield, pp. 317–33. Raven Press, New York.

Calder, A. A. (1981). The human cervix in pregnancy: a clinical perspective. In *The Cervix in Pregnancy and Labour*. Ed. D. A. Ellwood and A. B. M. Anderson, pp. 103–22, Churchill Livingstone, Edinburgh.

Calder, A. A. & Greer, I. A. (1992). Cervical physiology and induction of labour. In *Recent Advances in Obstetrics and Gynaecology*. Ed. J. Bonnar, vol. 17, pp. 33–56, Churchill Livingstone, Edinburgh.

Chwalisz, K. (1988). Cervical ripening and induction of labour with progesterone antagonists. *XI European Congress of Perinatal Medicine-Rome*. p. 60. CIC Edizioni Internaziolini, Rome.

Colditz, I. G. (1990). Effects of exogenous prostaglandin E_2 and actinomycin-D on plasma leakage induced by neutrophil-activating peptide-1/interleukin-8. *Immune Cell Biology*, **68**, 397–403.

Danforth, D. N. (1947). The fibrous nature of the human cervix and its relationship to the isthmic segment in gravid and nongravid uteri. *American Journal of Obstetrics and Gynecology*, **53**, 541–57.

Danforth, D. N. (1954). The distribution and functional significance of the cervical musculature. *American Journal of Obstetrics and Gynecology*, **65**, 1261–70.

Danforth, D. N. (1980). The anatomy and physiology of the cervix. In *Dilatation of the Uterine Cervix*. Ed. F. Naftolin and P. G. Stubbrield, pp. 3–15, Raven Press, New York.

Danforth, D, N. & Hendrick, C. H. (1977). *Obstetrics and Gynaecology*. 3rd edn, Harper and Row, Maryland.

Danforth, D. N., Buckingham, J. C. & Roddick, J. W. (1960). Corrective tissue changes incident to cervical effacement. *American Journal of Obstetrics and Gynecology*, **80**, 939–45.

Ekman, G., Maslmstrom, A. & Uldbjerg, N. (1986). Cervical collagen: an important regulator of cervical function in term labour. *Obstetrics and Gynecology*, **67**, 633–6.

Ellwood, D. A., Anderson, A. B. M., Mitchell, M. D. *et al.* (1981). Prostanoids, collagenase and cervical softening in sheep. In *The Cervix in Pregnancy and Labour: Clinical and Biochemical Investigations*. Ed. D. A. Ellwood and A. B. M. Anderson, pp. 57–73, Churchill Livingstone, Edinburgh.

Elstein, M. & Chantler, E. M. (1991). Functional anatomy of the cervix and uterus. In *Scientific Foundations of Obstetrics & Gynaecology*. Ed. Philipp, E. and M. Setchell, pp. 114–33, Butterworth, Oxford.

Frydman, R., Baton, C., Lelaidier, C., Vial, M., Bourget, Ph. & Fernandez, H. (1991). Mifepristone for induction of labour. *Lancet*, **337**, 488–9.

Golichowski, A. (1980). Cervical stromal interstitial polysaccharide metabolism in pregnancy. In *Dilatation of the Uterine Cervix*. Ed. F. Naftohn and P. G. Stubblefield, pp. 99–111, Raven Press, New York.

Hillier, K. & Karim, S. M. M. (1970). The human isolated cervix: a study of its spontaneous motility and responsiveness to drugs. *British Journal of Pharmacology*, **40**, 576–7.

Horton, E. W. & Poyser, N. (1976). Uterine luteolytic hormone: a physiological role for prostaglandin $F_{2\alpha}$. *Physiology Review*, **56**, 595–651.

Hughesden, P. C. (1952). The fibromuscular nature of the cervix and its changes during pregnancy and labour. *Journal of Obstetrics and Gynaecology of the British Empire*, **59**, 763–76.

Hunter, W. (1774). *The Anatomy of the Human Gravid Uterus*. Baskerville, Birmingham.

Ingraham, C. B. & Taylor, E. S. (1947). Spontaneous annular detachment of the cervix during labor. *American Journal of Obstetrics and Gynecology*, **53**, 873–7.

Jeffrey, J. J., Coffrey, R. J. & Eizen, A. Z. (1971). Studies of uterine collagenase in tissue culture II. Effect of steroid hormones on enzyme production. *Biochimica et Biophysica Acta*, **252**, 143.

Johnston, T. A., Hodson, S., Greer, I. A., Kelly, R. W. & Calder, A. A. (1993). Plasma glycosaminoglycan and prostaglandin concentrations before and after the onset of spontaneous labour. *Proceedings of 3rd European Congress, Prostaglandins in Reproduction*, Edinburgh.

Johnstone, F. D., Boyd, I. E., McArthy, T. G. & McClure-Brown, J. C. (1974). The diameter of the uterine isthmus during the menstrual cycle, pregnancy and the puerperium. *Journal of Obstetrics and Gynaecology of the British Commonwealth*, **81**, 588–91.

Junqueira, L. C. U., Zugaib, M., Montes, G. S. *et al.* (1980). Morphologic and histomechanical evidence for the occurrence of collagenolysis and for the role of neutrophilic polymorphonuclear leukocytes during cervical dilatation. *American Journal of Obstetrics and Gynecology*, **138**, 273–81.

Kelly, R. W. & Bukman, A. (1990). Antiprogestogenic inhibition of uterine prostaglandin inactivation: a permissive mechanism for uterine stimulation. *Journal of Steroid Biochemistry and Molecular Biology*, **37**, 97–101.

Lambert, H., Overstreet, J. W. & Morales, P. (1985). Sperm capacitation in the human female genital tract. *Fertility and Sterility*, **43**, 325.

Leppert, P. C. & Yu, S. Y. (1990). Elastic and collagen in the human uterus; biochemical and histological correlations. *Abstracts of the Society for Gynecologic Investigation*, 37th Annual Meeting, St Louis, Missouri, p. 357.

Liggins, G. C. (1981). Cervical ripening as an inflammatory reaction. In *The Cervix in Pregnancy and Labour*. Ed. D. A. Ellwood and A. B. M. Anderson, pp. 1–9, Churchill Livingstone, Edinburgh.

Lindahl, U. & Hook, M. (1978). Glycosaminoglycans and their binding to biological macromolecules. *Annual Review in Biochemistry*, **47**, 385.

MacLennan, A. H. (1981). Cervical ripening and induction of labour by vaginal prostaglandin $F_{2\alpha}$ and relaxin. In *The Cervix in Pregnancy and Labour*. Ed. D. A. Ellwood and A. B. M. Anderson, pp. 187–196. Churchill Livingstone, Edinburgh.

McMutry, J. P., Floerscheim, G. L. & Bryant-Greenwood, G. D. (1980). Characterization of the binding of ^{125}I-labelled succynylated porcine relaxin in human and mouse fibroblasts. *Journal of Reproduction and Fertility*, **58**, 43–9.

von Maillot, K., Weiss, M., Nagelschmidt, M. *et al.* (1977). Relaxin and cervical dilatation during parturition. *Archiv Gynakologie*, **223**, 323–31.

von Maillot, K., Stuhlsatz, H. W., Mohanaradhkrishan, V. *et al.* (1979). Changes in the glycosaminoglycan distribution pattern in the human uterine cervix during pregnancy and labour. *American Journal of Obstetrics and Gynecology*, **135**, 503–6.

MRC/RCOG Working Party on Cervical Cerclage (1993). Final report of the Medical Research Council/Royal College of Obstetricians and Gynaecologists Multicentre Randomised Trial of Cervical Cerclage. *British Journal of Obstetrics and Gynaecology*, **100**, 516–23.

Nixon, W. C. W. (1951). Uterine, activin, normal and abnormal. *American Journal of Obstetrics and Gynecology*, **62**, 964–84.

Norstrom, A. (1984). The effects of prostaglandins on the biosynthesis of connective tissue constituents in the non-pregnant human cervix uteri. *Acta Obstetrica et Gynecologica Scandinavica*, **63**, 169–73.

Novy, M. J., Hammond, J. & Nichols, M. (1990). Shirodkar cerclage in a multifactorial approach to the patient with advanced cervical changes. *American Journal of Obstetrics and Gynecology*, **162**, 1412–20.

Radestad, A., Bygdeman, M. & Green, K. (1990). Induced cervical ripening with mifepristone (RU 486) and bioconversion of arachidonic acid in human pregnant uterine cervix in the first trimester. *Contraception*, **41**, 283–92.

Rath, W., Adelmann-Girill, B. C., Pieper, U. *et al.* (1987). The role of collagenases and proteases in prostaglandin induced cervical ripening. *Prostaglandins*, **34**, 119–27.

Rath, W., Osmers, B. C., Adelmann-Grill, B. C., Stuhlsatz, H. W., Severenyi, M. & Kuhn, W. (1988). Biophysical and biochemical changes of cervical ripening. In *Prostaglandins for Cervical Ripening and/or Induction of Labour*. Ed. C. Egarter and P. Husslein, pp. 32–41.

Rodger, M. W. & Baird, D. T. (1990). Pretreatment with mifepristone (RU 486) reduces interval between prostaglandin administration and expulsion in second trimester abortion. *British Journal of Obstetrics and Gynaecology*, **97**, 41–5.

Schwarz, O. H. & Woolf, R. B. (1948). Cervical dystocia with special reference to the fibrous nature of the cervix. *American Journal of Obstetrics and Gynecology*, **55**, 151–68.

Scott, J. E. & Orford, C. R. (1981). Dermatan sulphate rich proteoglycan associates with rat tail tendon collagen at the d band in the gap region. *Biochemical Journal*, **197**, 213.

Szalay, S., Husslein, P. & Grunberger, W. (1981). Local application of prostaglandin E_2 and its influence on collagenolytic activity of cervical tissue. *Singapore Journal of Obstetrics and Gynecology*, **12**, 15.

Uldbjerg, N., Ekman, G. & Malstrom, A. (1983a). Ripening of the human uterine cervix related to changed in collagen, glycosaminoglycans and collagenolytic activity. *American Journal of Obstetrics and Gynecology*, **147**, 662–6.

Uldbjerg, N., Ulmsten, V. & Ekman, G. (1983b). The ripening of the human uterine cervix in terms of connective tissue biochemistry. *Clinical Obstetrics and Gynecology*, **26**, 14–26.

Wendell-Smith, C. P. (1954). The lower uterine segment. *Journal of Obstetrics and Gynaecology of the British Empire*, **61**, 87–93.

14

Initiation of labour: uterine and cervical changes, endocrine changes

J.-C. SCHELLENBERG AND G. C. LIGGINS

The mechanism of the onset of labour in man is unknown. No condition has been described in which labour is prevented from occurring, and no hormonal event is known to initiate labour in man. This is in contrast to other species such as sheep in which certain lesions of the hypothalamus prevent labour and specific hormonal changes induce labour. Even if an experiment of nature was found in man in which labour was consistently suppressed or advanced, thus allowing the proposal of an hypothesis for the mechanism of the onset of labour, the hypothesis would be difficult to test given the limitation of experimentation in man. Likewise, while determinations of biochemical compounds (e.g. hormones) in human plasma, amniotic fluid, placenta, or fetal membranes may suggest plausible hypotheses, testing of these hypotheses requires experimentation. Experimentation in man is restricted to tissue explants from the uterine wall, placenta, and fetal membranes obtained at vaginal delivery or Caesarean section ('before labour' and 'during labour') and the onset of labour is difficult to reproduce *in vitro* for obvious reasons. Elucidation of the mechanism of the onset of labour in man therefore represents an extraordinary challenge. In addition, although experimentation in whole animals is feasible, some doubt will always remain regarding the relevance for man of observations made in any animal species. For all of these reasons, the barriers to proving any hypothesis of the mechanisms of the onset of labour in man in a scientifically rigorous fashion are likely to be almost insuperable. However, the clinician may not find this a problem if strong circumstantial evidence suggests effective therapeutic strategies (e.g. for the prevention of pre-term delivery).

A number of hypotheses regarding the mechanisms of the onset of labour have been proposed over the past 20 years and some are listed in Table 1. None of these hypotheses has been proven but some are more likely to be true than others. A general assumption underlying most hypotheses is that prostaglandins play a pivotal role in the initiation of labour. Three principal questions regarding the

Table 1. *Hypotheses for the mechanism of the initiation of labour in man*

Origin	Mechanism	Main agents involved and effects	Evidence
Mother	Maternal hypothalamus/ pituitary	Oxytocin	−
Fetus	Endocrine	Fetal cortisol → Maternal progesterone↓ Maternal oestrogen↑	− −
	Endocrine Fetal kidneys → Amniotic fluid → Fetal membranes	Oxytocin → maternal circulation PAF Stimulators of PG synthesis	− − −
	Fetal lungs → Amniotic fluid	PAF Surfactant	− −
Amnion Chorion	Paracrine/ Autocrine	Oestrogen production↑ Progesterone production↓	+
Amnion	Endocrine/paracrine	Progesterone metabolism↑	− −
Decidua	Paracrine	Oestrogen↑, progesterone↓ → labilisation of lysosomes → liberation of phospholipases A$_2$	+
Chorion	Paracrine	Inactivation of phospholipase Inhibitor (gravidin)	+
Chorion	Paracrine	Stimulator of PG synthesis↑	+
Decidua	Paracrine/autocrine	Main source of PGF$_{2\alpha}$ Role of cytokines: 'inflammation'	+
Amnion	Paracrine	Main source of PGE$_2$	−
Myometrium	(Endocrine)	Oxytocin receptors↑ → contractions↑	+ +
Decidua	Paracrine	Oxytocin receptors↑ → PG synthesis↑	+ +

Evidence for major role: + likely; + + very likely; − unlikely; − − very unlikely.
PG = prostaglandins; PAF = platelet activating factor.

mechanisms of the onset of labour need resolving: (1) where does the message for the onset of labour originate, (2) by which route is the message for the onset of labour transmitted to the target organs (myometrium, cervix), and (3) which are the agents involved in the transmission of this message?

Preparation for labour: uterine and cervical changes

Labour is defined by the occurrence of coordinated uterine contractions leading to cervical dilatation and expulsion of the conceptus. To make labour possible,

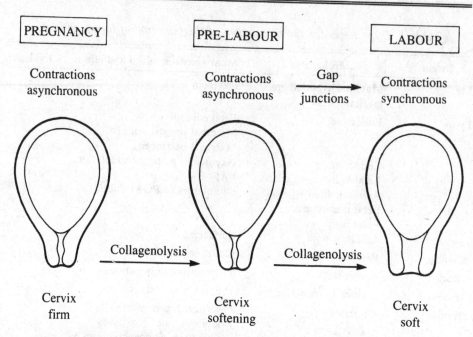

Fig. 1. Preparation for labour. The formation of gap junctions in the myometrium and remodelling of the connective tissue structure of the cervix are fundamental events in the preparation for labour.

the uterus must be capable of contracting in a synchronous manner and the cervix needs to be elastic to allow dilatation. The formation of gap junctions in the myometrium and changes in the properties of the connective tissue of the cervix are fundamental events in the preparation for labour.

For uterine contractions to become coordinated, the muscle fibres must be inter-connected electrically allowing excitation to spread throughout the myometrium; contraction of the uterus changes from asynchronous during pregnancy to synchronous during labour (Fig. 1). This is achieved by the formation of gap junctions between muscle fibres transforming the myometrium into a cohesive electrical and metabolic unit. Myometrial gap junctions are present in all species studied during term and pre-term labour (Garfield, 1988). In all species including man, gap junctions are present in higher numbers during labour than before labour. Labour in the absence of gap junctions has not been documented. On the other hand, the presence of gap junctions alone is not sufficient to initiate labour, at least not in rats (Garfield, 1988). In rabbits and rats, oestrogens promote and progesterone inhibits the formation of gap junctions. To what extent these steroids regulate gap junction formation in man is unknown; experiments are not feasible and there are no consistent changes in maternal plasma oestrogen and progesterone preceding labour. Prostaglandins modulate gap junction formation in rat, but their exact role is unknown. Inhibition of prostaglandin synthesis by non-steroid anti-inflammatory drugs inhibits gap junction formation in most instances, but under particular experimental conditions inhibition of prostaglandin synthesis increases gap junction formation (Garfield, 1988). In summary, reports on myometrial gap junctions in man are scarce but by analogy to other species there is little doubt that gap junctions play an important permissive role for the onset of labour.

The cervix is transformed in preparation for labour from a rigid organ occluding the uterine cavity to a stretchable and retractable part of the birth canal. The bulk of the cervix (about 85%) is made up of connective tissue, most of the fibrous component being collagen. Changes in the connective tissue play a major part in cervical ripening over the latter part of pregnancy and during labour. Compared to cervix from non-pregnant women, post-partum cervical biopsy specimens have a 12-fold lower mechanical strength, 50% lower concentrations of collagen and sulphated glycosaminoglycans, 35% lower concentration of hyaluronic acid, and five-fold increased collagenolytic activity (Rechberger, Uldbjerg & Oxlund, 1988). Biochemical correlates exist also for the clinical properties of cervices at term (Ekman *et al.*, 1986). Mean collagen concentrations in post-partum biopsy specimens are 30% higher in an 'unfavourable' cervix (firm and difficult to stretch) associated with slow progress of spontaneous labour compared to a 'favourable' (soft, stretchy) cervix associated with rapid progress of spontaneous labour (Ekman *et al.*, 1986). The proportion of non-extractable (highly cross-linked) collagen in an unfavourable cervix is twice that of a favourable cervix. Collagenolytic activity is significantly increased in the cervix of women treated intracervically with PGE$_2$ for cervical priming and induction of labour (Edkan *et al.*, 1986). Although not documented, it is likely that similar transformations of the connective tissue occur in the uterus, particularly in the lower segment.

The regulation of cervical ripening is not well understood and has received relatively little attention in the literature. A major role of prostaglandins is likely in view of the numerous clinical reports on the effectiveness of prostaglandins in inducing cervical ripening in the absence of increased uterine activity. Other compounds likely to be involved in cervical ripening are relaxin and oestrogens. Although porcine relaxin applied to the cervix has similar effects to prostaglandins, it is not known whether relaxin has any biological significance in this respect (MacLennan *et al.*, 1980). Relaxin is synthesized in the decidua from where it may diffuse into the cervical stroma and induce connective tissue changes (Bryant-Greenwood & Greenwood, 1988). Similar considerations apply to oestrogens which have also been used to induce cervical ripening (Lerner, 1980).

The origin of the signal for the onset of labour

The origin of the signal for the onset of labour is unknown. Although it makes sense that the conceptus (fetus, placenta, or fetal membranes) triggers the onset of labour when maturity is adequate for extra-uterine survival, the possibility that the mother determines the moment of birth has not been disproved. Direct evidence gained from several animal species including sheep and the intermediate lengths of gestation of pregnancies in animals crossed from breeds with different gestation lengths shows that the conceptus must influence the length of gestation (Liggins *et al.*, 1977; Challis & Olson, 1988). For these reasons most hypotheses revolve around the assumption that the conceptus determines the onset of labour.

Possible routes of signal transmission for labour

Assuming that the conceptus triggers labour, the following routes of transmission to the target organs (cervix, myometrium) are conceivable (Fig. 2). The signal could emanate from the fetus, the placenta, the amnion, or the chorion. A message of fetal origin could (1) be carried from the fetal circulation via the placenta to the uterus (directly or via the maternal circulation), (2) be secreted into the amniotic fluid by the fetal kidneys, or (3) be secreted by the fetal lungs and carried via the amniotic fluid and the membranes directly to the uterine wall (decidua, myometrium, cervix) with or without spillover into the maternal circulation. A message of placental origin would, in the haemochorial placenta, be most likely passed into the fetal or the maternal circulation. Finally, the triggering signal for labour could originate in the fetal membranes and act in a paracrine fashion, via the decidua, on the myometrium and the cervical stroma. This latter pathway may or may not entail leakage into the maternal circulation of agents involved in the mechanisms of the onset of labour. This putative paracrine pathway with the signal for labour originating in the fetal membranes is favoured by many investigators.

Does the fetus trigger labour via an endocrine signal?

The hypothesis that the fetus triggers labour by means of a pituitary-dependent endocrine signal was tested in fetal sheep following the observation that hypothalamic and pituitary malformations prevent labour in this species. It was demonstrated that labour is prevented by fetal but not maternal hypophysectomy and that labour can be induced by administration of ACTH or cortisol to intact or hypophysectomized fetuses at or before term (Fig. 3). Further experiments established that administration to the fetus of glucocorticoids increases the activity

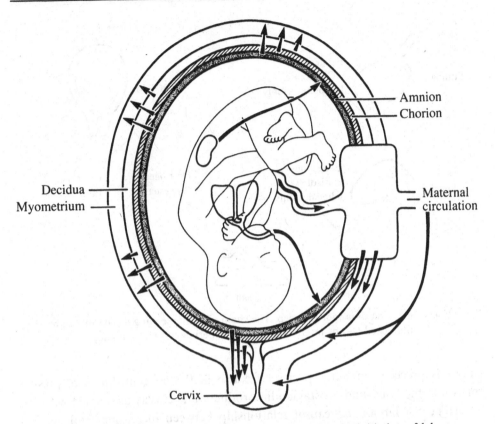

Fig. 2. Possible routes of transmission of the signal for the initiation of labour from the conceptus to the mother. Note the large area of contact between the chorion and the decidua which makes the paracrine route an effective way of signal transmission from conceptus to mother.

of placental enzymes (the most important being 17-alpha hydroxylase), resulting in increased synthesis of oestrogens and decreased synthesis of progesterone. As a consequence concentrations of progesterone decrease in maternal plasma and concentrations of oestradiol-17$_{\text{beta}}$ increase leading to increased activity of phospholipase A$_2$ in amnion and chorio-allantois, raised concentrations of prostaglandin F$_{2\text{alpha}}$ in utero-ovarian blood, and labour (Liggins *et al.*, 1977) (Fig. 3). A similar chain of events occurs naturally; increasing plasma concentrations of fetal cortisol are followed by increasing concentrations of oestrogens and decreasing concentrations of progesterone in maternal plasma, and increased uterine prostaglandin production and labour (Liggins *et al.*, 1977; Challis & Olson, 1988).

Man shares several features of the endocrinology of pregnancy with sheep but there are fundamental differences in regard to the onset of labour (Table 2). While

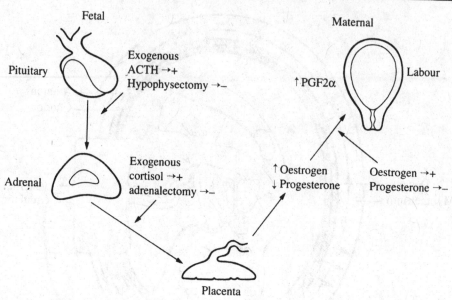

Fig. 3. Initiation of labour in sheep. The chain of events leading to labour can be mimicked (+) or interrupted (−) by experimental manipulation.

labour is preceded in both species by a rise in the concentrations of plasma cortisol in the fetus, and prostaglandin production is closely associated with the occurrence of labour, no causal relationship between increasing fetal cortisol concentrations and the initiation of labour has been established in man. The substrate for cortisol action in the ovine placenta (placental 17-alpha hydroxylase) is absent in the human placenta (Fig. 4). Consequently there cannot be any activation of placental 17-alpha hydroxylase nor switching of placental steroid production from progesterone to oestrogens. As expected there is no consistent rise in maternal plasma concentrations of oestrogens or any consistent decline of progesterone concentrations before the onset of labour in man (Flint, 1979). Hence, if fetal cortisol has a role in the mechanisms of the onset of labour in man, its mode of action must be different from that in sheep.

Further observations suggest that the fetal hypothalamo-pituitary-adrenal axis, and hence fetal cortisol, has no regulatory role in the initiation of labour in man (Table 1). Administration of glucocorticoids to the human fetus (via the maternal–placental route using glucocorticoids that cross the placenta) does not induce labour before term. Absence of the hypothalamus, the pituitary, or the adrenals is compatible with delivery at term in man (but not in sheep) (Tables 2 and 3). Mean gestational length in anencephalic fetuses without polyhydramnios is 40 weeks but the variance is greater than in normal fetuses, suggesting that the pituitary has a modulating effect on the duration of pregnancy (Honnebier

Table 2. *Common and distinctive features of the endocrinology of pregnancy and parturition in man and sheep*

	Man	Sheep
Common features		
Pregnancy not interrupted by ovariectomy after mid-pregnancy	+	+
Placenta major source of progesterone in second half of pregnancy	+	+
High plasma levels of progesterone	+	+
Fetal cortisol increases before labour	+	+
Fetal hypothalamic lesions disturb duration of pregnancy	+	+
Maternal hypophysectomy prolongs gestation	−	−
Prostaglandins induce labour	+	+
Oxytocin increases in maternal plasma at onset of labour	−	−
Uterine sensitivity to oxytocin increases towards term	+	?
Gap junctions increase in labour	+	+
Distinctive features		
Sharp pre-partum fall in progesterone	−	+
Administration of progesterone delays parturition	−	+
Sharp pre-partum rise of oestrogens	−	+
High maternal plasma levels of oestrogens	+	−
Administration of oestrogens induces labour	−	+
Fetal 16-steroid hydroxylation	+	−
Oestriol major oestrogen	+	−
Fetal zone in adrenal	+	−
Placental 17-alpha hydroxylase	−	+
Glucocorticoids induce labour before term	−	+
Absent fetal pituitary prolongs pregnancy	−	+

+ present, − not present, ? likely.

& Swaab, 1973). Further differences between man and sheep relate to the effects of exogenous oestrogen and progestins. In contrast to sheep, administration of progesterone to pregnant women does not delay labour and administration of oestrogens does not induce labour (at least not usually, see below).

Fetal concentrations of oxytocin increase in labour and, being higher in the artery than vein, there is a possibility of feto-maternal transfer (Chard, 1989). Whether the human placenta is permeable to oxytocin is not clear and whether fetal production rates would be able to influence maternal plasma concentrations is unknown. Similar considerations to fetal cortisol apply to fetal oxytocin in view of the normal gestational length of anencephalic fetuses; it is concluded that the hypothalamo-pituitary axis has a modulating but not a regulatory role for the initiation of labour in man.

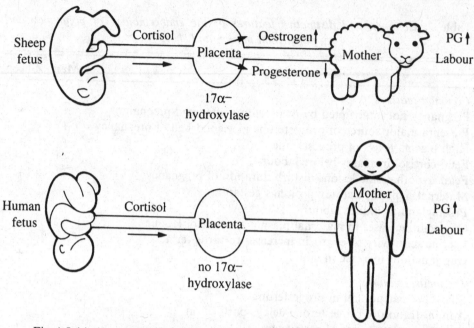

Fig. 4. Initiation of labour in sheep and man. Although concentrations of cortisol in fetal plasma rise in both species preceding labour and production of PGF$_{2alpha}$ is closely associated with labour, a causal relationship between the rise of fetal cortisol and the initiation of labour has been established only in sheep. Man lacks placental 17-alpha hydroxylase which in sheep is a crucial link in feto-maternal signal transmission for the onset of labour. PG = prostaglandins.

Fetal signals transmitted through the fetal kidneys

Stimulation and/or abolition of inhibition of prostaglandin production is thought to be fundamental to the initiation of labour (see section on prostaglandins and Fig. 5). Two reports describe chemically undefined substances that may represent fetal signals transmitted through the fetal kidneys. A protein-associated substance of apparent renal origin was found to stimulate PGE$_2$ synthesis in monolayer cultures of human amnion cells (Casey, MacDonald & Mitchell, 1983) (Table 1). Other authors reported that unextracted fetal urine in a concentration of 20% stimulated PGE$_2$ synthesis by microsomes from bovine seminal vesicles (Strickland *et al.*, 1983). The active compound was heat stable and had a molecular weight of less than 12 kD (Strickland *et al.*, 1983). A third putative stimulator of prostaglandin synthesis is fetal oxytocin. Median concentrations of oxytocin in amniotic fluid are 2.5 times higher in labour than before labour and oxytocin is present in high concentrations in newborn urine (Seppälä *et al.*, 1972). As oxytocin stimulates production of PGE$_2$ by amnion cells in culture (Moore *et al.*, 1988), it is possible that oxytocin released into the amniotic fluid has a role in the initiation or the maintenance of labour.

Table 3. *Experiments of nature which fail to support a major role of some of the suggested mechanisms of initiation of labour*

Defect	Consequence	Onset of labour
Anencephaly	No fetal ACTH, cortisol	Term, increased variability of gestation
Adrenal agenesis	No fetal cortisol	Slightly post-term
Tracheal atresia	No PAF, no surfactant stimulating PG synthesis in amnion	Term
Renal agenesis	No nephrogenic stimulators of PG synthesis in amniotic fluid	Term
Hypobetalipoproteinaemia	Very low plasma progesterone	Term
Placental sulphatase deficiency	Very low plasma oestrogens	Term
Amnion bands	Amnion (major source of PG) not in contact with uterine wall	Term
Maternal hypophysectomy	No or very low plasma oxytocin	Term

PAF = platelet activating factor; PG = prostaglandins.

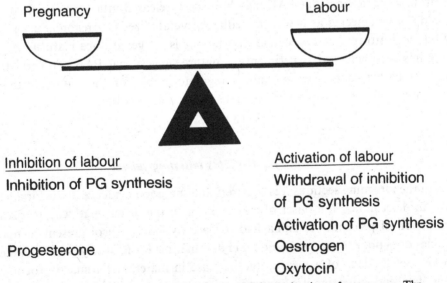

Pregnancy   Labour

Inhibition of labour
Inhibition of PG synthesis

Progesterone

Activation of labour
Withdrawal of inhibition
of PG synthesis
Activation of PG synthesis
Oestrogen
Oxytocin

Fig. 5. Factors underlying the maintenance and termination of pregnancy. The balance between inhibition and stimulation of prostaglandin production may be fundamental in the switching from pregnancy to labour. Progesterone, oestrogens, and oxytocin are thought to play major roles. A large number of other factors known to inhibit or stimulate prostaglandin synthesis are not shown (see text). PG = prostaglandins.

Any role of these stimulators of prostaglandin synthesis is likely to be modulating rather than regulatory in view of experiments of nature; fetuses with renal agenesis or total obstruction of the urinary tract deliver at term (Table 3).

Fetal signals transmitted through the fetal lungs

Two substances produced by the maturing fetal lung could function as signals for the onset of labour. Pulmonary surfactant stimulates production of PGE_2 by human amnion *in vitro* (Lopez Bernal *et al.*, 1988). Platelet activating factor (PAF) is produced in human fetal lung explants as glycogen stores decrease during lung maturation. The suggestion that increasing pulmonary PAF production coincides with (or is a feature of) lung maturation is supported by observations in rabbits in which increasing production of PAF in lung parallels increasing production of surfactant. PAF stimulates production of PGE_2 in human amnion *in vitro* and could, in theory, initiate labour with advancing lung maturation. These speculations are supported by the finding that, in one study, amniotic fluid from women before the onset of labour contained no measurable PAF but amniotic fluid from all labouring women (n = 10) contained PAF, while in another study, samples from about half of the labouring women contained PAF (Johnston, Bleasdale & Hoffman, 1987). Samples from women in labour without measurable PAF contained significant amounts of the PAF-inactivating enzyme, acetyl-hydrolase, suggesting that PAF may have been released into amniotic fluid but could not be detected as it was immediately metabolized (Johnston *et al.*, 1987). While it is attractive to speculate that labour is triggered once maturity of the lung has been achieved, experiments of nature suggest that PAF and surfactant have at best a supportive and not a regulatory role for the onset of labour; congenital bilateral pulmonary agenesis is associated with normal delivery at term (Claireaux & Ferreria, 1958) (Table 3).

Evidence for the fetus initiating labour

From the foregoing sections it is apparent that no good evidence exists for a fetal role in determining the onset of labour in man: the 'usual' pathway involving activation of placental 17-alpha hydroxylase by fetal cortisol present in many species does not exist in man; and an endocrine role for fetal oxytocin is unlikely in view of the lack of a measurable increase in maternal plasma oxytocin; no other fetal endocrine signal is known to exist in any other species; and a regulatory role for the onset of labour of fetal signals transmitted via the lungs or the kidneys is unlikely in view of the evidence available from experiments of nature. For these reasons it has been postulated that the initiation of labour in man is regulated by paracrine mechanisms occurring between the conceptus (fetal membranes, placenta) and the maternal tissues (decidua, myometrium, cervical stroma) (Fig. 3).

Agents likely to play a major role in the initiation of labour

Knowledge gained from sheep and other species suggests an essential role of oestrogens, progesterone, and prostaglandins in the events leading to labour; a biological role of these compounds for human parturition is therefore likely. In addition, oxytocin has long been suspected to play a crucial role in parturition. The following sections will highlight the physiology of these compounds.

Eicosanoids

Strong but inconclusive evidence suggests a central role for eicosanoids in the mechanism of the initiation of labour in man (Fig. 5). The crucial piece of evidence for a regulatory role of eicosanoids is unavailable. However, a release of eicosanoids immediately preceding labour would be difficult to demonstrate in view of the difficulty of predicting labour and the difficulty of obtaining samples from suitable sites. A number of clinical observations support the hypothesis that eicosanoids are essential for the onset of labour. Most observations relate to cyclooxygenase metabolites (prostanoids) rather than lipoxygenase metabolites (hydroxyeicosatetraenoic acid = HETE, leukotrienes = LTs, and others) which have received only recent attention (Fig. 6). Among the prostanoids, most research

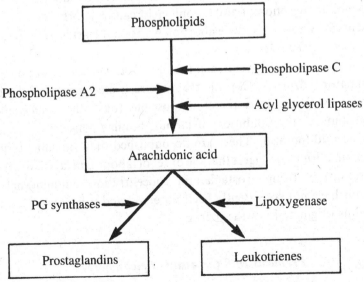

Fig. 6. A simplified pathway of eicosanoid synthesis.

has been directed towards PGF_{2alpha} and PGE_2 both of which elicit contractions in pregnant myometrium *in vitro* and are present in intra-uterine tissues in relatively large amounts.

Clinical observations suggesting a role of prostaglandin in the initiation of labour

The following observations have led to the belief that prostaglandins are essential for both maintenance and initiation of labour:

1. Administration of PGF_{2alpha} and PGE_2 is highly efficacious in causing abortion or labour at any stage of pregnancy from soon after implantation to term. Provided that dosage is low and that treatment is extended over a long enough period, all the clinical features of spontaneous labour are reproduced.
2. Prostaglandin antagonists inhibit labour even if the cervix is partly dilated. Labour resumes when the antagonist is withdrawn.
3. Ingestion of high doses of acetylsalicylic acid during the last six months of pregnancy prolongs pregnancy.
4. The concentrations of PGF_{2alpha}, PGE_2 and their metabolites in amniotic fluid and plasma increase progressively after the onset of labour.
5. Successful (but not unsuccessful) induction of labour at term with oxytocin is associated with a sustained increase in the concentration of PGFM (PGF_{2alpha} metabolite) in maternal plasma.
6. Infection (chorio-amnionitis) and trauma (amniotomy, stripping of membranes) that cause release of eicosanoids are often followed by labour.
7. Intra-amniotic injection of arachidonic acid causes abortion.
8. No agents are known to induce abortion without at least having the potential for stimulating the release of eicosanoids.

Qualification of some of these statements is in order. The effects of non-steroidal anti-inflammatory drugs (point 2) are not restricted to the inhibition of prostaglandin synthesis. It is therefore possible that other pharmacological effects contribute to the inhibition of labour. Similar considerations apply to acetylsalicylic acid (point 3). There are no published data on short-term use of aspirin or similar drugs to suggest that the onset of labour is delayed. Furthermore, the observations of rising prostaglandin concentrations in maternal plasma during labour have not consistently been observed and it is not proven that the prostaglandins originate from the uterus.

Problems with the assay of eicosanoids

Measurements of primary eicosanoids that accurately reflect concentrations *in vivo* are difficult to obtain. Many eicosanoids are not hormones in the classical sense but act in an autocrine or paracrine fashion. The presence of these eicosanoids in plasma appears to be fortuitous by 'leakage' from tissue into the circulation; conclusions regarding their concentrations in the target tissue are therefore tenuous. These considerations apply to PGF_{2alpha} and PGE_2 which are virtually completely metabolized when passing through the pulmonary circulation and consequently cannot have the function of a classical hormone. PGI_2 (prostacyclin) seems to act, at least in part, as a hormone. Eicosanoids are rapidly released from the tissues after synthesis rather than stored and, as a consequence, the tissue concentrations are low and difficult to detect. Even minor trauma stimulates the synthesis of eicosanoids which accumulate between harvesting and processing of the tissues. Prostaglandin E_2 and its metabolites are unstable and transformed into PGA_2 and PGB_2 during storage and assay. Prostaglandin E_2 and thromboxane A_2 are released by platelets retained in tissues and present in blood samples. Some of these problems have been overcome and more credible results have been obtained in recent studies. Examples of improved methodology include the addition of inhibitors of PG synthase (e.g. aspirin) to plasma on collection, assay of stable metabolites such as PGFM (13,14-dihydro-15-keto PGF_{2alpha}), bicyclo-PGE_2, thromboxane B_2, and 6-keto-PGF_{1alpha} (a metabolite of prostacyclin, or PGI_2) rather than the primary unstable prostaglandin, methoximation of the ketone group attached to the cyclopentane ring of PGE_2 and its metabolites and assay of the stable derivative. Finally, unrecognized cross-reactivity may occur in the immunoassays which have become the cornerstones of eicosanoid determination.

Concentrations of eicosanoids in maternal plasma

Reported plasma concentrations of PGF_{2alpha} differ considerably and may not reflect uterine PGF_{2alpha} production (Keirse, 1979). Concentrations of PGFM in maternal plasma are low and do not change during pregnancy; there is a rise in established labour, increasing progressively as cervical dilatation advances (Nagata *et al.*, 1987). Sequential sampling immediately preceding and during early labour has not been reported. Calculations of the amounts of PGF_{2alpha} needed to induce labour suggest that an increase in maternal plasma concentrations of PGF_{2alpha} and of PGFM is unlikely to occur; unchanged plasma levels of PGF_{2alpha} and PGFM preceding labour would therefore not disprove the hypothesis that increased production of uterine PGF_{2alpha} initiates labour (Casey & MacDonald, 1988). Measurements of PGF_{2alpha} in uterine venous plasma have not added to our understanding of uterine prostaglandin production preceding or during labour (Keirse, 1979). Concentrations of PGEM have been reported to double in labour (Husslein, 1984) but there is little or no increase in the concentrations of PGE_2 and bicyclo-PGE (a stable metabolite of PGE_2)

(Brennecke *et al.*, 1985). Similar conclusions regarding measurement of PGF_{2alpha} may apply to PGE_2. After delivery of the placenta, plasma concentrations of PGEM decline more rapidly than those of PGFM suggesting that the main source of PGE_2 is amnion, chorion or the placenta, and that of PGF_{2alpha} is decidua or myometrium (Husslein & Sinzinger, 1984).

Concentrations of eicosanoids in amniotic fluid

The concentrations of PGF and PGFM in amniotic fluid show a pattern similar to that in plasma, without change before the onset of labour (Keirse, 1979; Mitchell, 1984). Amniotomy is followed by a rapid rise of concentrations of PGFM and thromboxane B_2 (Keirse, 1979). The hypothesis that the release of PGF_{2alpha} plays a role in the initiation of labour and is not merely a consequence of uterine contractions is supported by the observation that the concentrations of PGFM in amniotic fluid (and in plasma) rise early in spontaneous labour but not until late in oxytocin-induced labour (Fuchs *et al.*, 1983). The concentrations of PGE_2 in amniotic fluid are similar and rise in parallel to those of PGF_{2alpha} (Keirse, 1979; Mitchell, 1984). The higher concentrations of lipoxygenase products in labour suggest that these eicosanoids may also play a role in the maintenance, and perhaps the initiation, of labour (Romero *et al.*, 1987). Concentrations of 12-HETE are comparable to those of PGE_2 and PGF_{2alpha} whereas those of 15-HETE and LTB_4 are much lower (Romero *et al.*, 1987).

Patterns of eicosanoid production in pregnancy in vitro

Eicosanoids are produced by the uterus, fetal membranes, and the placenta. The eicosanoid production is well documented although there are some discrepancies between authors in the exact pattern described. In studies using a tissue perifusion technique, amnion was the principal source of prostanoids and the principal product was PGE_2 (Mitchell *et al.*, 1978). All tissues examined (amnion, chorion, decidua, and placenta), produced less PGF_{2alpha} than 13,14-dihydro-15-keto-PGF_{2alpha} (Mitchell *et al.*, 1978). This contrasts with the finding of similar production rates of PGE_2, PGF_{2alpha}, and 6-keto-PGF_{1alpha} by dispersed cells from amnion, chorion, decidua, and placenta (Olson, Skinner & Challis, 1983). Relative production rates were placenta > decidua > chorion ⩾ amnion in this study in tissues obtained before labour; after labour production was highest in amnion and chorion (Olson *et al.*, 1983). A number of other studies has suggested that the principal prostanoid is PGE_2 in amnion, PGE_2 and PGF_{2alpha} in chorion, PGF_{2alpha} in decidua, and PGI_2 (prostacyclin) in myometrium (Bleasdale & Johnston, 1984; Fuchs & Fuchs, 1984; Mitchell, 1984; Challis & Olson, 1988; Lundin-Schiller & Mitchell, 1990).

Prostaglandin production in vitro by intra-muterine tissues in relation to labour

In decidua, production rates of PGF_{2alpha} by tissue obtained at Caesarean section were found to be higher in labour than before the onset of labour in one study (Fuchs & Fuchs, 1984); in another study, there was no difference in production rates of PGE, PGF, and 6-keto-PGF_{1alpha} by dispersed decidual cells from placentas delivered vaginally or at elective Caesarean section (Olson *et al.*, 1983). In the former study, production rates of PGE and PGF were lower in amnion obtained at Caesarean section in labour than before the onset of labour; the authors speculated that this may have been due to metabolism of prostaglandins (Fuchs *et al.*, 1984). In the Olson study (1983) production rates of PGE, PGF, and 6-keto-PGF_{1alpha} in both amnion and chorion were higher after labour than before labour. Mitchell and colleagues (1978*b*) showed a 2.5 fold increase in production rates of 6-keto-PGF_{1alpha} by superfused pieces of amnion but not by chorion, decidua or placenta. Production rates of PGE, PGF, and PGFM were similar in tissues obtained before and after labour (Mitchell *et al.*, 1978*a*). Manzai & Liggins (1984) showed that production rates of PGE but not PGF were higher in dispersed amnion cells harvested after labour than in those obtained before labour. These and other studies suggest that there is an increase in production rates of several species of eicosanoids during labour in amnion, and probably in decidua and chorion. A switch during or before labour from lipoxygenase metabolites of arachidonic acid to cyclooxygenase products is suggested by the observation that confluent cultures of amnion cells harvested before labour produced HETEs but no PGE_2 from intracellular pools of arachidonic acid; by contrast cultures established with cells obtained during labour released PGE_2 in addition to HETEs (Rose, Myatt & Elder, 1990).

The relative importance of PGE and PGF for the onset of labour

The question of which prostanoid plays the more important role in initiating parturition and which tissue is the major source remains unresolved. The hypothesis that PGE_2 synthesized by the amnion initiates labour was favoured by many workers as it is the major prostanoid formed by fetal membranes *in vitro*; the concentration of PGE_2 in amniotic fluid rises in labour; the rate of production of PGE_2 by amnion *in vitro* increases during labour; and PGE_2 is more potent than PGF_{2alpha} in inducing labour (Table 1). Recent work calls for a revision of this hypothesis; more reliable assays of PGE_2 metabolites show no increase in plasma concentrations during labour, while concentrations of PGF_{2alpha} increase (Brennecke *et al.*, 1985) and it is doubtful if significant amounts of non-metabolized PGE_2 pass through the membranes to reach the uterine wall. Experiments using a double-chamber perfusion system showed that less than 5% of radiolabelled

PGE_2 crossed the combined amnion and chorion in a 4 h period whereas more than 50% traversed the amnion alone from the fetal to the maternal side (McCoshen, 1988). Although another study found that PGE_2 traversed the amnio-chorion in either direction and the rate of passage was greater after than before labour (Nakla *et al.*, 1986), the importance of the amnion as a source of prostanoids for the onset and the maintenance of labour remains doubtful. A major role of amnion prostaglandins in the maintenance of labour is also unlikely since the amnion depends on uptake of arachidonic acid from amniotic fluid and the net content of arachidonic acid in amnion increases in the latter stages of labour in spite of a substantial increase in uterine prostaglandin production (as evidenced by increasing plasma concentrations of PGFM) (Casey & MacDonald, 1988). It is therefore unlikely that the amnion is a major source of prostaglandin production, even less so as PGE_2 rather than PGF_{2alpha} appears to be the major prostanoid produced by amnion, and there is no evidence for any significant transformation of PGE_2 to PGF_{2alpha}. A further argument against the amnion as a prime factor in the initiation of labour is the existence of pregnancies in which the amnion is detached from the chorion forming constricting bands that may amputate fetal limbs: labour occurs at term in these pregnancies provided there is no premature rupture of the membranes (Table 3).

An alternative hypothesis proposes the decidua as the primary source of prostanoids with PGF_{2alpha} as principal prostanoid for the initiation and maintenance of labour (Casey & MacDonald, 1988) (Table 1). Decidual stromal cells may function like macrophages in which cytokines such as tumour necrosis factor and interleukins stimulate prostaglandin synthesis (Casey & MacDonald, 1988).

In summary, the source of prostanoids contributing to the initiation of labour is unknown. Several sources and several eicosanoids might be involved; for example amniotic PGE_2 may affect the decidua (e.g. by stimulating PGF_{2alpha} production) and decidual PGF_{2alpha} may act on the myometrium and the cervix. There is little evidence for a major role of other eicosanoids such as PGI_2 and lipoxygenase products.

The control of prostaglandin synthesis

If it is accepted that inhibition of prostaglandin synthesis is essential for the maintenance of pregnancy, abolition of this inhibition with or without concomitant stimulation of prostaglandin synthesis is essential for labour to take place (Bleasdale & Johnston, 1984; Fuchs & Fuchs, 1984; Mitchell, 1984; Challis & Olson, 1988; Thorburn *et al.*, 1988; Lundin-Schiller & Mitchell, 1990; Olson *et al.*, 1990). In view of the popularity of this hypothesis, major efforts have been undertaken to study prostaglandin synthesis and metabolism in the amnion and decidua. Prostaglandins are released as they are synthesized; there are no intracellular stores. Increasing concentrations of prostaglandins in labour are the result of increased synthesis, not reduced degradation (Keirse, 1979). Tissue concentrations of prostaglandins are determined by the rate of release of arachidonic acid from the phospholipids of cell membranes and the rate of transformation of arachidonic acid into prostaglandins by prostaglandin H synthase (PGHS, or cyclooxygenase) (Fig. 6). Phospholipase A_2 releases arachidonic acid from the sn-2 position of phospholipids. In fetal membranes phospholipase A_2 activity is relatively specific for phosphatidylethanolamine, is Ca^{2+}-dependent, and is a microsomal enzyme. An alternative pathway of arachidonic acid release is initiated by phospholipase C. In fetal membranes, this enzyme is Ca^{2+}-independent, has specificity for phosphatidylinositol and therefore releases mainly inositol triphosphate. After inositol triphosphate is split off, diacylglycerol serves as a substrate for a diacylglycerol lipase. Diacylglycerol lipase catalyses the hydrolysis of the fatty acid in the sn-1 position, and a monoacylglycerol lipase liberates arachidonic acid from the sn-2 position. A synergism exists between phospholipase C and phospholipase A_2. Inositol triphosphate released from phosphatidylethanolamine by phospholipase C increases intracellular Ca^{2+} concentrations, which in turn activates phospholipase A_2. It is not known which pathway (phospholipase A_2 or phospholipase C) is more important for the liberation of arachidonic acid (Bleasdale & Johnston, 1984; Mitchell, 1984; Challis & Olson, 1988; Lundin-Schiller & Mitchell, 1991; Olson et al., 1990).

It is not certain whether prostaglandin synthesis in fetal membranes is rate-limited by the activity of phospholipases or by PGHS. The rapid release of prostaglandins associated with amniotomy near term suggests that PGHS is not rate limiting although it may limit production earlier in pregnancy (Keirse, 1979).

More than twenty defined agents stimulating or inhibiting prostaglandin synthesis in amnion are known (Bleasdale & Johnston, 1984; Fuchs & Fuchs, 1984; Manzai & Liggins, 1984; Mitchell, 1984; Challis & Olson, 1988; Thorburn et al., 1988; Lundin-Schiller & Mitchell, 1990; Olson et al., 1990). In addition, several undefined stimulators and inhibitors acting in a paracrine fashion have been described. One protein inhibitor, named gravidin, has been chemically defined (Wilson, Liggins & Joe, 1989). Gravidin isolated from chorion before labour inhibits arachidonate release from perifused human decidual cells and phospholipase A_2 activity in a cell-free system (Wilson et al., 1989). Gravidin obtained from human chorion after birth does not inhibit arachidonate release or phospholipase A_2 activity (Wilson et al., 1989). N-terminal amino acid sequencing shows homology between the 8–10 terminal amino acids of gravidin and the secretory component of IgA. Incubation of gravidin with antibodies to secretory component inhibits antiphospholipase activity, suggesting identity of gravidin and secretory component (Wilson & Christie, 1991). Serum concentrations of secretory IgA (a-IgA) in early pregnancy are lower in women who subsequently deliver pre-term than in women who deliver at term (Wilson & Gandendren, 1992) suggesting a role of gravidin for the maintenance of pregnancy and the onset of labour. These findings lend further support to the hypothesis that the regulation of prostaglandin synthesis is pivotal for the maintenance of pregnancy and the initiation of labour.

Oxytocin

Oxytocin is the most potent natural agent known to elicit uterine contractions. Before the introduction of prostaglandins in clinical practice oxytocin was the only agent known to induce labour. For these reasons oxytocin was thought to play a major role in the initiation of parturition until measurements of maternal and fetal plasma concentrations of oxytocin failed to show an unequivocal rise of oxytocin in early labour (see Chard, Chapter 12). In recent years, the findings of an increase in myometrial and decidual oxytocin receptors in man during pregnancy and labour and the possibility of a paracrine role of oxytocin have rekindled interest in this compound. In addition, there are several lines of evidence suggesting an interplay between ocytocin and prostaglandins.

Oxytocin antagonists may inhibit preterm labour (Akerlund *et al.*, 1987). The results of controlled clinical trials may confirm this, but the question as to whether oxytocin plays a role in the initiation of labour is unlikely to be resolved by these studies.

Plasma concentrations of oxytocin in the mother

Oxytocin is measurable in most women throughout pregnancy by specific radioimmunoassays and there is a weak trend towards increasing concentrations with advancing pregnancy (Chard, 1989). Oxytocin seems to be released in spurts, which may explain some of the discrepancies of results between authors most of whom did not take samples at sufficiently close intervals to detect spurts. Some authors reported that the frequency of spurts of oxytocin release increased throughout labour (Chard, 1989). These observations lend little support to the hypothesis that labour is triggered by increasing maternal plasma concentrations of oxytocin (Table 1).

Plasma concentrations of oxytocin in the fetus

Oxytocin concentrations are higher in umbilical artery than in vein suggesting fetal production. Concentrations in fetal blood increase during labour but it is not known when concentrations begin to rise (Chard, 1989). A regulatory role of oxytocin in the initiation of labour is improbable in view of experiments of nature (see sections on fetal signals for labour).

Uterine response to oxytocin

Intravenous infusion of oxytocin stimulates contractions throughout pregnancy. Uterine contractile response is low in early pregnancy and increases progressively until at least 34–36 weeks (Caldeyro-Barcia & Sereno, 1961). Oxytocin is able to induce labour only close to term and inconsistently unless amniotomy is performed concurrently (Theobald, Robards & Suter, 1969). Induction of labour is achieved with infusion rates of oxytocin (1–8 mU/min) that raise maternal plasma concentrations within physiological limits. Successful induction of labour is accompanied by a sustained increase in maternal plasma concentrations of PGFM (Fuchs & Fuchs, 1984).

Oxytocin receptors

Specific binding sites for oxytocin have been described by several authors. There is circumstantial evidence that these sites function as receptors. The evidence includes binding affinities of oxytocin analogues to these sites in the rank order of their biological potencies and a reasonable correlation between oxytocin receptor concentrations in myometrium and oxytocin sensitivity (Soloff, 1988).

The capacity of myometrium to bind oxytocin increases during pregnancy and early labour. Mean concentrations of myometrial oxytocin receptors were six-fold higher at 13–17 weeks gestation than in non-pregnant uteri and increased a further six times towards term (Fuchs *et al.*, 1984). In patients scheduled for elective Caesarean section who went into spontaneous labour (cervical dilatation ≤ 4 cm at operation) concentrations of oxytocin receptors were 2.5 times greater than in patients who underwent elective Caesarean sections before the onset of labour and 10 times higher than in parturients operated on in late labour (cervical dilatation 7–10 cm). Receptor affinity does not change during pregnancy and labour (Fuchs *et al.*, 1984). The extent to which the apparent decrease in receptor concentration during labour is due to receptor downregulation or to sampling from a more caudal site with advancing labour as the lower segment of the uterus is distended upwards has not been resolved. This question is relevant as the tissue was obtained from the Caesarean section wound and receptor concentrations are lower in the lower segment than in the upper part of the uterus (Fuchs *et al.*, 1984).

In decidua, similar changes in receptor concentration to those in myometrium occur during pregnancy and labour with the exception that concentrations are similar at term in patients in labour and not in labour (Fuchs *et al.*, 1984). The existence of oxytocin receptors in decidua is also suggested from experiments *in vitro*. Oxytocin leads to an immediate release of arachidonic acid and PGF_{2alpha} by dispersed decidual cells *in vitro* (Wilson, Liggins & Whittaker, 1988). The quantity of arachidonic acid released by cells obtained after spontaneous labour in response to a standard dose of oxytocin is twice that released by cells obtained at elective Caesarean section at term (Wilson *et al.*, 1988). These findings give support to the hypothesis that oxytocin has a dual effect on uterine contractions – by a direct action on the myometrium and an indirect action via stimulation of decidual PGF_{2alpha} production (Fuchs & Fuchs, 1984). Whether the greater response to oxytocin obtained in decidua harvested during labour (Wilson *et al.*, 1988) is due to increased concentrations of oxytocin receptors (which would contradict the findings by Fuchs *et al.*, 1984) or enhanced post-receptor responsiveness remains to be established. The observation that oxytocin stimulates prostaglandin release in decidua may offer an explanation for the clinical observation that infusion of oxytocin to patients with an unfavourable cervix eventually leads to cervical ripening and labour.

As increased concentrations of oxytocin receptors are one of the earliest events known to occur during (or preceding?) labour, knowledge of the regulation of oxytocin receptors becomes paramount in understanding the mechanisms of the initiation of labour. In rats (in which the concentrations in maternal plasma of oestrogens increase and those of progesterone decrease, as in sheep), oestrogen stimulates and progesterone inhibits the formation of oxytocin receptors (Fuchs & Fuchs, 1984). It is not known whether oestrogens and progesterone have similar effects in man (see sections on oestrogens and progesterone). In rats a close correlation exists between the concentrations of uterine oxytocin receptors and PGF_{2alpha}, and treatment with an inhibitor of prostaglandin synthase results in a marked reduction in receptor concentrations (Chan, 1987). Human myometrial strips show enhanced responsiveness to oxytocin after administrations of prostaglandins. This is in keeping with induction of oxytocin receptors by prostaglandins (Brummer, 1972). The observations of release of PGF_{2alpha} by oxytocin in decidua (Wilson *et al.*, 1988) and the enhancement of oxytocin action in myometrium after pretreatment with prostaglandins (Brummer, 1972) suggest a positive feed-back loop between oxytocin and prostaglandins (Fig. 7).

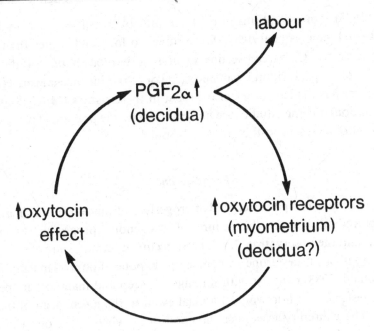

Fig. 7. The putative positive feed-back loop between prostaglandins and oxytocin in the uterus. Induction of oxytocin receptors in myometrium by prostaglandins has been demonstrated in rats (see text). PG = prostaglandin.

Is oxytocin obligatory for labour?

Women with diabetes insipidus can deliver normally at term. Whether this denies a pivotal role for maternal oxytocin in the onset of labour is uncertain as normal lactation and milk ejection occur in these women, and cases have been reported with normal plasma levels of oxytocin (Chard, 1989). The fact that hypophysectomized women given hormonal replacement therapy (glucocorticoids, thyroid hormones, and vasopressin) deliver at term also makes a major role for maternal oxytocin unlikely although small amounts of oxytocin sufficient to play a permissive role in parturition may enter the maternal circulation from various sources including the fetus. Fetal oxytocin is very unlikely to have an obligatory role in the initiation of parturition. A possible paracrine function of oxytocin is discussed in the following section.

Does oxytocin have a paracrine mechanism of action?

Recent findings of oxytocin mRNA in human chorion and, in very small quantities, in amnion suggest that these tissues synthesize oxytocin (Chibbar, Miller &

Mitchell, 1993). Concentrations of oxytocin mRNA in cultured chorio-decidual cells harvested after vaginal delivery are three- to four-fold higher than in cells obtained at elective Caesarean section suggesting that locally produced oxytocin may play a role in parturition by an autocrine or paracrine mechanism. However, these workers have failed to detect oxytocin in these tissues (Mitchell, personal communication). Further studies are needed to assess the potential for a paracrine contribution of oxytocin to the onset of labour.

Progesterone

The absence in man of a consistent fall of progesterone concentrations in maternal plasma preceding labour, the failure of exogenous progestins to prolong pregnancy, and the observation that labour occurs at term in spite of low plasma concentrations of progesterone in congenital hypobetalipoproteinaemia (Casey & MacDonald, 1988) contrast with findings in sheep and many other species in which progesterone withdrawal is a crucial event in the mechanism of the onset of labour. These discrepancies raise the question of whether the onset of labour in man is fundamentally different from that in animals possessing placental 17-alpha hydroxylase or whether the events at the tissue level are similar in all species. The importance of progesterone for the maintenance of human pregnancy seems to decline with increasing gestational age; the rate of successful termination of pregnancy after administration of a progesterone receptor blocker, mifepristone (RU 486), decreases from 93% to 70% between 5 and 7–8 weeks amenorrhea, unless prostaglandins are used in conjunction (mifepristone has glucocorticoid receptor blocking activity as well as progesterone receptor blocking activity) (Baulieu, Ulmann & Philibert, 1987). On the assumption that progesterone withdrawal is a necessary feature of initiation of labour in all species, the hypothesis has been proposed that progesterone acts in an autocrine or paracrine manner whereby changes in uterine progesterone concentrations are not detectable in maternal plasma (Challis & Mitchell, 1988). The hypothesis is based on the observation that extraplacental intra-uterine tissues can synthesize and metabolize progesterone and that the local concentration of this steroid can be independent of placental production. This may be achieved by some sort of compartmentalization. Pregnenolone and pregnenolone sulphate are taken up by chorion and decidua, and 20-alpha dihydroprogesterone by amnion, and converted to progesterone *in vitro* (Challis & Mitchell, 1988). Synthesis of progesterone is greater in amnion, chorion and decidua obtained at elective Caesarean section than after vaginal delivery (Challis & Mitchell, 1988). Fetal plasma concentrations of pregnenolone sulphate are sufficiently high in late pregnancy to provide the substrate for synthesis of progesterone by chorion and decidua. These findings support the hypothesis of a 'local progesterone withdrawal' occurring during (or before the onset of) labour (Challis & Mitchell, 1988).

Oestrogens

In women there is a slow and steady increase in maternal plasma concentrations of oestrogens throughout pregnancy but only one study, on highly selected patients, found a consistent and marked rise in oestrogen concentrations preceding labour while most other investigations did not detect any such increase (Flint, 1979). Oestrogens are therefore unlikely to exert a major effect on the uterus through endocrine mechanisms. Whether oestrogens have any regulatory role in parturition at all is doubtful in view of the following observations. Intravenous injections of dehydroepiandrosterone sulphate (DHEAS), the substrate for oestrogen synthesis in man, markedly increase circulating levels of oestradiol and oestriol at term but the onset of labour is not advanced. Conversely, administration of glucocorticoids at term depressed circulating oestrogen levels to about 10% of normal values by inhibiting fetal and maternal secretion of DHEAS but pregnancy is not prolonged. Oestrogen concentrations are similarly low in a sex-linked genetic disorder, placental sulphatase deficiency, which impairs the conversion of DHEAS to DHEA, but labour occurs at term (although in primigravidae, dystocia due to impaired cervical ripening may occur) (France, Seddon & Liggins, 1973) (Table 3). One controlled trial reported a significantly higher number of women commencing labour within seven days of a single intravenous dose of 200 mg oestradiol than after placebo but several other studies failed to detect any effect of even very large doses of oestrogens (Flint, 1979). In view of the ability of exogenous oestrogens to induce labour in other species, the failure of very high or very low plasma concentrations of oestrogens to exert any consistent effect on gestation length in women suggests that oestrogens have no regulatory role in human parturition (Flint, 1979).

There is a potential for a paracrine action of oestrogens. Chorion and decidua but not amnion contain steroid sulphatase capable of synthesizing oestrone, oestradiol, and DHEA from the biologically inactive oestrone sulphate and DHEAS (which are increasingly abundant in amniotic fluid towards term) (Challis & Mitchell, 1988). In tissue explants and in dispersed chorion cells, the conversion by steriod sulphohydrolase of oestrone sulphate into oestrone and further metabolism into oestradiol is greater in cells harvested after vaginal delivery than at elective Caesarean section before labour, lending support to the hypothesis that oestrogens play some role in the initiation or the maintenance of labour in man (Challis & Mitchell, 1988). These observations in intact cells contrast with

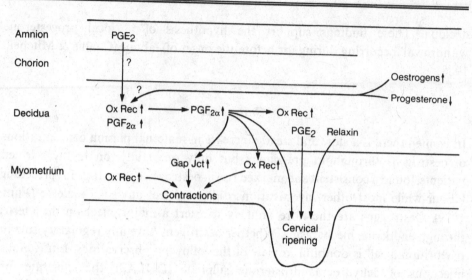

Fig. 8. A tentative model for the initiation of human parturition. The first measurable events are raised concentrations of PGF_{2alpha} in amniotic fluid and increased oxytocin receptor concentrations in myometrium and decidua. Oxytocin is available from the maternal circulation and possibly from chorion and decidua (not shown). PG = prostaglandin; Ox Rec = oxytocin receptors; Gap Jct = gap junctions.

findings on sulphohydrolase activity in microsomal preparations from chorion (the cell fraction in which the specified activity of this enzyme is highest); hydrolytic activity was no different whether the tissue was obtained at Caesarean section before labour or during labour (Chibbar & Mitchell, 1988). Further studies are needed to resolve these discrepancies and to elucidate the possible consequences of increased oestrogen production in man, which by analogy to other species could entail increased prostaglandin synthesis and the formation of oxytocin receptors and gap junctions.

Summary

A soundly based model for the initiation of labour in man is not yet available. The following proposal is speculative but may serve as a useful framework in which to incorporate future development (Fig. 8).

The earliest identifiable events in labour are increases in the production of PGF_{2alpha} and in the concentration of oxytocin receptors. It is not known which event occurs first but it is possible that a relatively small increase in prostanoid production, conceivably PGE_2 by amnion, stimulates oxytocin receptor formation. This could lead, in turn, to an enhanced response to circulating or locally produced oxytocin manifested in the myometrium by contractility and in the macrophage-like decidual stromal cells by PGF_{2alpha} production. As a consequence of prostaglandin production by decidua the myometrium is stimulated both directly and also by potentiation of the response to oxytocin. The connective tissue of the cervix and uterine body undergoes complex biochemical changes that lead to softening and distensibility similar to the changes in response to relaxin; locally formed relaxin is likely to act in synergy with prostanoids on connective tissues.

The signal to the foregoing events is unknown. No convincing evidence exists of fetal involvement either by a circulating hormone or by a substance entering the amniotic fluid. Available evidence points strongly to the mechanism initiating labour being an intra-uterine, paracrine system and consequently that the signal arises in the placenta/chorion. Various possibilities then arise; most favoured is the idea that local changes in oestrogen and progesterone metabolism alter the ratio of the two hormones to promote prostanoid release but evidence that this occurs *in vivo* and of how it is regulated is lacking. Alternatively, the initiating system may be activated by a chorionic genetic clock transduced by protein kinases yet to be identified.

References

Akerlund, M., Stromberg, P., Hanksson, A., Andersen, L. F., Lyndrup, J., Trojnar, J. & Melin, P. (1987). Inhibition of uterine contractions of premature labour with an oxytocin analogue. Results from a pilot study. *British Journal of Obstetrics and Gynaecology*, **94**, 1040–4.

Baulieu, E. E., Ulman, A. & Philibert, D. (1987). Contragestion by antiprogestin RU 486: a review. *Archives in Gynaecology and Obstetrics*, **241**, 73–85.

Bleasdale, J. E. & Johnston, J. M. (1984). Prostaglandins and human parturition: regulation of arachidonic acid mobilization. In *Reviews in Perinatal Medicine*. Ed. E. M. Scarpelli and E. V. Cosmi, vol. 5, pp. 151–91, AR Liss, New York.

Brennecke, S. P., Castle, B. M., Demers, L. M. & Turnbull, A. C. (1985). Maternal plasma prostaglandin E_2 metabolite levels during human pregnancy and parturition. *British Journal of Obstetrics and Gynaecology*, **92**, 345–9.

Brummer, H. C. (1972). Interaction of E prostaglandins and syntocinon on the pregnant human myometrium. *Journal of Obstetrics and Gynaecology of the British Commonwealth*, **78**, 305–9.

Bryant-Greenwood, G. D. & Greenwood, F. C. (1988). Postulated roles for luteal or decidual relaxins at parturition in the pregnant sow and woman. In *The Physiology and Biochemistry of Human Fetal Membranes*. (*Research in Perinatal Medicine*; vol. 6.) Ed. B. F. Mitchell, pp, 141–56, Perinatology Press, Ithaca.

Caldeyro-Barcia, R. & Sereno, J. (1961). The response of the human uterus to oxytocin throughout pregnancy. In *Oxytocin*. Ed. R. Caldeyro-Barcia and H. Heller, pp. 177–202, Pergamon Press, Oxford.

Casey, M. L., MacDonald, P. C. & Mitchell, M. D. (1983). Stimulation of prostaglandin E_2 production in amnion cells in culture by a substance(s) in human fetal and adult urine. *Biochemical and Biophysical Research Communications*, **114**, 1056–63.

Casey, M. L. & MacDonald, P. C. (1988). Decidual activation: the role of prostaglandins in labor. In *The Onset of Labor: Cellular and Integrative Mechanisms*. Ed. D. McNellis, J. Challis, P. MacDonald, P. Nathanielsz and J. Roberts, pp. 141–56, Perinatology Press, Ithaca. (*Reproductive and Perinatal Medicine*, **9**.)

Challis, J. R. G. & Mitchell, B. F. (1988). Steroid production by the fetal membranes in relation to the onset of parturition. In *The Onset of Labor: Cellular and Integrative Mechanisms*. Ed. D. McNellis, J. Challis, P. MacDonald, P. Nathanielsz and J. Roberts, pp. 233–36, Perinatology Press, Ithaca. (*Reproductive and Perinatal Medicine*, **9**.)

Challis, J. R. G. & Olson, D. M. (1988). Parturition. In *The Physiology of Reproduction*. Ed. E. Knobil and J. Neill, pp. 2177–215, Raven Press, New York.

Chan, W. Y. (1987). Enhanced prostaglandin synthesis in the parturient rat uterus and its effects on myometrial oxytocin receptor concentrations. *Prostaglandins*, **34**, 889–902.

Chard, T. (1989). Fetal and maternal oxytocin in human parturition. *American Journal of Perinatology*, **6**, 145–52.

Chibbar, R. & Mitchell, B. F. (1988). Steroid sulfohydrolase activity in human chorion. I. Interactions of other steroids with estrone sulfate as substrate. *Journal of Clinical Endocrinology Metabolism*, **66**, 1192–6.

Chibbar, R., Miller, F. D. & Mitchell, B. F. (1993). Synthesis of oxytocin in amnion, chorion and decidua may influence the timing of human parturition. *Journal of Clinical Investigation*, **91**, 185–92.

Claireaux, A. E. & Ferreira, H. P. (1958). Bilateral pulmonary agenesis. *Archive of Diseases of Childhood*, **33**, 364–6.

Ekman, G., Malmström, A., Uldbjerg, N. & Ulmsten, U. (1986). Cervical collagen: an important regulator of cervical function in term labor. *Obstetrics and Gynecology*, **67**, 633–6.

Flint, A. P. F. (1979). Role of progesterone and oestrogens in the control of the onset of labour in man: a continuing controversy. In *Human Parturition. New Concepts and Developments*. Ed. M. J. N. C. Keirse, A. B. M. Anderson and J. B. Gravenhorst, pp. 85–100. University Press, Leiden. (*Boerhaave Series for Postgraduate Medical Education*, **15**.)

France, J. T., Seddon, R. J. & Liggins, G. C. (1973). A study of a pregnancy with low oestrogen production due to placental sulfatase deficiency. *Journal of Clinical Endocrinology Metabolism*, **26**, 1–9.

Fuchs, A. R., Goeschen, K., Husslein, P., Rasmussen, A. B. & Fuchs, F. (1983). Oxytocin and the initiation of human parturition: III. Plasma concentrations of oxytocin and 13,14-dihydro-15-keto-prostaglandin F_{2alpha} in spontaneous and oxytocin induced labor at term. *American Journal of Obstetrics and Gynecology*, **147**, 497–502.

Fuchs, A.-R. & Fuchs, F. (1984). Endocrinology of human parturition; a review. *British Journal of Obstetrics and Gynaecology*, **91**, 948–67.

Fuchs, A.-R., Fuchs, F., Husslein, P. & Soloff, M. S. (1984). Oxytocin receptors in the human uterus during pregnancy and parturition. *American Journal of Obstetrics and Gynecology*, **150**, 734–41.

Garfield, R. E. (1988). Structural and functional studies of the control of myometrial contractility and labor. In *The Onset of Labor: Cellular and Integrative Mechanisms*. Ed. D. McNellis, J. Challis, P. MacDonald, P. Nathanielsz and J. Roberts, pp. 55–80, Perinatology Press, Ithaca. (*Reproductive and Perinatal Medicine*, **9**.)

Honnebier, W. M. & Swaab, D. F. (1973). The influence of anencephaly upon intrauterine growth of the fetus and placenta and upon gestation length. *Journal of Obstetrics and Gynaecology of the British Commonwealth*, **80**, 577–88.

Husslein, P. (1984). Concentrations of 13,14-dihydro-15-keto-prostaglandin E_2 in the maternal peripheral plasma during labour of spontaneous onset. *British Journal of Obstetrics and Gynaecology*, **91**, 228–31.

Husslein, P. & Sinzinger, H. (1984). Concentration of 13,14-dihydro-15-keto-prostaglandin E_2 in the maternal peripheral plasma during labour of spontaneous onset. *British Journal of Obstetrics and Gynaecology*, **91**, 228–31.

Johnston, J. M., Bleasdale, J. E. & Hoffman, D. R. (1987). Functions of PAF in reproduction and development: involvement of PAF in fetal lung maturation and parturition. In *Platelet-Activating Factor and Related Lipid Mediators*. Ed. F. Snyder, pp. 374–402, Plenum Publishing Corp., New York.

Keirse, M. J. N. C. (1979). Endogenous prostaglandins in human parturition. In *Human Parturition. New Concepts and Developments*. Ed. M. J. N. C. Keirse, A. B. M. Anderson and J. B. Gravenhorst, pp. 101–42, University Press, Leiden. (*Boerhaave Series for Postgraduate Medical Education*, **15**.)

Lerner, U. (1980). The uterine cervix and the initiation of labour: action of oestradiol-17 beta. In *Dilatation of the Uterine Cervix. Connective Tissue Biology and Clinical Management*. Ed. F. Naftolin and P. G. Stubblefield, pp. 301–16, Raven Press, New York.

Liggins, G. C., Fairclough, R. J., Grieves, S. A., Forster, C. S. & Knox, B. S. (1977). Parturition in the sheep. In *The Fetus and Birth*. Ed. J. Knight and M. O. Connor, pp. 5–25, Ciba Foundation Symposium, Vol. 47, Elsevier North-Holland, Amsterdam.

Lopez-Bernal, A., Newman, G. E., Phizackerley, P. J. R. & Turnbull, A. C. (1988). Surfactant stimulates prostaglandin E production by human amnion. *British Journal of Obstetrics and Gynaecology*, **95**, 1013–17.

Lundin-Schiller, S. & Mitchell, M. D. (1990). The role of prostaglandins in human parturition. *Prostaglandins, Leukotrienes and Essential Fatty Acids*, **39**, 1–10.

MacLennan, A. H., Green, R. C., Bryant-Greenwood, G. D., Greenwood, F. C. & Seamark, R. F. (1980). Ripening of the human cervix and induction of labour with purified porcine relaxin. *Lancet*, **i**, 220–3.

Manzai, M. & Liggins, G. C. (1984). Inhibitory effects of dispersed humam amnion cells on production rates of prostaglandin E and F by endometrial cells. *Prostaglandins*, **28**, 297–307.

McCoshen, J. A. (19). Associations between prolactin, prostaglandin E_2 and fetal membrane function in human gestation. In *The Physiology and Biochemistry of Human Fetal Membranes*. Ed. B. F. Mitchell, pp. 117–39, Perinatalogy Press, Ithaca. (*Research in Perinatal Medicine*, **6**.)

Mitchell, M. D., Bibby, J., Hicks, B. R. & Turnbull, A. C. (1978). Specific production of prostaglandin E by human amnion *in vitro*. *Prostaglandins*, **15**, 377–82.

Mitchell, M. D. (1984). The mechanism(s) of human parturition. *Journal of Developmental Physiology*, **6**, 107–18.

Moore, J. J., Dubyak, G. R., Moore, R. M. & Vaner Kooy, D. (1988). Oxytocin activates the inositol–phospholipid–protein-kinase-C system and stimulates prostaglandin production in human amnion cells. *Endocrinology*, **123**, 1771–7.

Nagata, J., Sunaga, H., Furuya, K., Makimura, N. & Kato, K. (1987). Changes in the plasma prostaglandin F_{2alpha} metabolite before and during spontaneous labor and labor induced by amniotomy, oxytocin and prostaglandin E_2. *Endocrinology Japan*, **34**, 153–9.

Nakla, S., Skinner, K., Mitchell, B. F. & Challis, J. R. G. (1986). Changes in prostaglandin transfer across human fetal membranes obtained after spontaneous labour. *American Journal of Obstetrics and Gynecology*, **155**, 1337–41.

Olson, D. M., Skinner, K. & Challis, J. R. G. (1983). Prostaglandin output in relation to parturition by cells dispersed from human intrauterine tissues. *Journal of Clinical Endocrinology Metabolism*, **57**, 694–9.

Olson, D. M., Zakar, T., Potestio, F. A. & Smieja, Z. (1990). Control of prostaglandin production in human amnion. *News Physiological Science*, **5**, 259–63.

Rechberger, T., Uldbjerg, N. & Oxlund, H. (1988). Connective tissue changes in the cervix during normal pregnancy and pregnancy complicated by cervical incompetence. *Obstetrics and Gynecology*, **71**, 563–7.

Romero, R., Emamian, M., Wan, M., Grzyboski, C., Hobbins, J. C. & Mitchell, M. D. (1987). Increased concentrations of arachidonic acid lipoxygenase metabolites in amniotic fluid during parturition. *Obstetrics and Gynecology*, **70**, 849–53.

Rose, M. P., Myatt, L. & Elder, G. (1990). Pathways of arachidonic acid metabolism in human amnion cells at term. *Prostaglandins, Leukotrienes, Essential Fatty Acids*, **39**, 303–9.

Seppälä, M., Aho, I., Tissari, A. & Ruoslahti, E. (1972). Radioimmunoassay of oxytocin in amniotic fluid, fetal urine, and meconium during late pregnancy and delivery. *American Journal of Obstetrics and Gynecology*, **114**, 788–95.

Soloff, M. S. (1988). The role of oxytocin in the initiation of labour, and oxytocin–prostaglandin interactions. In *The Onset of Labor: Cellular and Integrative Mechanisms*. Ed. D. McNellis, J. Challis, P. MacDonald, P. Nathanielsz and J. Roberts, pp. 87–110, Perinatology Press, Ithaca. (*Reproductive and Perinatal Medicine*, **9**.)

Strickland, D. M., Saeed, S. A., Casey, M. L. & Mitchell, M. D. (1983). Stimulation of prostaglandin biosynthesis by urine of the human fetus may serve as a trigger for parturition. *Science*, **220**, 521–2.

Theobald, G. W., Robards, M. F. & Suter, P. E. N. (1969). Changes in myometrial sensitivity to oxytocin in man during the last six weeks of pregnancy. *Journal of Obstetrics and Gynaecology British Commonwealth*, **76**, 385–93.

Thorburn, G. D., Hooper, S. B., Rice, G. E. & Fowden, A. L. (1988). Luteal regression and parturition: a comparison. In *The Onset of Labor: Cellular and Integrative Mechanisms*. Ed. D. McNellis, J. Challis, P. MacDonald, P. Nathanielsz and J. Roberts, pp. 185–206, Perinatology Press, Ithaca. (*Reproductive and Perinatal Medicine*, **9**.)

Wilson, T., Liggins, G. C. & Whittaker, D. J. (1988). Oxytocin stimulates the release of arachidonic acid and prostaglandin F_{2alpha} from human decidual cells. *Prostaglandins*, **35**, 771–81.

Wilson, T., Liggins, G. C. & Joe, L. (1989). Purification from incubated chorion of a phospholipase A_2 inhibitor active before but not after the onset of labour. *American Journal of Obstetrics and Gynecology*, **160**, 602–6.

Wilson, T. & Christie, D. L. (1991). Gravidin, an endogenous inhibitor of phospholipase A_2 activity, is secretory component of IgA. *Biochemical and Biophysical Research Communications*, 447–52.

Wilson, T. & Ganandren, R. (1992). Serum concentrations of secretory IgA in pregnancies delivering at term or preterm. *Prostaglandins*, **44**, 373–8.

15

Measurement of uterine contractions

C. ROMANINI

Introduction

The uterus is specialized, first, for the reception of the ovum by the endometrium and the continuous nourishment of the developing fetus and, second, for the eventual expulsion of the fetus, by means of the strong isometric contractions of the myometrium. The latter requires a massive increase in size and weight of the organ and considerable tissue differentiation. One of the enigmas of gestation is the ability of the uterus to grow without any large increase in muscle tension. Histological examination shows that this takes place almost entirely by an increase in size of the muscle cells, with only a small amount of cell division in early pregnancy. The phenomenon is accompanied by the synthesis of the contractile proteins and of the enzymes concerned in energy provision. These changes are stimulated by the ovarian oestrogens, which also determine the deposition of energy stores such as glycogen. In spite of its growth, the myometrium responds effectively to such stimuli as oxytocin only at the end of pregnancy, when the loss of amniotic fluid results in the shortening of the stretched muscle bundles. Parturition can then take place.

Studies of myometrial physiology provides basic knowledge which may be applied to clinical situations, such as the prevention of premature labour (the greatest single cause of human perinatal loss).

Anatomical and physiological background

Structure

The muscular coat or myometrium forms the greater part of the wall of the uterus. It is continuous with that of the tubes above and the vagina below. Bundles of superficial smooth muscle are prolonged into the various ligaments that attach

337

to the uterus. There is relatively less muscle, but more fibrous tissue in the isthmus and cervix.

The myometrium is composed of three inter-digitating muscle layers: an outer, mainly longitudinal, a middle and an inner, mainly circular. The middle forms the bulk of the organ and is composed of obliquely inter-digitating strands of muscle fibres.

The myometrial cell has the appearance of an elongated double cone, with a central nucleus. The greater diameter varies from 3 to 8 μm and the length from 15 to 200 μm, except in the pregnant uterus, where it may exceed 500 μm. The outline of the cells is indistinct in longitudinal views, but is easily seen in cross-section (Josimovich, 1973).

As the muscle cells differentiate, their exterior surface acquires an external lamina, which segregates them from the surrounding connective tissue. The plasma membrane is characterized by numerous caveolae, which protrude into the cytoplasm. Adjacent muscle cells form nexuses, or gap junctions, and here the external lamina is lacking and intimate membrane-to-membrane contact is achieved, providing a functional attachment between the cells. The modulation of gap junctions is one of the major mechanisms involved in control of myometrial activity in the human (Sakai *et al.*, 1992).

In these smooth muscle cells, mitochondria and rough endoplasmic reticulum are located at the nuclear pole as is the nearby Golgi apparatus. The cytoplasm is dominated by longitudinally aligned contractile filaments. The two major contractile proteins, actin and myosin, are contained in the filament systems of uterine muscle, but the most readily seen filaments are thin and composed of actin. Some workers have postulated that most of the myosin is present in an unaggregated form, while aggregation into visibly thick filaments occurs during tension production. The actin filaments often course obliquely in the cell, attaching in characteristic condensations along the inner surface of the plasmalemma. The tension is transmitted to these dense areas which form sites for interconnection between actin filaments.

Between the large bundles of smooth muscle cells are collagenous and elastic fibres. Smooth muscle cells are capable of synthesizing considerable amounts of collagen and elastin; this is particularly evident in the cervix where a decrease in elastin seems to be correlated with incompetence. The function of cervical elastin may be to maintain a closed cervix throughout gestation.

The mechanism of contraction in uterine muscle

The contraction of uterine smooth muscle is dependent upon interaction of thick and thin myofilaments. This interaction requires activation by calcium ions released into the cytoplasm followed by phosphorylation of light chain myosin. Actin (troponin) serves this function in skeletal muscles.

The contraction of myometrium is slow and sustained. The arrangement of the filaments, orientated obliquely to the axis of the muscle fibre containing them, allows these fibres to exert a relatively large force through a short distance. The functional result is a contraction that is very efficient, generating less heat for production of the same tension. This ultrastructural feature explains the ability of uterine muscle to sustain a forceful and prolonged contraction with minimal expenditure of energy and relatively low shortening velocity. It is also correlated with the facility for localized contraction.

Electrophysiology

Pacemakers and pacefollowers

As in all autorhythmic tissues, the frequency of the pacemaker sets the frequency of the activity of the tissue.

In the myometrium, two types of frequencies can be discerned. One type has a long period, of the order of several seconds to tens of seconds. The other type has a short period, 0.5–1 second, and is associated with repetitive activity. The long period determines the frequency, while the short period affects the intensity of each contraction (Harbert, 1992).

Not all myometrial cells are pacemakers; conduction probably results from spread of local current and the cells which are involved are termed pacefollowers. However, pacemakers and pacefollowers in the myometrium are not anatomically discrete, because each myometrial cell is capable of being either. However, in studies on the rat uterus, Crane showed that if the influence of pacemakers is permanently removed, new pacemakers do not develop (Crane & Martin, 1991).

In uterine muscle a small rapid stretch can cause depolarization (Coleman & Parkington, 1992). Under extreme stretch, discharges from a parturient uterus become continuous.

Membrane potential and ion fluxes

Excitable cells transmit signals via a set of pores that mediate rapid changes of membrane permeability. This has the effect of amplifying a small voltage change by an increase of sodium [Na]. An action potential is initiated by depolarization of a sensory receptor or a synapse. [Na] rises, then decays after a short time when potassium [K] increases. The result is an outward current of K^+.

Although no ions move through the membrane during current flow, the change in the distribution of the ions leads to a redistribution of charge on the membrane.

The first phase of this is a rearrangement of electrons along the lipid molecules that form the bulk of the membrane. The second and third components are movements of charged molecules attached to the membrane.

Ions flow through the membrane pores ('gates') in response to changes of membrane voltage; flow is controlled by dipolar molecules that rotate when the voltage is changed. The membrane potential steps from -63 mV (normal resting) to -26 mV (Lydrup, 1991), after a latent period of 200–300 ms. The concentration of intracellular free calcium in resting cells is 116–18.5 nM. The (K^+) of oestrogen-dominated myometrium is about 158 meq/litre cell water, while in progesterone-dominated tissue, it becomes about 132 meq (Josimovich, 1973).

Uterine muscle relaxation is associated with removal of calcium ions, by a Ca-pump. Inward current is carried through two types of Ca^{2+} channels: slow (L type) and fast (T type) Ca^{2+} channels. The fast inward current decays within 30 ms and depends on [Na]; the slow one depends on [Ca] or [Ca^{2+}]. The fast inward current is probably a fast Na^+ channel current and the slow current is a slow Ca^{2+} channel. The number of fast Na^+ channels increases during gestation because of an increase in the fraction of cells that possess fast Na^+ channels. Na^+ is involved in spread of excitation, whereas Mg^{2+} depresses it. Among the K^+ channels one is responsible for repolarization of the individual action potential and another for repolarization of the slow wave.

The duration of the relaxed period can be influenced by activation of K^+ channels (Lydrup, 1991); a fibre depolarized for some time becomes refractory, with Na gates closed and K activation gates open.

When a muscle has been inactive a long time the contractile activity is greatly reduced.

Effects of autonomic nerve stimulation

The sympathetic innervation of the uterus is carried through the presacral (hypogastric) nerves, which are represented in the human by a series of plexuses: the superior middle and inferior hypogastric plexuses, which contain both efferent and afferent fibres. The myometrial adrenergic fibres are most dense in the cervix. The ganglion cells supplying the myometrium are located at the utero-vaginal junction and along the hypogastric nerve. This implies lack of direct relations between nerve and muscle, spread of transmitter over larger volumes by diffusion and the necessity for myogenic spread of excitation from cell to cell. Stimulation of the hypogastric nerve may cause a uterine response mainly due to release of norepinephrine and epinephrine at the post-ganglionic nerve terminal. The hormonal factors that modify the response of the uterine muscle operate on the muscle itself. not the nerve terminal.

Catecholamines exert their action on one of several sites: the cell membrane, contractile proteins and cellular metabolism. In each case, alpha-excitatory and beta-inhibitory adrenergic receptors are involved. In animals, myometrial alpha adrenergic receptors are regulated by gonodal steroids. There are alpha1 and alpha2 adrenergic receptors. The affinity and number of alpha1 receptors is not affected by hormonal conditions, whereas the number of the alpha2 receptors increases with circulating plasma oestradiol levels; this effect is counteracted by progesterone (Bottari *et al.*, 1983). Beta2 receptors dominate in the progesterone primed uterus, while both beta1 and beta2 receptors can be found in oestrogen dominated uterus. Epinephrine acts on both adrenergic receptors, while norepine-phrine has only alpha receptor stimulating ability (Marshall, 1979). During the luteal phase of the menstrual cycle, or near term and in labour, there is an increase in the beta receptors, reflected in the predominant inhibiting effect of epinephrine, which can be reversed by a beta blocker.

Uterine activity may also be affected by two neuropeptides, galanin (GAL) and calcitonin gene-related peptide (CGRP), which are present in the fibres innervating the myometrium. In the rat, GAL immunoreactivity (GAL-I) and CGRP-I are localized in myometrial nerves (Shew *et al.*, 1992), in mesometrial smooth muscle, vascular structures and endocervix. GAL stimulates uterine activity in a dose-related manner; CGRP had no effect on basal uterine tension but reduced GAL stimulated uterine contraction by 92.5%.

Measurement of uterine contraction

The focus of this chapter is the techniques that are employed on human uterus *in vivo*.

In 1872, Schatz demonstrated the feasibility of studying contractile activity of the pregnant human uterus by means of an intra-cavitary fluid-filled bag. Since then a variety of non-invasive external or invasive internal techniques have been described.

External tocography uses a pressure sensor that detects changes in the antero-posterior diameter of the abdomen, resulting from uterine contractions. The recordings allow assessment of the frequency, duration and wave form of uterine contraction. The external method is simple and practical and can clearly reproduce the results obtained with an intra-uterine catheter (Oliva *et al.*, 1979a). When compared with internal monitoring, an external transducer detected 90.8% of uterine contractions with a specificity for uterine quiescence of 98.1%. The predictive value of external monitoring is excellent in circumstances such as pre-term pregnancies. However, because there are no units of measurement it is not suitable for quantifying uterine activity. Also, it is difficult to apply to obese patients (Romanini *et al.*, 1972). Abdominal tocography is not suitable as a research method.

Many variations of the internal technique have been described. In our experience, the use of an intra-amniotic catheter with multiple openings is the method of choice (Oliva *et al.*, 1979*a*). Compared with a balloon or sponge-tipped catheter, it is simpler and has a smaller incidence of artifacts than catheters with only one opening.

Inaccuracies may occur if the diaphragm of the pressure transducer is not placed exactly at the level of the catheter tip or if these relationships vary with patient movement. Also it cannot be used in pregnancy. An extraovular microballoon (Csapo, 1964) has been utilized in patients with an intact amniotic sac and the cervix partly dilated, but only when the effects of a possible rupture of the amniotic sac would not be serious.

Tocography provides a continuous measure of intra-uterine pressure. Via a carrier pre-amplifier this permits calculation of many parameters. Baseline pressure is the lowest pressure recorded between contractions; it usually ranges from 8–12 mm Hg, but it may fluctuate from values of <8 mm Hg (hypotonus) to values >30 mm Hg. Hypertonus can be distinguished in: weak (>20 mm Hg), medium (>20, <30 mm Hg) and strong (>30 mm Hg) forms. Another parameter is the intensity (or amplitude); this depends on the myometrial mass and on the number of excited cells. Amplitude detection may be difficult if elevation of basic tone occurs, or when the thickness of the abdominal wall and the amount of amniotic fluid are increased. Frequency is an expression of the average time of contraction intervals, generally measured in a 10 minute period. Contraction duration, is related to baseline pressure and amplitude. The latter is a non-linear correlation: an increase in duration results from a lengthened contraction and relaxation time, but not from an increase in the apparently invariant midportion of the contractile wave (Harbert, 1992).

The Montevideo Unit (MU) is the most widely used method of quantitation. It is the product of the average intensity (measured from the basic tone) multiplied by the number of contractions in 10 minutes. The Alexandria Unit (AU) was an attempt to overcome the limitations of MU, which do not allow for variable duration; AU is equal to the product of MU multiplied by the average duration. Finally, the active pressure area can be measured, that is the area above baseline pressure, reflecting a uterine activity integral (Romanini & Bompiani, 1970). Computer systems are now used to provide formal numeric evaluation.

Real time evaluation was originally performed with an on-line computer. The method had some limitations, such as the difficulty of identifying contractions only by changes of tocometric potential which could be biased by artifacts in the pressure signal. We have therefore investigated off-line analysis with a hybrid

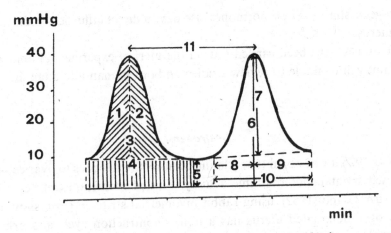

Fig. 1. Diagrammatic representation of the parameters examined by the programme: 1 AS = Area of pressure increase; 2 AD = Area of pressure decrease; 3 APA = AS + AD = Area of active pressure; 4 ATO = AS + AD + APA + Area covering the basal tone = Total area expressed by the contraction; 5 TB = Basal tone; 6 I = Total intensity; 7 A = Actual intensity; 8 TS = Duration of pressure increase; 9 TD = Duration of pressure decrease; 10 D = Total duration of contraction; 11 INT = Interval.

analog and digital computer. This off-line method produces a series of 11 parameters (Fig. 1). The values of each parameter are recorded on a screen and in hard copy at the end of every contraction, together with a graphic presentation of the contraction. A fast Fourier transform is used to analyse the morphology of contraction. These are, of course, research rather than routine procedures (Romanini *et al.*, 1982).

For clinical use, the trend of intensity values is the most suitable for routine application. Indeed, a human operator can easily identify the trend of individual values simply by watching the curve and its changes in relation to different physiological phases or to administration of different drug.

The physiological roles of hormones upon uterine contraction

The myometrium is quiescent during most of pregnancy. Since the description of the influence of the two ovarian hormones, oestrogen and progesterone, upon the contractility of the myometrium, many biochemical and physiological investigations have been carried out to explain this phenomenon. The studies of Csapo (1959) showed that oestrogens and progesterone cause hyperplasia and/or hypertrophy of myometrial smooth muscle cells, so that the effects of steroids can result in a 'formative' effect on the contractile elements, changing the response to neurogenic stimuli. These hormones also have a direct influence on the motility of the uterus.

Most studies have been carried out on the uteri of experimental animals but an attempt will be made to review studies on both human and animals.

Oestrogens

As early as 1925 it was noted that administration of oestrogens to ovariectomized rats caused spontaneous rhythmic activity. This phenomenon can be observed only *in vivo*. Csapo (1952), using rabbit myometrial strips *in vitro*, showed that the oestrogen-dominated uterus has a longer contraction cycle and exhibits a positive 'staircase' phenomenon.

Oestradiol in concentrations of 10–15 ng/ml reduces the frequency of contraction of human myometrium *in vitro* without changing the amplitude. Studies *in vivo* of the pregnant human uterus near term have shown an oxytocic effect, with an increase in myometrial activity, a rise of uterine tonus and intensity of contractions. Wilson reported that, in baboon, an elevated oestradiol-to-progesterone ratio coincides with the initiation of uterine contractions. It was hypothesized that the oestradiol induces contractions by oxytocin release and/or increase in uterine oxytocin receptors.

Maggi *et al.* (1991) also observed that oxytocin receptors rise sharply in the late luteal phase and during menstruation in human non-pregnant myometrium; conversely, the lowest oxytocin receptor density was found at mid-cycle and in menopause. But the effects of oestrogen administration on uterine activity varies with animal species: for instance, in the non-pregnant ovariectomized sheep myometrial contractility is inhibited by prolonged oestrogen supplementation.

The effect of these steroids can be seen not only in the increase of actomyosin concentration, but also in adenosinetriphosphatase activity. During pregnancy the content of actomysin in the myometrium rises as the pregnancy advances. Kelly & Verhage (1981) showed that oestradiol induces assembly of thick filaments in ovariectomized cats, while progesterone promotes thick filaments disassembly. In particular, animals which were treated for 14 days with oestradiol displayed in all cases a double array of thick (14–16 mm) myofilaments, whereas those which also received progesterone exhibited a single array of thick filaments only.

The uterine contractile response to adrenergic factors is controlled by the hormonal milieu. Oestrogens increase the alpha1 adrenergic sensitivity of rabbit myometrium. Whereas relaxation is mediated by beta-2-adrenoceptors, uterine contraction is promoted by alpha1 adrenoceptors. As cholinergic-stimulated production is not increased by oestrogen treatment, it seems probable that oestrogen enhancement of uterine adrenergic sensitivity is associated with increased post-receptor response. Some studies suggest the presence of parallel pathways for receptor activation of a common post-receptor response, while others suggest that at least one component of the adenylate cyclase beyond the beta adrenoceptor is a target for ovarian steroids: oestrogens will reduce beta adrenoceptor-mediated CAMP production (Riemer *et al.*, 1988).

Progesterone

That progesterone might have an inhibitory effect on the uterus has been known since 1926: Csapo (1959) postulated a localized myometrial block as a result of diffusion of this hormone from the placenta. During pregnancy the contractile response does not propagate from one cell to the other: when the uterus is dominated by progesterone, only the segment actually stimulated contracts. Unlike oestrogens a progesterone-dominated uterus exhibits a negative staircase phenomenon.

Progesterone can inhibit the spontaneous contractility of full-term pregnant or non-pregnant myometrial strips and also oxytocin-stimulated activity. There is no evidence for a decrease in plasma progesterone prior to the onset of human labour; there might, however, be a correlation between the progesterone level at term and the sensitivity to oxytocin. Women at term with low progesterone levels are more sensitive to oxytocin (Maggi *et al.*, 1992).

Some progesterone metabolites show little or no affinity for the progesterone receptor, but are potent modulators of the GABAA receptor system. Putnam tested 3beta-hydroxy-5beta-pregnan-20 one, 3alpha-hydroxy-5alpha-pregnan-20 one, 5beta-pregnan-3-20-dione, and progesterone. All inhibited spontaneous uterine contractions; however, when uterine tissues were exposed to a combination of steroid and antagonist, the action of the first two metabolites appeared to be mediated through the GABA system, while the others act through the progesterone receptor system. Lofgren, Holst & Backstom (1992) has shown that 5alpha-reduced progestins are not as potent inhibitors of contracting human term myometrium *in vitro* as progesterone. However, they are potent central nervous system depressants, so that 5alpha-pregnane-3alpha-ol-20-one has anaesthetic properties in man.

Progesterone also controls prostaglandin effect: Csapo showed that elevation of PGF-levels in rat induces labour only when the myometrial action of P is critically reduced (Csapo, Bernard & Eskola, 1980).

Oxytocin (OT)

The role of oxytocin in the control of human myometrial function is described in detail in Chapter 12 (Chard).

Circulating oxytocin concentrations are similar in men, non-pregnant women or pregnant women before labour. Husslein et al. (1983) noted that, plasma oxytocin is raised over pre-labour values reaching 12.6 μ U/ml during the third stage, and fall, to control levels 30 minutes post-partum. In spontaneous labour, there was no obvious relation between plasma oxytocin and the uterine contraction period, and no significant difference was found between the mean value in contraction periods (12.1 μ U/ml) and that in relaxation one (11.5 μ U/ml).

In myometrium oxytocin receptors mediate contractility, while in endometrium they mediate the release of other uterotonic substances, as endothelin (ET) (Maggi et al., 1991). Oxytocin also induces prostaglandin (PG) release. Corticotropin releasing hormone (CRH) potentiates the contractile response to oxytocin of human gestational myometrium, and this effect, in accordance with the study of Quartero et al. (1991), is dependent on prostaglandins.

Prostaglandins

Several authors have studied the effect of PG on the human non-pregnant or pregnant myometrium. PGF_{2a}, instilled into the uterine cavity of non-pregnant women, produces an increase in activity. PGE, has an inhibitory action on the isolated non-pregnant myometrium but stimulates the intact organ. Strips of non-pregnant human cervix are inhibited by PGE, while PGF has a more variable effect. Prostaglandins are probably involved in the process of menstruation through their myometrial stimulant action. PGE_2 and F_{2a} are thought to originate in the disintegrating endometrium, and might stimulate the myometrium either by local diffusion or by absorption via the circulation (Csapo et al., 1980).

During pregnancy there is little or no prostaglandin in amniotic fluid, but substantial amounts appear during spontaneous abortion or labour. Responses to PG can be greatly modified by the concentrations of hormones; this is reflected by the variation in sensitivity at different stages of the menstrual cycle. Thus progesterone decreases the inhibitory effect of PGE at the time of ovulation, but increases it during the early and middle proliferative phase. In constrast, oestradiol has no effect on PG activity (Csapo et al., 1989).

Prostaglandins may induce uterine contraction by promoting Ca^{2+} entry into the cell through specific receptors, coupled with calcium channels, while progesterone and 5-beta-reduced progestins promote smooth muscle relaxation by blocking calcium influx; progestins can therefore counteract PG-induced contraction. This phenomenon depends on external calcium, since extracellular calcium depletion abolishes the PG effect.

Prostaglandins may modify cyclic-AMP formation. Sodium increases adenyl cyclast activity and calcium has the opposite effect; thus, under PG stimulation, alteration of the $(Ca^{2+})-(Mg^{2+})$ ratio and Na^+ distribution would favour activation of adenyl cyclase.

Goureau *et al.* (1992) identified PG receptors in rat myometrium, where prostaglandins induced adenosine-3',5'-cyclic monophospate and inositol phosphates generation, reflecting a PGF_{2alpha} receptor-mediated process. Contractions, caused by PGF_{2alpha} were correlated to receptor activation and were also associated with the phospholipase C pathway.

Other hormones

Endothelin (ET) induces uterine contraction and myometrium may be a target organ for this hormone. Plasma ET level increased gradually during pregnancy being higher during labour (0.59 ± 0.006 p mol/l); a high level of ET is detected in amniotic fluid at term delivery. Two days post-partum ET reaches the non-pregnant level. In quiescent human myometrial cells, ET produces an increase in cytosolic free Ca^{2+}, in non-quiescent cells the ET-evoked Ca^{2+} was reduced and the response to OT was retained.

Vasoactive intestinal polypeptide (VIP) is localized in neurons which innervate vessels and non-vascular smooth muscle. This peptide inhibits myoelectrical activity and contractility of the uterine muscle, and increases myometrial blood flow (Clark *et al.*, 1981).

Parathyroid hormone (PTH) and PTH-related proteins can also inhibit uterine contraction (Shew *et al.*, 1991).

Clinical and pharmacological considerations

Efficient uterine action is essential for normal delivery. Pharmacological effects on the myometrium involve augmentation or depression (tocolysis) of contractility. The effects of a given hormone or drug are variable and related to the irritability of the myometrium at the time the hormone or drug is administered.

Tocolysis

Tocolytic treatment attempts to inhibit premature labour activity and to delay birth. The most widely used agents are calcium antagonists and beta-sympathomimetics.

Calcium antagonists

These drugs lower the activity of the myometrium. This can be demonstrated in the normal uterus, in patients with dysmenorrhoea, in the gravid uterus, and also on the ureter and the bladder (Andersson, 1988). The mechanism of action was elucidated by Fleckenstein (1971): calcium antagonists inhibit the slow, inward calcium current through the slow Ca channels. The opening of these is dependent on membrane potential and on the presence of specific agonists or antagonists.

Animal data suggest a teratogenic effect of nifedipine, but not at the doses (6×10 mg) used to inhibit labour (Roundtable, 1986). Verapamil shows no such effect. In isolated uterine horns in rats, Nifedipine is more potent ($p < 0.001$) than verapamil; diltiazem is least effective (Metro et al., 1987) (Fig. 2). Ca-antagonists may act on the cell membrane or within the cell. Thus, nifedipine receptors are found on the external surface, whereas verapamil receptors are found inside the cell.

The effect of verapamil and anaesthetics (especially enflurane) can be additive. Volatile anaesthetics also modify Ca^{2+} availability and depress contractility: general anaesthesia in patients being treated with Ca-antagonists may represent a high risk.

Non-steroid anti-inflammatory agents and beta-mimetic catecholamines

Aspirin prolongs pregnancy. Atad, David & Abramovic (1980) has shown the effect of indomethacin on uterine contractions, suppressing them completely after 1 h in threatened premature labour with minimal side effects. Melatonin has a similar effect.

The non-steroidal anti-inflammatory drug nimesulide does not affect active pressure or the direction and velocity of propagation of activity in non-pregnant women, though it alleviates pain significantly in dysmenorrhoeic patients (Pulkkinen et al., 1992).

Ritodrine and metaproterenol are the most powerful tocolytics, with complete inhibition of contractile activity after 30 minutes and some response even after 10 minutes (Figs. 3 and 4). Isosuprine is less effective and bufenin is intermediate (Oliva et al., 1979b). Intravenous isoprenaline and salbutamol inhibit spontaneous contractions of the rat uterus and increases the uterine cAMP; a desensitization to beta adrenergic agonists occurs after excessive stimulation.

cAMP increases significantly during the administration of uterine inhibitors, both in vivo and in vitro. It may indicate the degree of inhibition. Dibutyryl cAMP is also inhibitory.

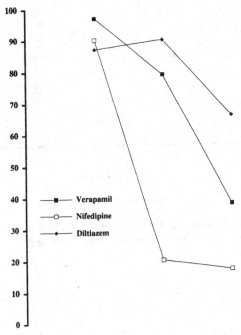

Fig. 2. Changes of contractility of rat uterine horn after administration of diltiazem, verapamil and nifedipine.

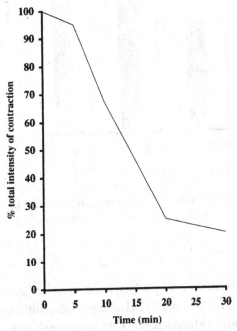

Fig. 3. Activity of ritodrine on uterine contractility in pre-term labour.

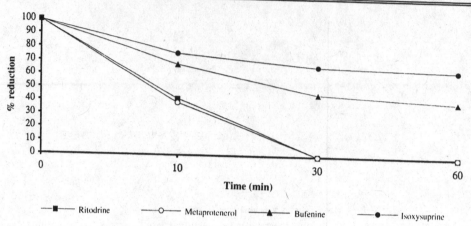

Fig. 4. Percentage of reduction (as compared with the initial value) of the area during the various tocolytic treatments.

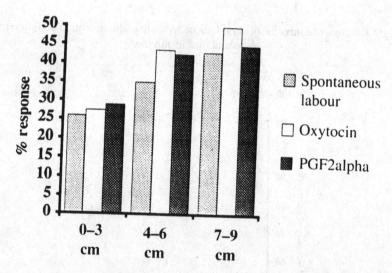

Fig. 5. Changes of intensity of contraction in spontaneous labour and after administration of oxytocin or prostaglandin F_{2alpha} (i.v.).

Intravenous nitroglycerin (NTG) has been used to allow replacement of a tightly contracted, inverted uterus. NTG also provides sufficient uterine relaxation to allow difficult twin extraction at Caesarean delivery and merits further evaluation as a uterine relaxant (Mayer & Weeks, 1992).

Induction of labour

Parenteral administration of a very dilute solution of oxytocin is the most widely used method for induction of labour. Oxytocin analogs have also been examined. For example, the effect of carbetocin, a long-acting oxytocin analogue, may offer advantages in management of the third stage of labour (Hunter, 1992).

The efficacy and safety of oral PGE_2 has been evaluated by several authors. Bremme *et al.* (1990), showed that the best interval between oral doses of PGE_2 is one hour. Following 1.0 mg PGE_2, the plasma concentration peaked after 45 to 60 minutes and had returned to approximately pre-treatment levels after 120 minutes. When the dose was increased to 2.0 mg, signs of overstimulation were observed. A comparative study of oral PGE_2 or OT by intravenous infusion showed that labour was established slightly earlier in the oxytocin group. Frequency and amplitude of contractions as well as uterine contractility were similar in both treatment groups (Romanini *et al.*, 1977) (Fig. 5). The frequency of atypical activity was lower in oxytocin-induced labour, but the need for analgesia was greater (Keirse *et al.*, 1980).

Unlike OT, which requires massive doses to cause the early pregnant uterus to contract, PGE_2 and PGF_{2alpha} stimulate the uterus in early gestation at doses only about tenfold those required at term. They are highly efficacious for cervical dilatation in the second trimester; all patients have a termination of pregnancy by 42 h after PG intramuscular injection (Bygdeman *et al.*, 1980).

Application of PGE_2 (intracervically in the form of gel and intravaginally in the form of a tablet), in patients with an immature cervix stimulates labour in 80% within 24 h.

The effect of analgesia on labour

Some believe that analgesia begun during the latent phase of the first stage may delay the progress of labour, often making it necessary to use OT. Others describe a brief period of decreased uterine activity following any form of analgesia. Eventually labour may accelerate presumably due to decreased maternal anxiety and serum concentration of catecholamines. Therapeutic doses of morphine may prolong labour. If the uterus is made hyperactive by OT, morphine tends to restore tone, frequency, and amplitude of contractions to normal (Petrie, 1976).

Meperidine may increase uterine activity during active labour. Other substances, such as pentazocine, have little or no effect. Meperidine can cause loss of cyclic variation of fetal heart rate and inhibition of myometrial contractility (Romanini, personal observation). Similar but smaller changes are induced by pentazocine.

Conclusions

The mechanism of uterine contraction at the molecular and cellular levels is similar to that of skeletal muscle, but the kinetics are different. This chapter collates information on these processes, their electrical and hormonal regulation. With more insight into biophysical and biochemical aspects of parturition, more effective treatment may be devised for abnormal states. Dysfunction of active labour is best analysed by measuring myometrial activity. This is an important diagnostic measure for the study of pharmacological actions and for selection treatment in patients. It is best evaluated by computerized tocography; this permits off-line evaluation of the area under the intra-uterine pressure waveform. This is an acceptable substitute for the more traditional parameters (amplitude, frequency and calculation of Montevideo or Alexandria Units) because it allows a more detailed study of the components and regulation of uterine contractility and of its modification by drugs.

References

Altabef, K. M., Spencer, J. T. & Zimberg, S. (1992). Intravenous nitroglycerin for uterine relaxation of an inverted uterus. *American Journal of Obstetrics and Gynecology*, **166**(4), 1237–8.

Anderson, K. E. (1988). Calcium antagonists and dysmenorrhea. *The New York Academy of Sciences*, Ed. Govoni, pp. 747–56, New York.

Atad, J., David, A. & Abramovic, H. (1980). Classification of threatened premature labor related to treatment with a PG inhibitor: indomethacin. *Biology of the Neonate*, **37**, 291–6.

Bernestein, P. (1991). PGE2 gel for cervical ripening and labor induction: a multicentre controlled trial. *Canadian Medical Association Journal*, **145**, 1249–54.

Bottari, S. P. *et al.* (1983). Differential regulation of alpha adrenergic receptor subclasses by gonadal steroids in human myometrium. *Journal of Clinical Endocrine Metabolism*, **57**, 937–41.

Breeme *et al.* (1990). Induction of labor by oral PGE2 administration: evaluation of different dose schedules. *Acta Obstetrica et Gynecologica Scandinavica*, Suppl. **92**, 5–10.

Bygdeman, M. *et al.* (1980). Mid-trimester abortion by vaginal administration of 9-deoxo-16, 16-dimethyl-9-methylene-PGE2. *Contraception*, **22**, 153–64.

Chan, W. Y. (1980). The separate uterotonic and PG-releasing actions of OT. Evidence and comparison with angiotensin and methacholine in the isolated rat uterus. *Journal of Pharmacological Experimental Therapy*, **213**, 575–9.

Clark, K. E. *et al.* (1981). Effects of vasoactive polypeptides on the uterine vasculature. *American Journal of Obstetrics and Gynecology*, **139**, 182–8.

Coleman, H. A. & Parkington, H. C. (1992). Propagation of electrical and mechanical activity in uterine smooth muscle. *Japan Journal of Pharmacology*, **38**, Suppl. 2, 369.

Crane, L. H. & Martin, L. (1991). Pacemaker activity in the myometrium of the oestrous rat: *in vivo* studies using video-laparoscopy. *Reproduction and Fertility Developments*, **3**, 519–27.

Csapo, A. (1952). The antagonistic effects of estrogen and progesterone on the staircase phenomenon in uterine muscle. *Endocrinology*, **51**, 378–85.

Csapo, A. (1959). Myometrial contractions related to estrogenes and progesterone. *American NY Academy of Science*, **75**, 790.

Csapo, A. (1964). Extraovular pressure. Its diagnostic value. *American Journal of Obstetrics and Gynecology*, **90**, 493.

Romanini, C. & Biomplani, A. (1970). L'integrazione elettronica del tracciato tocografico. Risultati preliminari. Atti 54. *Congr. Naz. Soc. It. Ost. Ginec.*, p. 508, Milano, B. Mattioli publ.

Csapo, A. T., Bernard, A. & Eskola, J. (1980). The biological meaning of PG levels. *Prostaglandins*, **19**, 385–90.

Flecklenstein, A. (1971). Specific inhibitors and promoters of calcium action in the excitation-contraction coupling of heart muscle and the role in prevention or production of myocardial lesions. In *Calcium and the Heart*. Ed. P. Harris and L. H. Opie. pp. 135–88, Academic Press, London.

Goren, H. S., Geonzon, R. M. *et al.* (1980). OT action: lack of correlation between receptor number and tissue responsiveness. *Journal of Super Structure*, **14** (2), 129–38.

Goureau, O., Tanfin, Z. & Harbons, M. S. (1992). Diverse prostaglandin receptor active distinct signal transduction pathways in rat myometrium. *American Journal of Physiology*, **263**, 257–65.

Harbert, G. M. Jr. (1992). Assessment of uterine contractility and activity. *Clinical Obstetrics and Gynecology*, **35** (3), 546–58.

Haut, J. C. *et al.* (1986). Uterine contraction pressure with OT induction/augmentation. *Obstetrics and Gynecology*, **68**, 305–9.

Heaton, R. C. (1992). The effects of intracellular and extracellular alkalinization on contractions of the isolated rat uterus. *Plüfers Archive*, **422**, 24–30.

Hunter, D. J., Schulz, P. & Wasserman, W. (1992). Effect of carbetocin, a long acting oxytocin analog on the postpartum uterus. *Clinical Pharmaceutical Therapy*, **52**, 60–7.

Husslein, P. *et al.* (1983). OT and PG plasma concentration before and after spontaneous labor. *Wien Klinic Woch*, **95**, 367–71.

Insel, T. R. (1992). Oxytocin: a neuropeptide for affiliation. *Psychoneurology*, **17**, 3–35.

Josimovich, J. B. (1973). Physical forces acting upon the gravid uterus. In *Uterine Contraction, Side Effects of Steroidal Contraceptives*. Ed. J. B. Josimovich, pp. 1–8. Wiley-Interscience publication, New York, London, Sydney, Toronto.

Keirse, M. J. *et al.* (1980). Comparison of oral PGE2 and intravenous OT for induction of labor in hypertensive pregnancies. *European Journal of Obstetrics and Gynecology Reports Biology*, **10**, 231–7.

Kelly, R. E. & Verhage, H. G. (1981). Hormonal effects on the contractile apparatus of the myometrium. *American Journal of Anatomy*, **161**, 375–82.

Leake, R. D., Weitzman, R. E. & Glatz, T. H. (1981). Plasma OT concentration in men, nonpregnant women, and pregnant women before and during spontaneous labor. *Journal of Clinical Endocrine Metabolism*, **53**, 730–3.

Lofgren, M., Holst, J. & Backstom, T. (1992). Effects *in vivo* of progesterone and two 5-alpha reduced progestins on contracting human myometrium at term. *Acta Obstetrica et Gynecologica Scandinavica*, **71**, 28–33.

Lydrup, M. L. (1991). Role of K$^+$ channels in spontaneous electrical and mechanical activity of smooth muscle in the guinea pig mesotubarium. *Journal of Physical Condition*, **433**, 327–40.

Maggi, M. *et al.* (1991). Steroid modulation of oxytocin/vasopressin receptors in the uterus. *Journal of Sterility Biochemistry and Molecular Biology*, **40**, 481–91.

Maggi, M. *et al.* (1992). Sex steroid modulation of neurohypophysial hormone receptors in human nonpregnant myometrium. *Journal of Clinical Endocrine Metabolism*, **74**, 385–92.

Marshall, J. M. (1979). Motility in cell function. In *Symposium in Cell Biology*. Ed. F. A. Pepe, J. W. Sanger & V. T. Nachmias, pp. 415–17, Academic Press, New York, Sydney, Toronto, San Francisco.

Mayer, D. C. & Weeks, S. K. (1992). Antepartum uterine relaxation with nitroglycerin at caesarean delivery. *Canadian Journal of Anaesthetics*, **39**, 166–9.

Metro, D., Rizzo, G. & Arduini, D. (1987). Differential effect of calcium antagonists on isolated uterine horn in the rat. *European Journal of Physiology*, **408**, 551.

Oliva, G. C., Arduini, D., Bompiani, R., Gaglione, R. & Romanini, C. (1979a). Quantitative study of the activity of some drugs on the human myometrium *in vivo*. *Acta Medica Roma*, **17**, 238–46.

Oliva, G. C., Arduini, D., Bompiani, R. & Romanini, C. (1979b). Betamimetics drugs during pregnancy. *Acta Medica Roma*, **17**, 147–254.

Otsuki, Y. *et al.* (1983). Serial plasma OT levels during pregnancy and labor. *Acta Obstetrica Gynecologica Scandinavica*, **62**, 15–18.

Paul, M. J. & Smeltzer, J. S. (1991). Relationship of measured external tocodynamometry with measured internal uterine activity. *American Journal Perinatology*, **8**, 417–20.

Petri, R. H. *et al.* (1976). The effect of drugs on uterine activity. *Obstetrics and Gynecology*, **48**, 431.

Pulkkinen, M., Monti, T. & Maciocchi, A. (1992). Analysis of uterine contractility after administration of the N-SAI drug mimesulide. *Acta Obstetrica Gynecologica Scandinavica*, **71**, 181–5.

Putnam, C. D., Bran, D. W., Kolbeck, R. C. & Mahesh, V. B. (1991). Inhibition of uterine contractility by P and P-metabolites. *Biology of Reproduction*, **45**, 266–72.

Quartero, H. W., Noort, W. A., Fry, C. H. & Keirse, M. J. (1991). Role of PG and leukotrienes in the synergistic effect of OT and CRH on the contraction force in human gestational myometrium. *Prostaglandins*, **42**, 137–50.

Riemer, R. K. *et al.* (1988). Estrogen reduces B receptor mediated cAMP production and the concentration of the guanyl nucleoide-regulatory protein G (S) in rabbit myometrium. *Molecular Pharmacology*, **33**, 389–95.

Romanini, C., Oliva, G. C. & Bompiani, A. (1972a). A new method for automatic evaluation of uterine activity. In *Labour in Perinatal Medicine*. Ed. Bossart, p. 354, Bern.

Romanini, C. & Bompiani, A. (1972b). Il monitoraggio elettronico della contrazione uterina-valutazione mediante integratore digitale. *Acta Medica Roma*, **10**, 49.

Romanini, C. *et al.* (1977). Ia farmacologia nel traaglio di parto: atti 53A. *Congr. Naz. Soc. Ital. Ostet. Ginecol.*, Catania-Taormina, p. 93.

Romanini, C., Oliva, G. C., Aruduini, D., Gagione, R. & Bompiani, A. (1982). Automatic analysis of uterine contraction. Methodological possibilities and clinical results. In *Uterine Contactility, VI FRESER Symposium*, Bruxelles.

Rosenwaks, Z. & Seegar, J. G. (1980). Menstrual pain: its origin and pathogenesis. *Journal of Reproductive Medicine*, **25**, 207–12.

Roundtable. (1981). Calcium antagonists in cardiovascular therapy: experience with verapamil. *Excerpta Medica Amsterdam*, pp. 405–13.

Rubig, A. & Broer, K. H. (1991). Administration of PGE2 in premature rupture of the membranes. *Zeitschrift Geburtshilfe Per*, **195**, 159–62.

Sakai, N., Tabb, T. & Garfield, R. E. (1992). Modulation of cell to cell coupling between myometrial cells of the human uterus during pregnancy. *American Journal of Obstetrics and Gynecology*, **167**, 472–80.

Shew *et al.* (1992). Galanin and calcitonin gene-related peptide immunoreactivity in nerves of the rat uterus. *Peptides*, **13**, 273–9.

Shew *et al.* (1991). PTH-related protein inhibits stimulated uterine contraction *in vitro*. *Journal of Bone Minor Research*, **6**, 955–9.

Shew, *et al.* (1984). Direct effect of PTH on rat uterine contractions. *Journal of Pharmaceutical Experiments*, **230**, 1–6.

Thornton, S., Gillespil, J. I. & Greenwell, J. R. (1992). Mobilization of calcium by the brief application of oxytocin and PGE 2 in single cultured human myometrial cells. *Experimental Physiology*, **77**, 293–305.

Tsukamoto *et al.* (1991). Intracellular calcium of longitudinal muscle isolated from pregnant rat myometrium cell. *Biological International Reports*, **15**, 637–44.

Wilson, L. Jr, Parson, M. T. & Flouret, (1991). Forward shift in the initiation of nocturnal estradiol surge in the pregnant baboon: is this the genesis of labor? *American Journal of Obstetrics and Gynecology*, **165**, 1487–98.

16

Uterine activity in labour

S. ARULKUMARAN

Introduction

Uterine contractions are a prerequisite for vaginal delivery. Unless there are mechanical difficulties such as disproportion or malposition, efficient contractions and expulsive efforts of the mother should result in unassisted vaginal delivery. In most centres uterine contractions are assessed by external palpation at regular intervals and the clinical outcome with such practice is generally satisfactory. However, much research has been devoted to the identification of better methods of measuring uterine activity. It is now possible to perform on-line quantification of uterine activity, but the appropriate use of this technology has not been defined. This chapter discusses whether uterine contractions should be measured, the reliability of the methods used, the uterine activity in normal, augmented and induced labour and in women with a Caesarean scar.

Is there a need to measure uterine contractions in labour?

Uterine contractions temporarily impede replenishment of the retroplacental pool of blood necessary for oxygen transfer to the fetus. Uterine contractions may also compress the cord. To detect deleterious effects caused by these events, the fetal heart rate is auscultated intermittently or observed continuously by electronic fetal heart rate monitoring. Any changes are interpreted in relation to uterine contractions. If there are no fetal heart rate changes suggestive of hypoxia and the rate of cervical dilatation is satisfactory, there may be little need to monitor uterine contractions in labour. But normal or abnormal progress of spontaneous labour cannot be predicted prospectively. If progress is abnormal, recorded information about preceding uterine contractions is of undoubted value.

Methods of measurement

This chapter deals with studies based on external tocography and internal tocography. Quantification is based on uterine activity integral units (UAI).

External tocography

Equipment is available that can prepare on-line graphical records of the duration, frequency and strength of contractions. External tocograph recorders use a transducer placed near the uterine fundus to detect changes in the anteroposterior diameter of the abdomen resulting from uterine contractions. The transducer is a plastic plunger on a membrane which, although sometimes uncomfortable, is non-invasive. External tocographic recordings provide a good measure of contraction frequency, a fair estimate of contraction duration and an approximation of contraction intensity. External tocography may be suitable for studies of the action of drugs on the uterus where a major effect is anticipated (Embrey, 1940) or where uterine activity is observed in the antenatal patient in an attempt to predict pre-term labour (Bell, 1983). It is sufficient for most patients in labour, but for quantifying uterine activity during labour in high risk situations and for scientific work, internal tocography is more accurate.

Internal tocography

Steer *et al.* (1978) introduced the transducer-tipped catheter (Sonicaid–Gaeltec Ltd, Quarry Lane, Chichester), which obviated the technical problems of a fluid-filled device. This catheter is simple to use, unlikely to cause trauma and is ideal for use in the ambulant patient. The pressure transducer is a bridge strain gauge deposited on a thin metal pressure-sensing surface. It is mounted on the end of a 90 cm catheter, with a sensing area which is recessed (Fig. 1), thus minimizing accidental damage and enabling lateral pressure measurements without impact of head or end-on pressure. The transducer tip lies in the amniotic cavity, and all transmission is then electronic through the catheter via a 2 metre flexible extension cable connected to the contraction module of a standard fetal monitor. The ease of use and reliability of this catheter have been well documented (Steer, 1979; Gibb & Arulkumaran, 1985). Recently, a fibre optic catheter (Fig. 1) has been introduced. It is more robust than the transducer tipped Gaeltec catheter and can be kept in the uterus during the second stage of labour (Svenningsen, Jensen & Dogson, 1986). The reliability compares favourably with that of the Gaeltec catheter (Tham *et al.*, 1991). More recently, catheters with transducers to measure pressure as well as facilities to perform amnioinfusion are combined

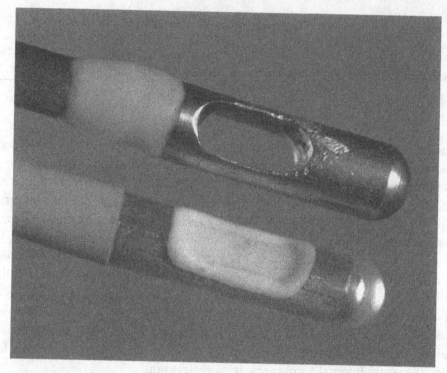

Fig. 1. The tip of fibre optic catheter with a smooth dome and distal fenestration housing the mirror arrangement is shown alongside the tip of the Gaeltec catheter with a recessed area behind the rounded tip.

into one device. The reliability and usefulness in cases of meconium stained or in situations of reduced amniotic fluid is now well-established (Arulkumaran *et al.*, 1991*a*; Owen, Henson & Hauth, 1990).

Reliability of intra-uterine pressure measurements

The advantages of intra-uterine pressure measurements over external tocography, especially in restless or obese patients, and those with abnormal progress of labour, have been documented (Csapo, 1970; Caldeyro-Barcio & Poseiro, 1950; Lacroix, 1968), but concern has been expressed about the validity of intra-uterine pressure measurements. Knoke *et al.* (1976) recorded intra-uterine pressure with three fluid-filled intra-uterine catheters (FFIUC) simultaneously in each of nine women in labour. They concluded that the variation in recorded pressure due to the random nature of catheter placement and loculations of amniotic fluid was approximately 5–10 mm Hg. They found a 25% measurement uncertainty. However, the discrepancies in measured pressure were not systematic, and over a period of several hours gross measurements of total uterine activity were comparable with all three catheters.

Steer *et al.* (1978) compared the measurement of intra-uterine pressure using a fluid-filled intra-uterine catheter with that measured using the transducer tipped catheters (Sonicaid–Gaeltec) in four women in labour. They showed only slight differences between the two methods. The small systematic under-reading of uterine pressure by the fluid-filled catheter was attributed to blockage. Neuman *et al.* (1972) comparing pressures derived from fluid-filled catheters with that from an intra-uterine sensor found a coefficient of variation similar to that noted by Steer *et al.* (1978).

Recent studies (Arulkumaran *et al.*, 1991a; Tham *et al.*, 1991; Chua *et al.*, 1992) confirm that while there may be contraction by contraction differences in recordings of intra-uterine pressures from two catheter tip pressure transducers in the same uterus, overall there is little systematic difference. The observed measurement differences between intra-uterine pressure transducers and the fluid-filled catheters obtained by Neuman *et al.* (1972) and Steer *et al.* (1978) were explained by the inherent inaccuracy of fluid-filled intra-uterine catheters due to blockage and compression. It is tempting to suppose that persistent differences in measured active pressure in two catheters is due to loculation of fluid so that different compartments develop different active pressures. However, the difference in the peak pressures obtained when two catheters are tied together and hence in the same pocket of amniotic fluid demonstrates that this is not the explanation. The reasons for the individual variations from contraction to contraction remain obscure, but may be due to mechanical (direct force) rather than fluid pressure acting on the transducer. Minor variations in contraction-to-contraction pressure do not influence clinical management of labour. Cumulative active pressure over the whole labour or over certain time segments (every 10 or 15 min) will have some bearing on the management of labour. Cumulative active pressure generated by the two catheters in the same or different pockets in individual women in labour did not show significant differences (Arulkumaran *et al.*, 1991a; Chua *et al.*, 1992).

Quantification of uterine activity

The elements of uterine contractions which relate to efficiency are frequency, active pressure, duration and coordination (Fig. 2). Amplitude or active pressure is easy to measure and is the difference between the pressure at the peak of a contraction and basal pressure; frequency is calculated over 10 min intervals and duration is the time between onset and offset of a contraction. The latter may be difficult to define especially when the decreasing pressure drops slowly to the

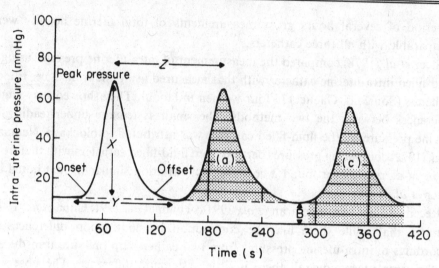

Fig. 2. Elements and terminology of uterine contractions. X: active pressure or amplitude, Y: duration, Z: contraction interval related to frequency, (a): active contraction area, B basal tone, (c): total contraction area.

basal level. Basal tone is the pressure at the lowest point of the tracing between contractions; this may also be difficult to establish if contractions have a tendency to merge or couple.

In the trend towards Système International (SI) units, Steer (1977) used the SI unit of pressure (the Pascal) instead of millimetres of mercury (mm Hg) (1 kilopascal = 7.52 mm Hg). One kilopascal of pressure over a duration of one second is 1 kilopascal second (1 k Pas). The active contraction area is usually quantified over 15 minutes and hence the uterine activity is expressed in kilopascal seconds/15 minutes (k Pas/15 min). Fifteen minutes was selected because of the time taken by the uterus to respond to changes in the rate of oxytocin infusion and because of short-term variations in the frequency of contractions.

Steer, Carter & Beard (1984) compared the levels of UAI in spontaneous labour with the traditional measures of uterine activity, i.e. frequency, active pressure and Montevideo units (MU). He confirmed the earlier suggestion (Steer, 1977), that UAI showed the closest correlation with rates of cervical dilatation in the active phase of labour. But whether managing labour using UAI measurements rather than simply frequency of contractions will significantly alter the obstetric outcome needs further evaluation.

Equipment has been developed which incorporates a uterine activity module in a conventional fetal monitor. This module, using the information obtained from the transducer tipped or fluid filled catheter, computes the active contraction area every 15 minutes and shows it in a display window on the module. The

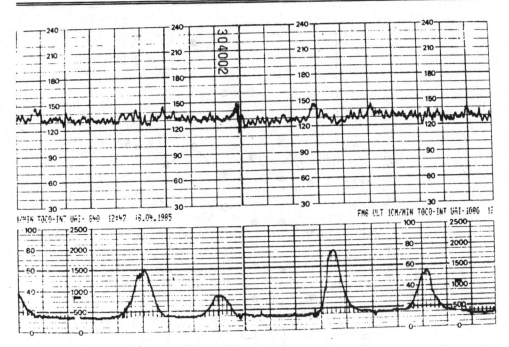

Fig. 3. Recording of UAI as a short dark line against a vertical axis from 0 to 2500 k Pas and the numerical printout of the UAI in addition to mode of recording, paper speed and time.

same value is printed in figures and is marked on the two channel chart recording paper against a vertical scale marked from 0 to 2500 k Pas/15 min (Fig. 3). This equipment is available at a cost no greater than that of a conventional fetal monitor.

Uterine activity in spontaneous normal labour

In nulliparae

Uterine activity in spontaneous labour varies according to the physical characteristics of the patient, the fetus, the presentation and the rate of progress. Most authors (Beazley & Kurjak, 1972; Philpott & Castle, 1972; O'Driscoll, Stronge & Minogue, 1973) have used a cervical dilatation rate of 1 cm/h to distinguish normal from abnormal labour. The uterine activity profile of normal labour defined as a rate of cervical dilatation of 1 cm/h or within a line drawn 2 h parallel and to the right of that line in a Singaporean Chinese population is shown in Fig. 4. This population had no oxytocic augmentation and all had unassisted vaginal delivery (Gibb *et al.*, 1984). In this population normal progress was associated with a minimum uterine activity of 855 k Pas/15 min and with an

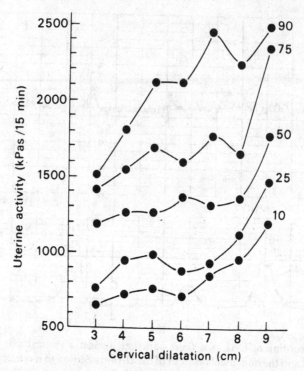

Fig. 4. Cervical dilatation specific uterine activity in k Pas/15 min in nulliparous
spontaneous normal labour.

overall median level of 1440 k Pas/15 min. Similar studies done in different
population groups (Cowan, Van Middlekoop & Philpott, 1982; Steer *et al.*, 1984,
Al-Shawaf, 1987; Fairlie *et al.*, 1988) have shown the wide range of uterine activity
associated with normal progress of labour. The range of uterine activity varied
from study to study based on the selection criteria for the study population.
Inclusion of population with slower labour gave lower uterine activity profiles
(Steer *et al.*, 1984); inclusion of women who were shorter or who had forceps
delivery had a higher uterine activity profile (Cowan *et al.*, 1982); when the criteria
were similar the profiles were similar (Fairlie *et al.*, 1988).

There was marked variation in amplitude, duration and incoordination of
contractions associated with normal labour and this was reflected by the wide
range of uterine activity observed. Because of the wide range of uterine activity
it is difficult to predict the rate of cervical dilatation prospectively. The efficiency
of contractions has to be assessed retrospectively based on cervical dilatation.
Uterine activity measurements are unlikely to give additional information if
partographic labour progess is normal.

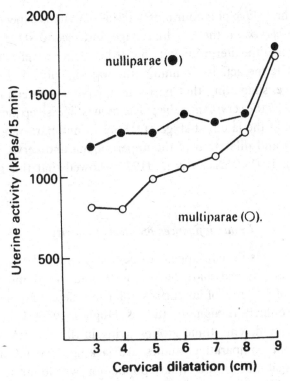

Fig. 5. Comparison of uterine activity in nulliparous and multiparous labour (median values, 50th centiles).

In multiparae

The multiparous woman with a previous vaginal delivery is more likely to have an easy labour than her nulliparous counterpart. This may be due to more advanced cervical dilatation on admission, more efficient uterine action, reduced cervical and pelvic tissue resistance or a combination of these factors. The functional difference between nulliparous and multiparous labour has been studied for many years. Turnbull (1957) observed lower pressures associated with faster progress in the multiparous patient compared with the nulliparous and proposed that this was due to the lower cervical and pelvic tissue resistance. Uterine activity in multiparae controlled for the physical characteristics of height of mother, weight of the newborn and the rate of progress of labour was studied by Arulkumaran *et al.* (1984). There was a wide range of uterine activity associated with normal labour. The overall median value was 1130 k Pas/15 min in multiparae compared with 1440 k Pas/15 min observed in nulliparous labour (Fig. 5). Similar observations have been made by Al-Shawaf *et al.* (1987) and Fairlie *et al.* (1988).

Until the late first stage of labour most uterine activity is expended on effacing and dilating the cervix. In the late first stage and second stage descent of the head takes place and the uterine activity needed is higher as reflected by the steep rise in activity. Uterine activity in multiparae was significantly lower only until the late first stage, suggesting that parity may have a greater influence on the resistance offered by the cervix than the pelvic tissues. The steep increase in uterine activity observed in the late first stage of labour in nulliparae and multiparae is due to stretching and dilatation of the upper vagina and cervix, the 'Ferguson reflex' (Ferguson, 1941). Vasicka et al. (1978) showed that this is mediated by oxytocin release.

Ethnic influences on uterine activity

Physiological functions in man appear to be uninfluenced by ethnic differences when controlled for physical characteristics of the individual and environmental factors. The rate of progress of labour is similar in different ethnic groups living in the same environment (Duignan, Studd & Hughes, 1975). Uterine activity in normal labour for different ethnic groups living in different environments has been described but comparative studies are lacking. The uterine activity in spontaneous normal labour in a Malay population was found to be similar to that of a Chinese population controlled for parity, maternal characteristics and the rate of progress (Arulkumaran et al., 1989a), thus lending support to the hypothesis that the human uterus acts in a similar way in different races. Short maternal stature, abnormal pelvic shape, fetal macrosomia and other 'pathological variables' such as uterine fibroids may lead to ethnic differences which are more apparent than real.

Uterine activity in breech presentation

Uterine activity in women with breech presentation is similar to that in vertex presentation when matched for parity, physical characteristics in the mother, the fetus and the progress of labour (Arulkumaran et al., 1988).

Uterine activity in augmented labour

The practice of augmentation is based on observed cervimetric progress of labour in the first stage and descent of the head in the second stage in conjunction with the assessment of uterine contractions. Prior to augmentation, malpresentation, fetopelvic disproportion and evidence of fetal compromise are excluded. When oxytocic augmentation is undertaken the question arises as to the target uterine activity that has to be reached to achieve optimal obstetric outcome. A contraction frequency of 3 to 4 in 10 min (Arulkumaran *et al.*, 1991*b*) appears to be essential for good trial of labour. Oxytocin titration to achieve preset uterine activity values measured by active contraction area does not lead to better outcome than achieving a target frequency of 4 to 5 contractions every 10 mins (each lasting >40 s) (Arulkumaran *et al.*, 1989*b*). There also appears to be no advantage in titrating oxytocin using intra-uterine catheters to quantify uterine activity or desired frequency of contractions compared with oxytocin titration based on external tocography in dysfunctional labour (Chua *et al.*, 1990).

Uterine activity in induced labour

Induction of labour is common in modern obstetric practice. The frequency varies from as low as 3% to as high as 30% in different units even in the same country. Artificial rupture of membranes and oxytocin infusion is the commonest method employed. Generally, oxytocin is titrated to achieve 4 contractions in 10 min after rupture of the membranes. Uterine activity in induced labour is higher than that in normal labour (Arulkumaran *et al.*, 1986). In order to regulate the oxytocin to achieve optimal levels of uterine activity, and to avoid ill effects to the fetus, oxytocin infusion has been titrated to achieve the 50th centile of uterine activity in normal labour according to parity (Gibb, Arulkumaran & Ratnam, 1985). The obstetric outcome with this approach was no better than in a group who had oxytocin titrated to achieve frequency of contractions of 4 to 5 in 10 min. In many patients who had oxytocin to achieve 50th centile activity, the progress of labour was slow and escalation of the oxytocin dose was necessary to achieve optimal frequency and acceptable progress. When oxytocin was titrated to achieve 75th centile activity, the two methods gave equally good outcome. Thus this quantification of uterine activity offers no advantage in induced labour (Arulkumaran, Ingemarsson & Ratnam, 1987). In a recent randomized study, uterine activity was quantified using an intra-uterine catheter in one group and by external tocography in the second group (Chia *et al.*, 1993). The obstetric outcome was similar in the two groups suggesting no advantage to the intra-uterine catheter in induced labour.

A uterus has to perform a given quantum of activity in order to effect delivery in induced labour (Arulkumaran *et al.*, 1985) (Fig. 6). The total uterine activity (TUA) is a reflection of the cervical and pelvic tissue resistance. If the expected total uterine activity for the given parity and cervical score is exceeded with little progress, it suggests cephalopelvic disproportion or failed induction.

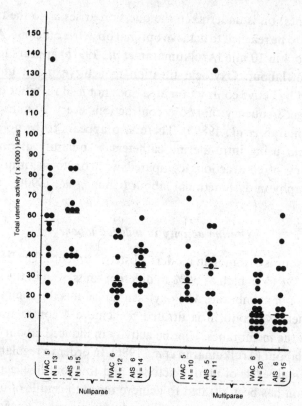

Fig. 6. Total uterine activity in induced labour according to parity, cervical score and two modes of oxytocin infusion – one mode to achieve 50th centile uterine activity of spontaneous normal labour (IVAC – manual infusion system) and the other to achieve 75th centile activity (AIS – automatic infusion system).

Uterine activity in patients with a Caesarean scar

Women with a Caesarean scar have lower activity levels if they had a previous vaginal delivery than if they had no vaginal delivey (Arulkumaran et al., 1989c). Those who had the Caesarean electively or in the latent phase of labour have higher uterine activity than women who had surgery in the active phase of labour. Women who are augmented have higher uterine activity than those who have normal labour (Arulkumaran et al., 1989d). Those who are likely to deliver vaginally show satisfactory progress in the first few hours of augmentation compared with those who need Caesarean section for poor progress in labour (Silver & Gibbs, 1987; Arulkumaran et al., 1989d). With careful selection and a limited period of augmentation, a satisfactory outcome can be achieved in most women with a Caesarean scar (Chua et al., 1989).

The classical signs of rupture, notably maternal tachycardia, hypotension and vaginal bleeding are late signs of scar rupture. Internal tocography may help in early identification of loss of integrity of scar in some cases but cannot predict impending rupture. Rodriquez *et al.* (1989) concluded that use of an intrauterine catheter was not of value in detecting early rupture of the uterus but two other groups (Beckley, Gee & Newton, 1991; Arulkamaran, Chua & Ratnam, 1992) have presented evidence that it may help. A breach in the scar affects wall tension and reduces the build up of intra-uterine pressure (Gee, Taylor & Hancox, 1988). This is reflected in a decline in the amplitude of the contractions once the scar gives way (Fig. 7). The frequency of contractions is usually not reduced with the scar rupture. In cases where uterine activity was not reduced, the catheter may have been introduced posterior to the head and be in an isolated pool of fluid. A posterior approach is the commonest and may have been used in the series (Rodriquez *et al.*, 1989) in which no reduction in uterine activity was observed with rupture of the uterus. Fig. 7 shows a case in which a reduction in uterine activity was noticed. It was believed that the catheter had slipped into the cervix as the patient had no signs or symptoms of scar rupture. On reinsertion of the catheter posterior to the head, contractions were observed (Fig. 8). Subsequently a uterine rupture involving the bladder was noted when the patient had a Caesarean for failure to progress. The location of the catheter and the extent of loss of integrity of the scar may determine the change in uterine activity observed.

Another reason for no reduction of uterine activity is incomplete rupture of the uterus. Paul, Phelan & Yeh (1985) found a similar incidence of incomplete rupture in those with a Caesarean scar whether they had a trial of labour and an emergency CS or an elective CS without trial of labour. With contractions there may have been a build up of pressure with the intact peritoneum which was not sufficient to cause cervical dilatation. At the time of CS for failure to progress the incomplete rupture would have been noticed. Such patients will not show a sudden reduction in uterine activity. Reduction in uterine activity may be more easily monitored by internal tocography than external tocography where a sudden reduction may be attributed to loosening of the belt or alteration in the position of the patient. Prolonged bradycardia is another sign associated with scar rupture (Arulkumaran *et al.*, 1992). Use of an intra-uterine catheter and continuous electronic monitoring of the fetal heart rate may help in early identification of the loss of scar integrity.

Incoordinate uterine contractions

Incoordinate uterine contractions are defined by irregular frequency or shape on the tocographic tracings. Incoordinate activity can be associated with normal

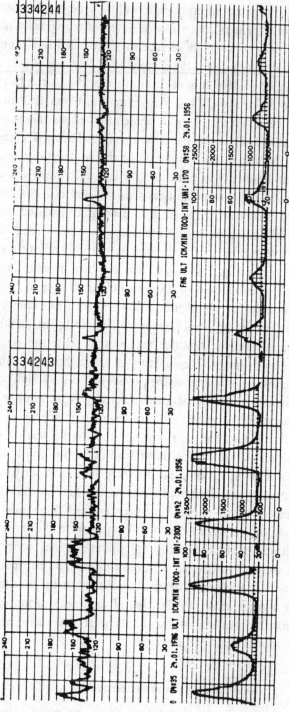

Fig. 7. Cardiotocographic trace showing sudden decline in the uterine activity – affecting only the amplitude of contractions and not the frequency, baseline pressure or fetal heart rate.

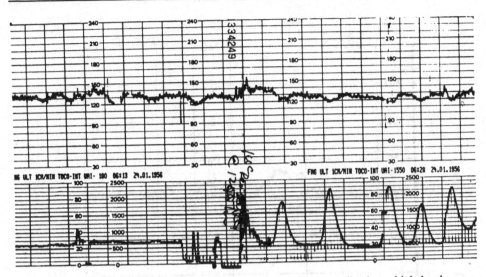

Fig. 8. Cardiotocographic trace showing return of the amplitude to high levels whilst the other parameters remain the same after reinsertion of the catheter posterior to the head.

progress of labour (Gibb *et al.*, 1984) and are not synonymous with inefficient contractions. Similarly, coordinate contractions need not always be efficient. In many patients minor degrees of incoordination are found in early labour, and the pattern of incoordination generally persists throughout the labour.

Incoordinate uterine contractions are not an indication for oxytocics unless they are also inefficient. The use of oxytocics may or may not correct the incoordination but should increase the efficiency. In addition, the use of oxytocin may cause incoordinate uterine contractions while improving their efficiency. Though internal tocography is likely to delineate incoordinate uterine activity better than external, it is not essential because the phenomenon is not directly linked to efficiency of contractions. Various degrees of incoordinate uterine activity during labour in women who progressed normally are shown in Figs. 9, 10 and 11.

Tetanic contractions, hypertonic uterine activity and hyper- or poly-systole

Contractions which merge to form a sustained contraction lasting for >3 min are a 'tetanic' contraction. Such contractions are usual in the third stage after administration of oxytocic. They are not seen in normal labour and are due to the use of oxytocics (Fig. 12). When the contractions do not merge but the baseline pressure is elevated by more than 20 mm Hg for more than 3 min they are called 'hypertonic' (increased tone of the uterus) (Fig. 13). A tetanic contraction will cut off the perfusion to the retroplacental pool of blood while hypertonic activity

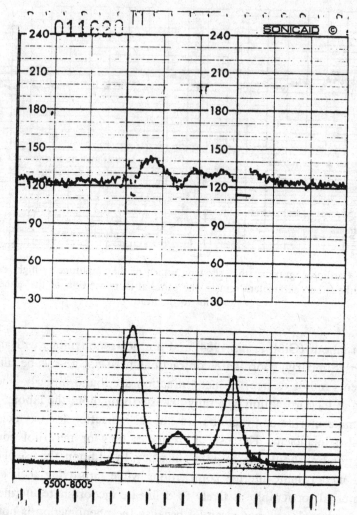

Fig. 9. Minor degree of incoordination of contractions.

will reduce perfusion. This causes fetal heart rate changes unless remedial action is taken by stopping the oxytocin and/or by giving a uterine relaxant (Ingemarsson *et al.*, 1985). A contraction frequency greater than one every 2 min is referred to as polysystole or hypersystole and is usually caused by higher than necessary levels of oxytocin. If remedial action is not taken it usually progresses to hypertonic activity and eventually tetanic contraction. Such hyperstimulation can occur without an increase in the dose of oxytocin due to the increase in sensitivity of the uterus with advancing labour (Sica Blanco & Sala, 1961).

Polysystole is also observed in some patients with abruptio placentae. A woman with bleeding, abdominal pain, polysystolic contractions of small amplitude and

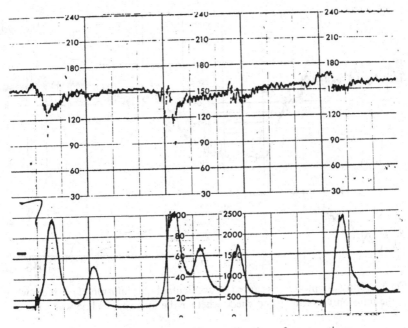

Fig. 10. Moderate degree of incoordination of contractions.

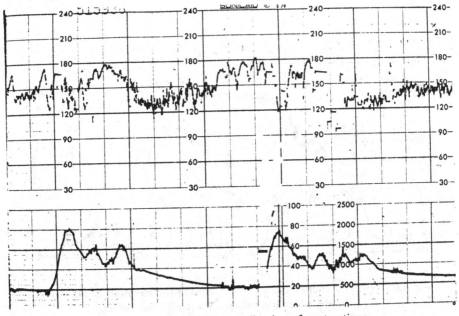

Fig. 11. Severe degree of incoordination of contractions.

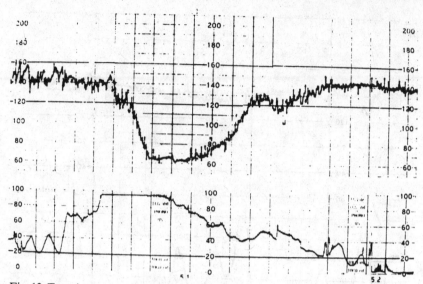

Fig. 12. Tetanic contractions caused by accidental bolus infusion of oxytocin when the infusion was run fast to check whether the intravenous line was patent.

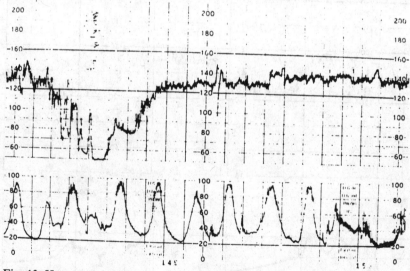

Fig. 13. Hypertonic uterine contractions, showing the elevation of the baseline pressure, which has caused a transient bradycardia.

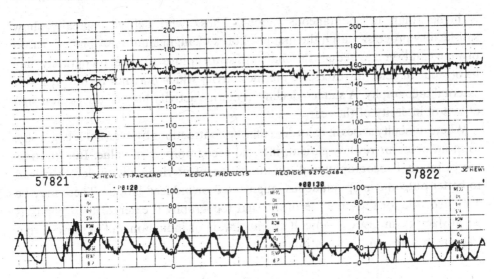

Fig. 14. Polysystolic contractions of low amplitude due to *abruptio placentae* in a patient who presented with continuous abdominal pain and bleeding per vaginam with the cervix 1 cm dilated. There is associated fetal tachycardia.

an abnormal fetal heart rate pattern may have abruptio placentae (Fig. 14). The polysystolic contractions are a result of the uterine irritability caused by seeping of blood into the myometrium.

Summary

Internal tocography and quantification of uterine activity by active contraction area measurements is of little value in spontaneous normal labour. In augmented labour, the use of internal tocography is not associated with improvement in duration of labour, dose of oxytocin, incidence of operative deliveries or neonatal outcome compared with external tocography. Whether internal tocography offers any advantage over external tocography in difficult cases of augmentation, i.e. those which do not show satisfactory progress in the first few hours, needs further study. Obstetric outcome has not improved with the use of internal tocography and quantification of uterine activity in induced labour. However, knowledge of total uterine activity (TUA) from internal tocography may be of value in selected cases in which fetal heart rate changes are observed with high uterine activity or in those who fail to progress despite having achieved adequate total uterine activity. The cases likely to benefit from such an exercise are too few to justify routine internal tocography in induced labour.

In those with a Caesarean section scar, uterine activity in augmented labour is higher than in spontaneous labour. Those who deliver vaginally show satisfactory progress within the first few hours of augmentation. A limited period of augmentation may reduce the chance of scar rupture. Internal tocography may be of value in detecting excessive uterine activity which may not be obvious with external tocography. A sudden decline in uterine activity may be the earliest sign of loss of integrity of the scar.

Where difficulty arises in recording uterine contractions by external tocography, as in an obese or restless patient, internal tocography is of value. But 'routine' use of internal tocography and quantification of uterine activity does not lead to better outcome in spontaneous, augmented or induced labour. There may be a limited role for selective use of internal tocography if external tocography is unsatisfactory, in cases of difficult augmentation or induction and in those with a Caesarean scar and oxytocin infusion.

References

Al-Shawaf, T., Al-Mogharaby, S. & Akiel, A. (1987). Normal levels of uterine activity in primigravidae and woman of high parity in spontaneous labour. *Journal of Obstetrics and Gynecology*, **8**, 18–23.

Arulkumaran, S., Gibb, D. M. F., Heng, S. H., Lun, K. C. & Ratnam, S. S. (1984). The effect of parity on uterine activity in labour. *British Journal of Obstetrics and Gynaecology*, **91**, 843–8.

Arulkumaran, S., Gibb, D. M. F., Ratnam, S. S., Heng, S. H. & Lun, K. C. (1985). Total uterine activity in induced labour – an index of cervical and pelvic tissue resistance. *British Journal of Obstetrics and Gynaecology*, **92**, 693–7.

Arulkumaran, S., Gibb, D. M. F., Heng, S. H., Lun, K. C. & Ratnam, S. S. (1986). Uterine activity in oxytocin induced labour. *Asia Oceania Journal of Obstetrics and Gynecology*, **12**, 533–40.

Arulkumaran, S., Ingemarsson, I. & Ratnam, S. S. (1987). Oxytocin titration to achieve preset active contraction area values does not improve the outcome of induced labour. *British Journal of Obstetrics and Gynaecology*, **94**, 242–8.

Arulkumaran, S., Ingemarsson, I., Gibb, D. M. F. & Ratnam, S. S. (1988). Uterine activity in spontaneous labour with breech presentation. *Australian and NZ Journal of Obstetrics and Gynaecology*, **28**, 275–8.

Arulkumaran, S., Gibb, D. M. F., Chua, S., Piara S. & Ratnam, S. S. (1989a). Ethnic influences on uterine activity in spontaneous normal labour. *British Journal of Obstetrics and Gynaecology*, **96**, 1203–6.

Arulkumaran, S., Yang, M., Ingemarsson, I., Piara, S. & Ratnam, S. S. (1989b). Augmentation of labour: does quantification of active contraction area to guide oxytocin titration produce better obstetric outcome. *Asia Oceania Journal of Obstetrics and Gynecology*, **15**, 47–51.

Arulkumaran, S., Gibb, D. M. F., Ingemarsson, I., Kitchener, C. H. & Ratnam, S. S. (1989c). Uterine activity during spontaneous normal labour after previous lower segment Caesarean scar. *British Journal of Obstetrics and Gynaecology*, **96**, 933–8.

Arulkumaran, S., Ingemarsson, I. & Ratnam, S. S. (1989*d*). Oxytocin augmentation in dysfunctional labour after previous Caesarean scar. *British Journal of Obstetrics and Gynaecology*, **96**, 939–41.

Arulkumaran, S., Yang, M., Chia, Y. T. & Ratnam, S. S. (1991*a*). Reliability of intrauterine pressure measurements. *Obstetrics and Gynecology*, **78**, 800–2.

Arulkumaran, S., Chua, T. M., Chua, S., Yang, M., Piara, S. & Ratnam, S. S. (1991*b*). Uterine activity in dysfunctional labour and target uterine activity to be aimed with oxytocin titration. *Asia Oceania Journal of Obstetrics and Gynecology*, **17**, 101–6.

Arulkumaran, S., Chua, S. & Ratnam, S. S. (1992). Symptoms and signs with scar rupture – value of uterine activity measurements. *Australian and NZ Journal of Obstetrics and Gynecology*, In press.

Beazley, J. M. & Kurjak, A. (1972). Influence of a partograph on the active management of labour. *Lancet*, **ii**, 348–51.

Beckley, S., Gee, H. & Newton, J. R. (1991). Scar rupture in labour after previous lower segment Caesarean section; the role of uterine activity measurement. *British Journal of Obstetrics and Gynaecology*, **98**, 255–69.

Bell, R. (1983). The prediction of preterm labour by recording spontaneous antenatal uterine activity. *British Journal of Obstetrics and Gynaecology*, **90**, 884–7.

Caldeyro-Barcia, R. & Poseiro, J. J. (1960). Physiology of uterine contractions, *Clinical Obstetrics and Gynecology*, **3**, 386–408.

Chia, Y. T., Arulkumaran, S., Soon, S. B., Norshida, S. & Ratnam, S. S. (1993). Induction of labour: does internal tocography result in better obstetric outcome than external tocography? *Australian and NZ Journal of Obstetric and Gynaecology*, **33**, 159–61.

Chua, S., Arulkumaran, S., Piara S. & Ratnam, S. S. (1989). Obstetric outcome in patients with previous Caesarean section. *Australian and NZ Journal of Obstetrics and Gynaecology*, **29**, 12–17.

Chua, S., Kurup, A., Arulkumaran, S. & Ratnam, S. S. (1990). Augmentation of labour; does internal tocography result in better obstetric outcome than external tocography. *Obstetrics and Gynecology*, **76**, 164–7.

Chua, S., Arulkumaran, S., Steer, P. J., Yang, M. & Ratnam, S. S. (1992). The accuracy of catheter tip pressure transducers for the measurement of intrauterine pressure in labour. *British Journal of Obstetrics and Gynaecology*, **99**, 186–9.

Cowan, D. B., Van Middlekoop, A. & Philpott, R. H. (1982). Intrauterine pressure studies in African nulliparae; normal labour progress. *British Journal of Obstetrics and Gynaecology*, **89**, 364–9.

Csapo, A. I. (1970). The diagnostic significance of the intrauterine pressure. *Obstetric and Gynecology Survey*, **25**, 403–35.

Duignan, N. M., Studd, J. W. W. & Hughes, O. A. (1975). Characteristics of normal labour in different racial groups. *British Journal of Obstetrics and Gynaecology*, **82**, 593–601.

Embrey, M. P. (1940). External hysterography. A graphic study of the human parturient uterus and the effect of various therapeutic agents on it. *Journal of Obstetrics and Gynaecology of the British Commonwealth*, 371–90.

Fairlie, F. M., Philips, G. F., Andrews, B. J. & Calder, A. Al. (1988). An analysis of uterine activity in spontaneous labour using a microcomputer. *British Journal of Obstetrics and Gynaecology*, **95**, 57–64.

Ferguson, J. K. W. (1941). A study of the motility of the intact uterus at term. *Surgery Gynaecology and Obstetrics*, **73**, 359–66.

Gee, H., Taylor, E. W. & Hancox, R. (1988). A model for the generation of intrauterine pressure in the human parturient uterus which demonstrates the critical role of the cervix. *Journal of Theory Biology*, **133**, 281–92.

Gibb, D. M. F., Arulkumaran, S., Lun, K. C. & Ratnam, S. S. (1984). Characteristics of uterine activity in nulliparous labour. *British Journal of Obstetrics and Gynaecology*, **91**, 220–7.

Gibb, D. M. F. & Arulkumaran, S. (1985). Uterine activity. In *Management of Labour*. Ed. J. Studd, pp. 235–51, Blackwell Scientific Publications Ltd, Oxford.

Gibb, D. M. F., Arulkumaran, S. & Ratnam, S. S. (1985). A comparative study of methods of oxytocin infusion for induction of labour. *British Journal of Obstetrics and Gynaecology*, **92**, 688–92.

Ingemarsson, J., Arulkumaran, S. & Ratnam, S. S. (1985). Bolus injection of terbutaline in term labour. 2. Effect on uterine activity. *American Journal of Obstetrics and Gynecology*, **153**, 865–9.

Knoke, J. D., Tsao, L. L., Neumen, M. Rl & Roux, J. F. (1976). The accuracy of intrauterine pressure during labour: a statistical analysis. *Comparative Biomedical Research*, **9**, 177–86.

La Croix, G. E. (1968). Monitoring labour by an external tocodynamometer. *American Journal of Obstetrics and Gynecology*, **101**, 111–19.

Neuman, M. R., Jordan, J. A. & Knoke, J. D. (1972). Validity of intra-uterine pressure measurements with trancervical intra-amniotic catheters and an intra-ammiotic transducer during labour. *Gynecology and Obstetric Investigations*, **3**, 165–75.

O'Driscoll, K., Stronge, J. M. & Minogue, M. (1973). Active management of labour. *British Medical Journal*, **iii**, 135–8.

Owen, J., Henson, B. V. & Hauth, J. C. (1990). A prospective randomized study of saline solution amnioinfusion. *American Journal of Obstetrics and Gynecology*, **162**, 1146–9.

Paul, R. H., Phelan, J. P. & Yeh, S. H. (1985). Trial of labour in the patient with a prior Caesarean birth. *American Journal of Obstetrics and Gynecology*, **151**, 297–304.

Philips, G. F. & Calder, A. A. (1987). Units for evaluation of uterine contractility. *British Journal of Obstetrics and Gynaecology*, **94**, 236–42.

Philpott, R. H. & Castle, W. M. (1972). Cervicographs in the management of labour in primigravidae. *Journal of Obstetrics and Gynecology British Commonwealth*, **79**, 592–8.

Rodriquez, M. H., Masaki, D. T., Phelan, J. P. & Diaz, F. G. (1989). Uterine rupture: are intrauterine pressure catheters useful in diagnosis? *American Journal of Obstetrics and Gynecology*, **161**, 666–9.

Sica Blanco, Y. & Sala, N. L. (1961). In *Proceedings of an International Symposium*, p. 127, Pergamon Press, London.

Silver, K. R. & Gibbs, R. S. (1987). Predictors of vaginal delivery in patients with a previous Caesarean section who require oxytocin. *American Journal of Obstetrics and Gynecology*, **156**, 57–60.

Steer, P. J. (1977). The measurement and control of uterine contractions. In *The Current Status of Fetal Heart Rate Monitoring and Ultrasound in Obstetrics*. Ed. R. W. Beard and S. Campbell, pp. 48–68, RCOG publication.

Steer, P. J., Carter, M. C., Gordon, A. J. & Beard, R. W. (1978). The use of catheter tip pressure transducers for the measurement of intrauterine pressure in labour. *British Journal of Obstetrics and Gynaecology*, **85**, 561–6.

Steer, P. J. (1979). Uterine activity in labour and the effects and regulation of oxytocin infusion. *Sonicaid Operating Handbook*, pp. 21–45, Sonicaid Ltd.

Steer, P. J., Carter, M. C. & Beard, R. W. (1984). Normal levels of active contraction area in spontaneous labour. *British Journal of Obstetrics and Gynaecology*, **91**, 211–19.

Svenningsen, L., Jensen, O. & Dodgson, M. S. (1986). A fibreoptic pressure transducer for intrauterine monitoring. In *Fetal and Neonatal Physiological Measurements*, Ed. P. Rolfe, pp. 15–21, Butterworths, London.

Tham, K. E., Arulkumaran, S., Chua, S., Anandakumar, C., Singh, P. & Ratnam, S. S. (1991). A comparison between fibreoptic and catheter tip bridge strain gauge transducers for measurement of intrauterine pressure in labour. *Asia Oceanic Journal of Obstetrics and Gynecology*, **17**, 83–7.

Turnbull, A. C. (1957). Uterine contractions in normal and abnormal labour. *Journal of Obstetrics and Gynaecology of the British Empire*, **64**, 321–32.

Vasicka, A., Kumaresan, P., Han, G. S. & Kumaresan, M. (1978). Plasma oxytocin in initiation of labour. *American Journal of Obstetrics and Gynecology*, **130**, 263–73.

Index